Pharmacy and the U.S. Health Care System

Third Edition

Pharmacy and the U.S. Health Care System

Third Edition

Michael Ira Smith, PhD
Albert I. Wertheimer, PhD, MBA
Jack E. Fincham, PhD
Editors

informa

healthcare

New York London

Informa Healthcare USA, Inc.
52 Vanderbilt Avenue
New York, NY 10017

© 2009 by Informa Healthcare USA, Inc. (original copyright 2005 by The Haworth Press, Inc.)
Informa Healthcare is an Informa business (cover design by Lora Wiggins)

No claim to original U.S. Government works
Printed in the United States of America on acid-free paper
10 9 8 7 6 5 4 3

International Standard Book Number-10: 0-7890-1875-6 (Hardcover)
International Standard Book Number-13: 978-0-7890-1875-5 (Hardcover)

Library of Congress Cataloging-in-Publication Data

Pharmacy and the U.S. health care system / Michael I. Smith et al., editors--3rd ed.
    p. cm.
    Includes bibliographical references and index.
    ISBN-13: 978-0-7890-1875-5 (hard : alk. paper)
    ISBN-10: 0-7890-1875-6 (hard : alk. paper)
    1. Pharmaceutical policy--United States. 2. Pharmaceutical services--United States.
[DNLM: 1. Pharmaceutical Services--United States. 2. Delivery of Health Care--United
States.] I. Smith, Michael I. II. Wertheimer, Albert I. III. Fincham, Jack E.

RA401.A3P43 2005
362.1'782'0973--dc22   2005000344

Visit the Informa Web site at
www.informa.com

and the Informa Healthcare Web site at
www.informahealthcare.com

MIS: To Rita, Neil, Bethany, and Mason

AIW: To Joaquima, Lia, and Debbie

JEF: To Melinda, Derek and Joni, and Kelcie
for making it all possible

CONTENTS

ABOUT THE EDITORS

Michael Ira Smith, PhD, RPh, is Founder and President of MIS Pharmaceutical Consultants, Inc., a management consulting firm for the pharmaceutical and health care industries. In 2002 he was elected as a Trustee for the American Pharmaceutical Association. He is also a member of the Pharmaceutical Business Intelligence Group, the Pharmaceutical Management Sciences Association, and the Pharmaceutical Marketing Research Group. He has been awarded such honors as the University of Minnesota Foundation Doctoral Dissertation Grant, the University of Minnesota Leadership Award, the Harold R. Popp Leadership Award, the John Y. Brekenridge Memorial Book Award, and the Pharmacists Mutual Award. Dr. Smith's work has been published in the *Journal of Health Politics, Policy, and Law.*

Albert I. Wertheimer, PhD, RPh, MBA, is Professor and Research Center Director at Temple University School of Pharmacy. He is a former Director of Outcomes Research and Management at Merck & Co., Inc., in West Point, Pennsylvania, and a former Vice President of Pharmacy Managed Care at First Health Service Corporation in Glen Allen, Virginia. Prior to his work with pharmaceutical companies, he held academic appointments at the University of Minnesota and the Philadelphia College of Pharmacy where he served as Dean. He has also served as a consultant to governmental and international agencies, such as the World Health Organization, United States Congress, and the World Bank, as well as to pharmaceutical manufacturers, managed care organizations, and professional societies. He is the author or co-editor of 13 books and the author or co-author of 300 journal articles as well as being a reviewer or editorial board member of 13 journals. Dr. Wertheimer has lectured and consulted in more than 40 countries. His current research interests are pharmacoeconomics and outcomes related to disease state management.

Jack E. Fincham, PhD, RPh, is the Albert W. Jowdy Professor of Pharmacy Care at the Department of Clinical and Administrative Pharmacy at the University of Georgia College of Pharmacy. Dr.

Fincham is a widely published researcher and author whose research includes postmarketing surveillance of pharmaceuticals, health outcomes of tobacco use, medication compliance, drug use in the elderly, and the U.S. health care system. He was a Kellogg Fellow at the University of Minnesota, where he received his PhD in Social and Administrative Pharmacy, and a Lilly Teaching Fellow at the University of Georgia. Dr. Fincham previously served as editor of the *Journal of Pharmacoepidemiology* and associate editor of the *Journal of Pharmacy Teaching.*

CONTRIBUTORS

Robert J. Amend, PharmD, Ortho Biotech Products, LP, Bridgewater, New Jersey.

Nicholas Bartone, RPh, PhD, Vice President, Ortho Bioscience, Raritan, New Jersey.

Richard J. Bertin, RPh, PhD, Board of Pharmaceutical Specialties, Washington, DC.

Richard R. Cline, PhD, Assistant Professor, University of Minnesota College of Pharmacy, Minneapolis, Minnesota.

Charles E. Daniels, PhD, Professor and Associate Dean for Clinical Affairs, Skaggs School of Pharmacy and Pharmaceutical Sciences, University of California, San Diego, California.

Robert I. Field, JD, MPH, PhD, Associate Professor and Director at Graduate Program in Health Policy, University of Sciences in Philadelphia, Philadelphia, Pennsylvania.

Ronald S. Hadsall, PhD, Professor, University of Minnesota College of Pharmacy, Minneapolis, Minnesota.

Richard S. Hurd, PharmD, Ortho Biotech Products, LP, Bridgewater, New Jersey.

Tanya C. Knight-Klimas, PharmD, CGP, FASCP, Clinical Assistant Professor, Temple University School of Pharmacy, Philadelphia, Pennsylvania.

Lon N. Larson, PhD, Professor, Drake University College of Pharmacy, Des Moines, Iowa.

Tom A. Larson, PharmD, Professor, University of Minnesota College of Pharmacy, Minneapolis, Minnesota.

Earlene E. Lipowski, PhD, RPh, Associate Professor, College of Pharmacy, University of Florida, Gainesville, Florida.

Patrick McKercher, RPh, PhD, Former Executive Director, Corporate Policy Initiatives, The Upjohn Company, Kalamazoo, Michigan.

Eucharia E. Nnadi, RPh, PhD, JD, Vice President for Program Planning and Personnel, University of Southern Nevada, Henderson, Nevada.

Somnath Pal, BS(Pharm), MS, MBA, PhD, Professor, St. Johns University, College of Pharmacy and Allied Health Professions, Jamaica, New York.

Craig A. Pedersen, RPh, PhD, FAPhA, Associate Professor and Director of Graduate Studies in Pharmaceutical Administration, The Ohio State University, Columbus, Ohio.

Kenneth W. Schafermeyer, PhD, Professor and Director of Graduate Studies, St. Louis College of Pharmacy, St. Louis, Missouri.

Jon C. Schommer, PhD, Associate Professor, University of Minnesota College of Pharmacy, Minneapolis, Minnesota.

Stephen W. Schondelmeyer, PhD, Professor, University of Minnesota College of Pharmacy, Minneapolis, Minnesota.

David M. Scott, MPH, PhD, RPh, Associate Professor, College of Pharmacy, North Dakota State University, Fargo, North Dakota.

Sandip Singh, PharmD, Ortho Biotech Products, LP, Bridgewater, New Jersey.

Richard G. Stefanacci, DO, MGH, MBA, CMD, Medical Director, St. Agnes Medical Center-Living Independently for Elders, Philadelphia, Pennsylvania.

Maria Marzella Sulli, PharmD, CGP, Assistant Clinical Professor, St. Johns University, College of Pharmacy and Allied Health Professions, Jamaica, New York.

Sheryl L. Szeinbach, PhD, RPh, Professor, College of Pharmacy, Ohio State University, Columbus, Ohio.

Joseph Thomas III, PhD, Professor, Purdue University School of Pharmacy, West Lafayette, Indiana.

Damary Castanheira Torres, PharmD, BCOP, Assistant Clinical Professor, St. Johns University College of Pharmacy and Allied Health Professions, Jamaica, New York.

Donald L. Uden, PharmD, Professor, University of Minnesota College of Pharmacy, Minneapolis, Minnesota.

William A. Zellmer, MPH, Deputy Executive Vice President, American Society of Health-System Pharmacists, Bethesda, Maryland.

Foreword

Much has changed in pharmacy and in health care over the past thirteen years, since the first edition was published in 1991. All pharmacists now graduate with the doctor of pharmacy (PharmD) degree and complete a minimum of one year of direct patient care experience. Instead of a surplus of pharmacists that was predicted to come after 2000, we have experienced a shortage of pharmacists. This has led to two significant changes: the first, in the mid-1990s the Pharmacy Technician Certification Board (PTCB) was established and has certified over 170,000 technicians to support the pharmacist, patient care, and drug distribution responsibilities. Second, there has been an increase of greater than 20 percent in the number of pharmacy schools. At last count, we have over ninety-five schools of pharmacy, either as candidates or Accreditation Council for Pharmacy Education (ACPE) approved.

The United States health care system has experienced a significant number of changes. New technology has allowed most surgery to be completed and patients sent home in one day. The number of hospital beds has been reduced sharply, and the system relies more heavily on medication to improve the quality of our lives, control chronic diseases, or to eradicate acute diseases.

According to the Organization for Economic Cooperation & Development Report,

> The U.S. in 2004 spent more on drugs: $556 per person than France at $473, Canada $385, and Australia $252. But because the U.S. spends even more on health care, drugs are an even lesser share of healthcare spending elsewhere—12.4 percent of all healthcare spending in the U.S. versus 21 percent in France, 16.2 percent in Canada, and 13.8 percent in Australia.

The cost of health care in the United States was paid for primarily by employers as an employee benefit when the first edition of this book was written. Now this health care coverage benefit is being deleted because the increasing cost affects the employer's ability to stay competitive in a global marketplace. It is said that General Motors spends more on health care for its workers than it does for steel in its cars. Recently, there have been several major union-led work stoppages primarily because employers were unwilling to reimburse 100 percent of health care coverage. The federal government just extended Medicare coverage for prescription drugs, which will commence in January of 2006.

The lack of a U.S. government-mandated health care system has led to over 44 million Americans having no health care coverage. A recently conducted survey by the Commonwealth Fund identified that one in four Americans said that he or she did not fill a prescription during the past year because of cost, while only one in eight Canadians said the same.

Today, the successful pharmacist must know more than therapeutics, understanding the environment in which pharmacy is practiced and the forces at work both within and outside the profession that are critical to being successful. This book is the single place where one can gain the data and the perspective on the forces that are currently affecting the profession. In addition, it can also give the pharmacist a perspective on the forces facing other professions.

Today, pharmacists are changing their practices. An example is that they routinely immunize patients. This was accomplished by observing the low adult immunization rates in the United States, with pharmacists understanding these needs and modifying their practices to meet the needs of society and public health authorities.

What other services can be delivered by pharmacists because of their training and accessibility? We are currently studying to identify areas where the pharmacist can fill gaps that exist. Medications have become a primary source of treatment. Once an individual is diagnosed with diabetes and prescribed medications to control blood sugar, the quality of that patient's life and the outcomes of therapy are not in the hands of the physician or the pharmacist, but in the hands of the patient. Pharmacists have developed training programs to help patients modify their behavior and improve their medication utilization skills. This has led to dramatic improvement in the quality of care. Several recently completed studies have demonstrated and documented the improvement in patient care that can occur when pharmacists train patients to self-manage their diseases.

If this profession has consistently made one strategic error over the years, it has been viewing itself in isolation. This book provides perspectives and information, which will help end this isolationist mind-set.

Pharmacy's future is extraordinarily bright. The big question for readers of the third edition is whether or not we will become health care providers who are compensated for the quality of care that our patients administer to themselves with the medications, monitoring, and training we provide them.

John A. Gans, PharmD
Executive Vice President,
American Pharmacists Association

Preface

We believe that one major difference between the successful pharmacist and the unsuccessful pharmacist in the future will be that successful pharmacists will have knowledge of and a connection with the overall health care delivery system beyond the four walls of their pharmacies. Unsuccessful pharmacists will be misinformed and less connected.

Consider a talented major-league baseball pitcher who is skilled, disciplined, and reliable; we'd say he is an expert pitcher, but unless he knows what to do and what possibilities might occur under different eventualities, he is destined for mediocrity.

Pharmacy is but one, albeit an important component of the health care delivery system. Decisions are made every day about policy, financing, quality control, rationing, pricing, access to services, and regulations. Although many such decisions do not directly impact pharmacy, nearly all do, to some extent, indirectly.

If a patient asks us about managed care formularies, we should either immediately share the correct answer or quickly find the source of a correct, factual answer. There is no second chance here. The patient will either consider the pharmacist to be a valuable neighbor or an irrelevant individual who need not be consulted in the future. When interfacing with the public, each of us is an ambassador for the entire profession.

Leaders in the pharmacy profession must have a vision of where overall health care delivery is headed in the next ten to twelve years and help guide us to offer services in a way that is compatible with and contributory to the expected practice mode.

Moreover, we cannot afford to wait for the impressions of others. We must be proactive and learn about the financing and organization of care trends to enable us to be prepared for future events and changes. In order to optimally practice, it is incumbent upon us to know the facts and pro and con arguments for different alternative modalities. For example, we should be able to explain our feelings about positive versus negative formularies to managed care organization administrators; and we should always be able to make a clear, concise recommendation with supporting documentation.

Every pharmacist should know about the environment in which he or she practices. It is critical to know what you can expect from a podiatrist or optometrist, or what types of services are provided at different types of hospitals or clinics.

The health care field changes rapidly, driven by new technology solutions and the pressures to increase efficiency and lower costs from managed care organizations and other insurers. To remain viable, we must perform an R&D function in which we perfect more precise, more efficient systems and techniques that keep us ahead of the competition. Technicians, robotics, and other methods of dispensing pharmaceuticals will be looking for opportunities to demonstrate their value.

We have tried to create a book that prepares the pharmacist for independent practice in an unpredictable environment. The pharmacist may be confronted with a dermatology question one moment, and the next question may be about carbohydrate diets or a request for a dental referral. If the practitioner understands the structure and financial aspects of the health system and knows who all of the other actors are, that pharmacist can be of immense value to his or her patients.

We are indebted to the assistance of our expert, chapter authors, and for the production help from Janet Malkowski and Thomas Santella. Readers with suggestions or other comments are welcome to contact the editors.

Chapter 1

Health and Health Care in the United States

David M. Scott

HEALTH AND DISEASE

Although the purpose of health care is to promote health, the U.S. health care system is mostly concerned about the diagnosis and treatment of disease, not with the goal of promoting health. The primary focus of a health professional's (e.g., pharmacist, physician) education is on the pathophysiology of disease and drug treatment, rather than promoting health. However, this situation is changing. As costs continue to rise, the health care system has been undergoing increased scrutiny by consumers, employers, health professional groups, and policymakers.

What Is Health?

Merriam-Webster's Collegiate Dictionary defines health as "the condition of being sound in body, mind, or spirit, especially from physical disease or pain."[1] The World Health Organization (WHO) in 1958 defined health as "a state of complete physical, mental and social well-being, and not merely the absence of disease or infirmity."[2] This definition has been criticized as an ideal state. Other definitions of health have emphasized life functioning, such as H. David Banta and Steven Jonas, who defined health as "a state of well-being, of feeling good about oneself, of optimum functioning, or the absence of disease, and of the control and reduction of both internal and external risk factors for both disease and negative health conditions."[3] Risk factors include environment, living conditions, or personal habits that increase the possibility of developing a disease or negative health condition in the future.[4]

The U.S. Public Health Service in 1979 published *Healthy People: The Surgeon General's Report on Health Promotion and Disease Prevention.*[5] In 2000, the Department of Health and Human Services (HHS) published the third edition of this work, *Healthy People 2010,* which represents the third time that the HHS has developed ten-year objectives for the United States, with 467 objectives in 28 focus areas (see Exhibit 1.1).[6] Healthy People 2010 is a valuable asset to pharmacists, physicians, health planners, and educators who seek to improve health in the United States. Highlighting major health priorities for the nation are the ten leading health indicators: physical activity, overweight and obesity, tobacco use, substance abuse, responsible sexual behavior, mental health, injury and violence, environmental quality, immunization, and access to health care. Some exam-

EXHIBIT 1.1. Healthy People 2010 Focus Areas

1. Access to quality health services
2. Arthritis, osteoporosis, and chronic back conditions
3. Cancer
4. Chronic kidney disease
5. Diabetes
6. Disability and secondary conditions
7. Educational and community-based programs
8. Environmental health
9. Family planning
10. Food safety
11. Health communication
12. Heart disease and stroke
13. HIV
14. Immunization and infectious disease
15. Injury and violence prevention
16. Maternal, infant, and child health
17. Medical product safety
18. Mental health and mental disorders
19. Nutrition and overweight
20. Occupational safety and health
21. Oral health
22. Physical activity and fitness
23. Public health infrastructure
24. Respiratory diseases
25. Sexually transmitted diseases
26. Substance abuse
27. Tobacco use
28. Vision and hearing

Source: U.S. Department of Health and Human Services. *Healthy People 2010:* Volume 1. International Medical Publishing, McLean, Virginia, 2000.

ples of objectives to be attained by the year 2010 are to reduce the proportion of children, adolescents, and adults who are overweight or obese; to increase the proportion of adults who engage in regular, moderate physical activity for at least 30 minutes per day; and to reduce cigarette smoking by adolescents.[7] Although some progress has been made to attain healthy lifestyles, much more remains to be accomplished.

Health Problems: Impact of Public Health and Lifestyle

The ten leading causes of death changed significantly between 1900 and 2000 (see Table 1.1). In 1900, the leading causes of death in descending order were: influenza and pneumonia, tuberculosis, gastritis, heart disease, senility, stroke, chronic kidney disease, accidents, cancer, and diphtheria.[8] In 2000, the ten leading causes of death in descending order were: diseases of the heart; cancer; cerebrovascular disease; chronic lower respiratory dis-

TABLE 1.1. Leading Causes of Death, United States, 1900 and 2000

1900		2000	
Causes of death	% of all deaths	Causes of death	% of all deaths
Influenza and pneumonia	11.8	Cardiovascular disease	29.6
Tuberculosis	11.3	Cancer	23.0
Diarrhea, colitis, enteritis, and gastritis	8.3	Stroke	7.0
Heart disease	8.0	Chronic lower respiratory diseases	5.1
Senility, ill-defined, or unknown	6.8	Unintentional injuries (accidents)	4.1
Stroke	6.2	Diabetes mellitus	2.9
Renal disease	4.7	Influenza and pneumonia	2.7
Unintentional injuries (accidents)	4.2	Alzheimer's disease	2.1
Cancer	3.7	Renal disease	1.5
Diphtheria	2.3	Septicemia	1.3
All other causes	32.6	All other causes	20.7

Sources: 1900 data: U.S. Bureau of the Census. Washington, DC; 2000 data: U.S. Department of Health and Human Services. Centers for Disease Control, National Center for Health Statistics, Monitoring the People's Health, Health, United States, 2002, Mortality tables. Available online at <http://www.cdc.gov/nchs/>.

eases; accidental injuries; diabetes mellitus; influenza and pneumonia; Alzheimer's disease; nephritis, nephrotic syndrome, and nephrosis; and septicemia, and accounted for nearly 80 percent of all deaths occurring in the United States.[9] Five of the ten leading killers in 1900 were infectious diseases; this dropped to three in 2000. Of the five leading killers in 2000, alcohol abuse and/or cigarette smoking is a major risk factor.

There have been major improvements in U.S. health levels since 1900. Between 1900 and 1999, the overall (crude) death rate declined by 50 percent and the infant mortality rate (IMR) declined by 90 percent. The major contributor of this decline is the remarkable drop in mortality that occurred in younger age groups. In 1999, the IMR was a record low of 7.0 deaths for infants under one year of age per 1,000 live births. The IMR for white infants declined to 5.8, while the rate for black infants declined only to 14.0, which has widened the gap in infant mortality between the two races.[10] About two-thirds of all infant deaths occur during the neonatal period (first twenty-seven days of life) and the neonatal mortality for black infants was 2.4 times greater than that for white infants.[11] This suggests that both prenatal and postnatal care, especially for black infants, needs to be improved.

Life expectancy from birth rose from 47.3 years in 1900 to 76.7 years in 1999, a record high. Life expectancy at birth for the white population is 77.3 years, 5.9 years longer than that for the black population.[12] Lifestyle factors account for some of this difference in life expectancy. However, health care access, quality care, and environmental factors also contribute.

America's reliance on sophisticated technology for the diagnosis and treatment of disease has overwhelmed the ability to pay for it. In 1960, about 5 percent of the gross domestic product (GDP) paid for health care services and in 2002 it is estimated at 13.8 percent (Note: 13.2 percent average annual increase from 1995 to 2000).[13] Many of the leading causes of death are preventable and, given the escalating costs of health care, an economic imperative is to renew interest in disease prevention.

In efforts to improve U.S. health status, Victor Fuchs concluded that "the greatest current potential for improving the health of the American people is to be found in what they do or don't do for themselves."[14] Dr. Lester Breslow showed that life expectancy and better health are significantly related to a number of simple basic health habits. These habits include

1. three meals a day at regular times instead of snacking;
2. breakfast every day;
3. moderate exercise two or three times a week;
4. seven to eight hours of sleep a night;

5. no smoking;
6. moderate weight;
7. no alcohol, or use in moderation.[15]

Breslow's health habits provide the background for *Healthy People 2010*'s objectives concerning healthy lifestyles. Although these health habits appear to be common sense, they are not common practice. Some policymakers feel the primary barrier to good health is lack of financial access to quality health care. Although the need for quality health care for all Americans is an important issue, the primary cause of poor health and premature death in the United States today is primarily due to the unhealthy lifestyle practices of many American citizens.

Health is largely a result of the complex interaction between genetic factors, environmental factors, lifestyle, and health care.[16] Genetic makeup certainly plays an important role and has been linked to diseases such as alcoholism and obesity. Environment also plays a key role in determining health and disease. A fertile area for continued research is to investigate the interrelationships between genetic factors and the environment in producing disease. Risk factors such as diet, pollution, occupational hazards, and smoking are also related to the genesis of chronic disease.

Most of the improvement in reducing the death rate from infectious diseases such as tuberculosis was not due to effective drug therapy but to improvements in nutrition, water supply, sewage disposal, and other hygienic measures. Tuberculosis mortality rates had fallen from approximately 250 per 100,000 in 1890 to 35.6 in 1938.[17] However, specific antituberculosis drug treatment was not in general use until 1938. Tuberculosis and other communicable disease mortality rates were greatly reduced without effective drug therapy measures and apparently were related to improvements in nutrition and hygienic measures.[18]

In addition to environmental and genetic factors, important social and psychological factors have a significant impact on disease and health. America's health care system is primarily focused on treating disease rather than promoting health. The United States spends billions of dollars to prolong the lives of elderly citizens near the end of their lives, while spending very little to promote healthy lifestyles of elderly citizens and the general population. The United States spends enormous sums on high-tech machines to save low-birth-weight babies, yet spends very little to reduce the incidence of low-birth-weight babies.[19] From a societal standpoint, America's economic resources are not providing the most health benefit for the least cost.

HISTORICAL EVOLUTION OF HEALTH SERVICES

1850 to 1900

From colonial times, most of the sick were treated at home by the family using medicinal herbs, relying on friends and family for advice, and later by use of medical guides for lay people. Most physicians were trained under an apprenticeship system and were also referred to as apothecaries. The first medical school was established in 1756 at the College of Philadelphia, which later was renamed the University of Pennsylvania.[20] Later, the apothecary role evolved into being solely the compounder and dispenser of medications, although people frequently sought medical advice from the apothecary, as they do from today's pharmacist. The first college of pharmacy was established at the Philadelphia College of Pharmacy in 1821. Students were pharmacy apprentices who worked full-time and attended classes at night.

Acute infectious diseases were the most critical health problems for the majority of Americans during the period 1850 to 1900.[21] Many of these diseases, such as cholera and tuberculosis, were associated with inadequate sewage disposal, contaminated water, and impure food. As Boston, New York City, Philadelphia, and other cities developed sewage systems, water purification systems, and improved standards for milk and food, diseases such as cholera and tuberculosis declined.

1900 to 1945

The period from 1900 to the conclusion of World War II was an era of rugged individualism and a pay-as-you-go system for health services. Communicable disease epidemics were largely brought under control due to improved nutrition and improved environmental conditions. In 1906, the Food and Drugs Act was passed, which established guidelines to prevent the adulteration and misleading labeling of drugs and foods in the United States. Most of the act's impact was on food rather than drugs. In 1910, the Flexner Report,[22] published by the Carnegie Foundation, provided a scathing review of U.S. medical school education. This report brought about necessary changes in the formal training of physicians and established Johns Hopkins School of Medicine and its four-year curriculum as the preferred model for medical education. As a consequence of the Flexner Report, many schools closed and others revised their curricula. State licensing boards were empowered to raise practice standards and were encouraged to establish rigorous licensure. Physician training remained largely general practice, which met most health care needs of the time.

Notable therapeutic breakthroughs included the discovery of insulin in 1922 by Banting and Best, and in 1928 Alexander Fleming made the first of several discoveries that led to the use of penicillin. The discovery of penicillin began the "era of antibiotics," and this "miracle drug" revolutionized the treatment of infectious diseases. Now, instead of long-term disability and possible death, a patient could be given an injection of penicillin and sent home. With the eventual decline of many infectious diseases by penicillin and other antibiotics, people lived to be older, and chronic illnesses became the predominant problem of elderly American citizens.

Community pharmacies were relatively small independent pharmacies; most medicinal products were compounded and dispensed. As pharmaceutical companies manufactured an increasing number of pharmaceutical products, the number of products compounded by community pharmacists declined. Hospitals began to assume a more important role as technology developed (e.g., anesthesia and aseptic surgical techniques) and better-trained health professionals provided inpatient care.

1945 to 1999

As acute infectious diseases further declined with the arrival of the antibiotic era, chronic illnesses began to dominate as the major problems in health. Although healthy lifestyle practices can help prevent the onset of chronic illnesses, these habits must be implemented long before the signs and symptoms of chronic disease are manifested. Once chronic disease is diagnosed, it is not typically cured by medical or drug treatment and stays with the patient forever. Progression to later stages of chronic diseases is affected by nutrition, smoking, alcohol use, sedentary lifestyle, obesity, and other debilitating lifestyle habits.

From the end of World War II to about 1980, hospitals experienced a major growth period. The Hill-Burton Act (1946) stimulated hospital renovation and construction of new facilities in both urban and rural areas. The development of Blue Cross/Blue Shield plans and expansion of commercial health insurance groups also fueled this expansion. In 1965, with Medicare and Medicaid passage, health benefits were extended to the elderly and the poor, also increasing the use of inpatient hospital facilities.[23] In 1965, 25 percent of the health care dollar was consumed by hospitals, increasing to 36.5 percent in 2000.[24] Hospital costs remain the largest category of health spending, and also remain the primary target to control costs.

Hospitals' desire to have the latest technology has been a major force in driving up health care costs. While computerized axial tomography (CAT) scanners, magnetic resonance imaging (MRI), and positron emission technology (PET) scanners have advanced the diagnosis of some diseases, these advancements have also contributed to the high cost of health care.

During this time period, America's viewpoint on health switched from rugged individualism to "health care as a right." It was also felt that government should assume greater responsibility for solving health care problems for all American citizens. Examples of greater government involvement included Medicare and Medicaid passage in 1965, which used public funds to provide health care. As health care expenditures continue to soar, policymakers and employers began to exert pressure for cost control. Recent attempts have been made to restrain inpatient health care by emphasizing ambulatory health care.

Some of the strategies employed by the federal government to control the rising cost of health care include hospital planning, changing the amounts and methods of reimbursement for services, and encouraging the development of managed care systems.[25] One of the efforts that met with some success was President Nixon's Health Maintenance Organization (HMO) Act of 1973, which sought a new health delivery system that could be implemented at a reasonable cost. HMOs have been in existence for most of the twentieth century, although only a few of them have flourished. The HMO Act established financial incentives for the development of HMOs (a prepaid health delivery system), and encouraged their use by employers with twenty-five or more employees. HMOs and other forms of managed care have grown substantially since the passage of the HMO Act. Managed care systems, such as HMOs and preferred provider organizations (PPOs), should continue to grow at a rapid rate.

Another cost-containment measure that has met with some success was the development of the 1983 Medicare prospective payment system, which paid hospitals based on a preset diagnosis-related group (DRG) amount that is independent of the length of stay and services provided to the individual patient.[26] Given the government's success with prospective payment, other third-party payers, such as Blue Cross/Blue Shield and commercial health insurance carriers, have also converted to a prospective payment system.

2000 and Beyond

The health care delivery system in the United States has been marked by three distinct evolutions; it is now in its fourth period. From the era of rugged individualism to greater centralization of control by the federal government, America's health care system has certainly undergone dynamic changes. Our health care system has been described as the best and the worst in the world. The "best" when we speak of the freedom to choose the physician, hospital, and pharmacist and having access to the latest surgical and treatment techniques, which are paid for by our private insurance plans. The "worst" in the world when we speak of lacking access to quality health care by millions of Americans who have no health insurance or are underinsured, individuals who are on expensive prescription drugs but cannot afford them, and the disparity in life expectancy between Caucasians and other racial groups in the United States. The U.S. system is characterized by the overlapping, unplanned, and wasteful use of personal and public financial resources. The country's health care system has been described as the best and worst in the world, but the reality resides somewhere in between these polar perspectives.

Although it is difficult to categorize the American health care system, the next two sections will review health care delivery as one of two models: the private health care system and the public health care system. In reading this section, it should be kept in mind that these are somewhat arbitrary classifications.

THE PRIVATE HEALTH CARE SECTOR

Employed, Insured, Middle-Income America

When most Americans think of the U.S. health care system, they are usually employed, middle-income families with health insurance provided through their employment.[27] Ambulatory care services are provided by physicians in private practice or managed care settings. Each individual chooses a physician or managed care program to meet his or her own or family's health care needs. This informal set of services is paid for directly by the consumer or through a private health insurance plan. The coordination of this system is dependent on the customer or a primary care physician (e.g., family practice physician). When a specialist referral is needed, this is orchestrated by that gatekeeper physician. When medications are prescribed, the individual decides which community pharmacy will be used. Dependent upon insurance coverage, these ambulatory services may or may not be covered. Increasingly, prescription drug coverage is being included in insurance plans. Typically, the individual pays out-of-pocket for most of these services until a certain deductible is met and then the health insurance plan takes over the majority of further payments. When inpatient hospital services are needed, the physician sends the patient to a community hospital where that physician has medical-staff privileges. Typically, the majority of hospital care is covered under most health insurance plans. Therefore, the payment shifts from the individual to the insurance plan.

Approximately 55 percent of the total health care expenditures are spent by the private sector.[28] Examples of private sector health insurance plans include Blue Cross/Blue Shield plans, commercial health insurance companies, HMO and PPO plans, and employer self-insurance programs. Public sector spending currently comprises about 44 percent and will continue to increase unless funding cutbacks for health care are implemented by the federal and state governments.[29]

Long-Term Care

If long-term care is needed, a continuum of services is available; some of these services are covered by health insurance plans. Most health insurance plans provide little or no coverage for nursing home costs, causing the individual or family to personally cover costs (or obtain Medicaid coverage). Gradually more nursing home plans (MediGap plans) are being sold by private insurance companies. Much of long-term care has shifted away from hospital and nursing home settings to home health care groups with the assistance of a visiting nursing service.

Mental Health Services

Mental health services are increasingly being covered by the family's health insurance plan. However, with a long-term diagnosis, there may be a shift from the private sector to the public sector for additional services. Substance abuse treatment may be a part of an individual's private health insurance plan. Although the family practice physician is trained to handle minor emotional problems, if the problem becomes more complex or severe, the patient is usually referred to a psychiatrist or mental health facility for further evaluation and treatment.

Managed Care

Managed care is a network of providers formed to offer cost-effective services. An HMO is a prepaid health plan in which enrollees pay a fixed fee (often with copayment) for designated health services. Managed care is the use of a planned and coordinated approach to providing health care— the goal being quality care at the lowest cost, including emphasis on preventive care. With HMOs, payment is usually prepaid to the provider for services on a per-member, per-month (PMPM) basis. Thus, a provider is paid the same amount of money every month for a member regardless of whether that member receives services, and despite the cost of those services (a service contract). A PPO is an insurance plan in which the managed care organization contracts with health providers to provide health services under a discounted-fee schedule. This health care plan is prepaid, and the member or family is usually enrolled for a one-year period and is entitled to certain agreed-upon services. Health care services usually include physician visits, hospital services, prescription drugs, mental health services, and home health care services. Typically, a primary care physician (gatekeeper) is chosen or assigned to coordinate an individual or family's health care services. When a specialist referral or hospital service is required, the gatekeeper physician must approve the need for these services. If an individual or family goes outside the plan for these services, these services are usually not fully reimbursed, or may not be reimbursable at all. Strong incentives are built in to encourage members to stay within the system. Managed care plans now comprise about three-fourths of the U.S. health care marketplace.

Pharmaceutical Care

Greater emphasis is being placed on pharmaceutical care that has been defined by Doug Hepler and Linda Strand as the "responsible provision of drug therapy for the purpose of achieving definite outcomes that improve a patient's quality of life."[30] These outcomes are

1. cure of a disease,
2. elimination and reduction of a patient's symptomatology,
3. arresting or slowing of the disease process, and
4. preventing a disease or symptomatology.

Traditionally, pharmacists have been primarily concerned with the process of care. They ensure if the correct drug and the right dose at the right time are provided. With the focus on outcomes, the pharmacist is also responsible for what happens to the patient when the drug is given (outcome or result of care). Examples of outcome criteria include improved medication compliance, improved medication therapy, decreased adverse reactions, and patient satisfaction. As more and more community pharmacies are facing closure due to steadily declining gross margins and increasing competition by pharmacy superstores and mail-order centers, there is increasing impetus for pharmacists to adopt the pharmaceutical care role. To assume this role, community pharmacists will need to complete pharmaceutical care training programs (see, e.g., the American Pharmacists Association and the National Institute for Pharmaceutical Care Outcomes). Emphasis in these training programs is to encourage the community pharmacist to assume the role of the drug therapy expert and be responsible for the reduction of drug-related problems. These training programs assume that getting the pharmacist more involved in patient care will result in improved outcomes and the reduction of more expensive services, such as hospitalization and unnecessary physician visits, thereby reducing the overall cost of health care.

Summary

The distinctive feature of the private health care system is that the consumer has the ability to choose the physician and pharmacist. If satisfied, they maintain that relationship. The major limitation with the traditional fee-for-service system is that the emphasis is on overutilization of resources by the provider and the lack of incentives to encourage healthy lifestyles and reduction of high-tech care. With managed care, these incentives are reversed.

THE PUBLIC HEALTH CARE SYSTEM

Federal Government-Provided Care

Military Medical Care

The military medical care system is a general term that refers to the separate systems of the U.S. Army, Navy, and Air Force. This system has the responsibility of providing health care for active-duty military personnel, both in the United States and throughout the world, where care is needed for service-connected problems. It is a well-organized system in which there is no direct cost to the individual. There is considerable emphasis on promoting wellness and prevention of injuries, so this system of care is rather unique in that it promotes health and does not just provide for sickness care. Medical corpsmen (medics) are nonphysician personnel with special training who perform many of the routine ambulatory care services, and refer more complicated cases to physicians. Acute care services are provided at base dispensaries, sick bays aboard ship, or base hospitals on various military installations. Regional military hospitals provide more complicated services.

If a serviceperson receives a medical discharge, medical care is generally provided at the Veteran's Administration (VA) facilities. The VA system also operates for disabled and retired veterans of previous U.S. military service. The VA system operates hospitals and outpatient clinics throughout the United States, focusing largely on ambulatory care, hospital care, mental health services, and long-term care. Most of the patients are male veterans with multiple-system problems. The VA system is funded by the federal government. Although recent efforts have been made to privatize the VA system, it is unlikely that these efforts will be successful. Veterans Affairs medical centers have been among the leaders in the development of pharmacist's roles in ambulatory care. Pharmacists have been involved in VA primary care clinics in pharmacist-managed anticoagulation clinics, where they have provided benefits over standard care in the form of desired therapeutic control with fewer adverse effects.[31]

Indian Health Service

Treaties signed between American Indian Tribes and the U.S. government stipulated that American Indians would be provided certain medical and hospital services, and this precedent continues today. Management of the Indian Health Service (IHS) is provided by the U.S. Department of Health and Human Service's Public Health Service (PHS), and the majority of IHS pharmacists are PHS Commissioned Corps. Health care and pharmacy services are provided to 1.4 million American Indians and Alaska natives living on or near reservations in 34 states. IHS programs are carried out through 46 hospitals, 137 ambulatory health centers, and 201 other treatment locations. Pharmacists as PHS officers were first assigned to hospitals in 1953 to establish dispensing policies and practices. During the 1960s, several IHS innovations set the stage for an active clinical pharmacist role. The first innovation was the replacement of the traditional prescription blank with the patient's medical record as the primary document used to fill all prescriptions. The second innovation was that IHS pharmacists were the first to use private consultation rooms. The third major innovation was the provision of primary care to ambulatory patients with both acute and chronic health problems. These programs were developed under the leadership of Dr. Allen J. Brands, IHS pharmacist from 1955 through 1981, and remain an important part of pharmacy practice today. This unique primary care role has evolved due to a physician shortage and the needs of the underserved American Indian population, and is well suited for rural areas. Although the pharmaceutical care role has been advocated in the ambulatory setting, most of these innovations were first developed in the Indian Health Service.

Community Health Centers (CHCs)

In 1965, to stimulate societal growth and decrease poverty, Congress funded the Neighborhood Health Centers (NHC) as part of the Equal Opportunity Act of 1964, to provide comprehensive health care to low-income populations in urban and rural areas of the United States.[32] In 1973, the NHC program was transferred to the U.S. Public Health Service and the freestanding ambulatory care facilities were designated CHCs.[33] In 1974, the CHCs required provision of diagnostic treatment and other services by a physician or physician extender, laboratory services, well-child care, dental services, social services, and pharmaceutical services. The 1978 amendments to Sections 329 and 330 of the Public Health Service Act changed the "supplemental" services designation and made pharmacy a "primary" service. All CHCs are required to provide or arrange for pharmacy services for their patients; however, some CHCs provide pharmaceuticals through contracted arrangements with an off-site pharmacy, while other CHCs provide on-site licensed pharmacies. For instance, the Siouxland Community Health Center (SCHC) in Sioux City, Iowa, provides in-house pharmacy services. Given the rising costs of drug therapy and growing evidence of the cost of ineffectively managed drug therapy, demonstration projects such as SCHC were funded by the Health Resources and Services Administration (HRSA) to deliver progressive clinical pharmacy services (i.e., diabetes disease state management services to patients with diabetes at SCHC). SCHC and the University of Nebraska's College of Pharmacy were one of the first seven CHCs to receive funding from the U.S. Bureau of Primary Care to develop and deliver clinical pharmacy services.[34]

Unemployed, Uninsured, Low-Income America
(Local Government Health Care)

According to the Kaiser Family Foundation, in 2003, nearly 45 million Americans under the age of 65 had no health insurance. About one-fourth of the U.S. population will lose health insurance coverage for some period during the next two years. Losing a job often results in losing insurance coverage. Becoming ill or living with a chronic medical condition can also result in losing insurance coverage or not being able to obtain it.[35] When uninsured and underinsured Americans need health care, they often rely upon public hospitals, teaching hospitals, public health clinics, and community health centers. With proposed cutbacks in Medicaid, these providers will be requested to provide more services with fewer financial resources.

Medicaid

Medicaid is a jointly operated federal and state program designed to provide health care for the poor. Medicaid recipients include the blind and disabled, the aged poor, and families with dependent children (if one parent is absent, unemployed, or unable to work). Services for Medicaid recipients include inpatient and outpatient hospital care, physician visits, laboratory services, radiology services, and nursing facility care. Federal funding to states is set on a cost-sharing basis, based upon the state's per capita income, where wealthier states would get less than 50 percent and poorer states get more than 50 percent of the federal distribution. Although an outpatient prescription program is not mandated by federal regulations, it is an option provided by most states.

Passage of the Omnibus Budget Reconciliation Act of 1990 (OBRA 1990) mandated that pharmacists must offer to counsel Medicaid patients on outpatient prescription drugs. It also required pharmacists to document patient counseling and drug utilization review (DUR) activities. Although OBRA 1990 presented an opportunity to expand the pharmacist's role in health care, it is still unclear what impact has been made on changing counseling practices. Pharmacists objected to this mandate because there is no additional compensation, not enough time, and greater liability.[36] Many states have extended this legislative counseling mandate to include not only Medicaid patients but also non-Medicaid patients. Hence, some states now require that pharmacists offer to counsel all ambulatory care patients. Again, little research has been done to measure the impact of this legislation and boards of pharmacy have been lax in enforcing compliance with these regulations.

Medicare and Medicaid account for nearly three-fourths of public expenditures for personal health services. Medicaid expenditures have increased rapidly in recent years, causing budget overruns for many states. Increasingly, states are turning toward managed care programs in an attempt to control expenditures. In theory, managed care systems reduce costs by allowing providers to manage treatment of their patients, reducing unnecessary care and focusing on preventive care. In practice this is not always the case, and despite the growth in managed care plans most of the Medicaid dollars are still spent for traditional fee-for-service medicine. Medicaid expenditures account for 46.3 percent of the total nursing home expenditures and represent the largest category of Medicaid spending (44.1 billion dollars in 1998). The U.S. Congress and most states are examining strategies to reduce spending for Medicaid. Although cutbacks are inevitable, the impact on access to quality patient care is a major concern.

Medicare

Medicare beneficiaries are covered by the Social Security Amendments passed in 1965, which extended health care services to all persons sixty-five years of age and older. Medicare Part A coverage includes inpatient hospital care, skilled nursing facility care, hospice, and home health care, with deductibles and limits placed on each area. Medicare beneficiaries are also eligible for Medicare Part B coverage, which, for a relatively small health insurance premium, allows senior citizens to obtain extended coverage for physician services, outpatient hospital services, home health care services, and a limited number of outpatient drugs (e.g., hepatitis B vaccine, immunosuppressant drugs, epoetin, pneumococcal and influenza vaccine, and some oral cancer drugs).

Medicare Prescription Drug Benefit (Part D)

Medicare Part D and the Prescription Discount Card were passed by the U.S. Congress to provide a prescription drug benefit as part of Medicare. Intended as a transitional assistance program to help seniors pay for prescription drugs for 2004-05, enrollment in the Discount Cards has been slow and disappointing. Instead, elderly have purchased their drugs through traditional distribution channels (e.g., community pharmacies, mail order) and also through Canadian mail-order pharmacies.

Part D of Medicare was passed by the U.S. Congress in 2003 and will be implemented in 2006; this will establish a prescription drug benefit for the elderly. Beneficiaries' out-of-pocket costs for prescription drug coverage include: Part B premium, a $250 deductible, 25 percent coinsurance rate from $250 to $2,250, and no coverage from $2,250 to $5,100. Proponents of Part D have proclaimed Part D as a good plan and others suggest that it is a good start. The author's personal opinion is the Part D program combines limited prescription drug coverage with high out-of-pocket costs, and is a pathetic attempt to control prescription drug costs. Initial cost estimates of the plan were $400 billion over ten years and this estimate has grown in early 2005 to $800 billion.

Federal Government Agencies

The public health care sector also includes various agencies at the federal level, including the Department of Health and Human Services (DHHS). The FDA is within the DHHS and is responsible for the approval and regulation of new drug products in the American marketplace. The HRSA is involved in providing health care to health-manpower-shortage areas, to medically underserved populations, and to special service populations. HRSA is the administrative agency for the National Health Services Corps Programs and recruits practitioners for inner-city and rural areas that are designated as health-manpower-shortage areas. Another DHHS agency is the Centers for Medicare & Medicaid Services (CMS) that administers both the Medicare program and the Medicaid program. The Centers for Disease Control and Prevention (CDC) is another DHHS department and is responsible for the control and prevention of infectious and some chronic diseases. Other agencies within the federal government have health-related programs, but they are too numerous to list.

HEALTH CARE: RIGHT OR PRIVILEGE?

Within the framework of President Lyndon B. Johnson's "Great Society" era, the 1965 passage of the Medicare and Medicaid programs was accompanied by the belief that health care is a "right" and not a "privilege." Since the early 1900s, the United States has periodically examined the need for a nationalized health care program, but each time this type of health care reform has been defeated.[37] Health care costs are rising much faster than other sectors of the economy. About 14 percent of our GDP was spent on health care in 2002, and this double-digit rate is expected to continue for health care spending. The idea of universal coverage, a belief held by most American citizens, holds that every citizen should have access to health care coverage. However, the majority of American society does not want to pay for other people's health care. With recent congressional attempts to reduce funding for both the Medicare and Medicaid programs, combined with reduced expenditures for other health-related programs, the gap between "right" and "privilege" will undoubtedly become wider.

Although federal legislation did not pass, both the problems of our health care system and the efforts to reform the system continue. However, these efforts do not have the capability to appropriately address the problems of access, quality, and cost. Eventually, the federal government will again be faced with the issue of health care reform and the American people will accept major changes in their health care system only when the conditions are right. As David Banta and Steven Jonas concluded,

> the underlying problems of the U.S. health care delivery system are not access and cost. Those are simply outcomes of in-built and long-standing system difficulties. . . . If the money the American people are spending on health care bought the kind of health and health care

product it easily could buy, then we would be among the healthiest people in the world, and there would probably be little concern about the amount of money being spent.[38]

The United States spends much more of its GDP on health care than any other country in the world. One reason for this is that the United States spends huge amounts of dollars to prolong unhealthy life at the end of the life span and spends very little on health promotion.[39]

Methods proposed to change this situation include managed care and a Canadian-style, single-payer plan. The American system prides itself on high-quality, high-tech health care. Unfortunately, very few of the high-tech interventions have clearly shown to be of benefit. Brook and Lohr estimate that the United States spends 30 to 50 percent of health care expenditures to support services that produce little or no demonstrable benefit.[40] American society will need to examine societal benefit versus individual benefit in determining what types of technologies, new drugs and services will be used, and who will pay the cost. Issues of cost-effectiveness will play an increasingly important role in health and pharmaceutical care. These cost issues need to be examined according to ethical considerations and balancing individual benefit with societal benefit, so that appropriate decisions are made for American citizens.

CONCLUSION

This chapter provided a brief overview of the U.S. health care system and its historical evolution, the private and public health care systems, and issues that are associated with health care utilization. Although the purpose of health care is to promote health, the American system is mostly concerned about the diagnosis and treatment of disease, and not with the goal of promoting health. Our health care paradigm needs to change to one that values and rewards health promotion.[41] For this to happen, it will be necessary to redesign the U.S. health care system.

NOTES

1. *Merriam-Webster's Collegiate Dictionary,* Eleventh Edition. Springfield, MA: Merriam-Webster, Inc., 2003, p. 574.

2. World Health Organization. *The World Health Organization: A Report on the First Ten Years.* Geneva, Switzerland, 1958.

3. Banta, H.D. and Jonas, S. Health and Health Care. In Jonas, S. (ed.), *Health Care Delivery in the United States.* New York: Springer Publishing Company, 1995, pp. 11-33.

4. Ibid.

5. U.S. Department of Health, Education, and Welfare. *Healthy People: The Surgeon General's Report on Health Promotion and Disease Prevention.* Washington, DC: DHEW Pub. No. (PHS) 79-55071, 1979.

6. U.S. Department of Health and Human Services. *Healthy People 2010:* Volume 1. McLean, Virginia: International Medical Publishing, 2000.

7. Ibid.

8. Ibid.

9. U.S. Department of Health and Human Services, Centers for Disease Control and Prevention. *National Vital Statistics Reports,* 50:16 (September 16), 2002, p. 8.

10. U.S. Department of Health and Human Services. Centers for Disease Control and Prevention, National Center for Health Statistics. Health, United States, 2002, Mortality Tables. Available online at <http://www.cdc.gov/ nchs/>.

11. Ibid.

12. U.S. Department of Health and Human Services. Centers for Disease Control and Prevention, National Center for Health Statistics. Health, United States, 2002, Life Expectancy Table. Available online at <http://www.cdc.gov/nchs/>.

13. U.S. Department of Health and Human Services. Centers for Disease Control and Prevention, National Center for Health Statistics. Health, United States, 2002, National Health Expenditures Tables. Available online at <http://www.cdc.gov/ nchs/>.

14. Fuchs, W. *Who Shall Live?* New York: Basic Books, 1974.

15. Berkman, L.F. and Breslow, L. *Health and Ways of Living: The Alameda County Study.* New York: Oxford University Press, 1983.

16. LaLonde, M. *A New Perspective on the Health of Canadians.* Ottawa, Canada: Government of Canada, 1974.

17. Sigerist, H. *Medicine and Human Welfare.* College Park, MD: McGrath Publishing Company, 1970.

18. McKeown, T. *The Role of Medicine: Dream, Mirage, or Nemesis.* London: The Nufield Provincial Hospitals Trust, 1976.

19. Banta and Jonas, Health and Health Care.

20. Raffel, M.W. and Raffel N.K. History of Medical Education and Medical Practice in America. In Raffel, M.W. and Raffel, N.K. (eds.), *The United States Health System: Origins and Functions.* Albany, NY: Delmar Publishers, 1994, pp. 1-35.

21. Torrens, P.R. Historical Evolution and Overview of Health Services in the United States. In Williams, S.J. and Torrens, P.R. (eds.), *Introduction to Health Services.* Albany, NY: Delmar Publishers, Inc., 1993, pp. 3-28.

22. Flexner, A. *Medical Education in the United States and Canada:* Bulletin Four. In The Carnegie Foundation for the Advancement of Teaching. New York, 1910. Available online at <http://www.carnegiefoundation.org/elibrary/index.htm>.

23. Kovner, A.R. Hospitals. In Jonas, S. (ed.), *Health Care Delivery in the United States.* New York: Springer Publishing Company, 1995, pp. 162-193.

24. U.S. Department of Health and Human Services. Centers for Disease Control and Prevention, National Center for Health Statistics.

25. Eng, H.J. The U.S. Health Care System. In Fincham, J.E. and Wertheimer, A.I. (eds.), *Pharmacy and the U.S. Health Care System.* Binghamton, NY: The Haworth Press, 1991, pp. 8-29.

26. Balinsky, W. and Starkman, J.L. The Impact of DRGs on the Health Care Industry. *Health Care Manage. Rev.* 1987 Summer, 12(3):61-74.

27. Torrens, Historical Evolution and Overview.

28. U.S. Department of Health and Human Services. Centers for Disease Control and Prevention, National Center for Health Statistics.

29. Ibid.

30. Hepler, C.D. and Strand L.M. Opportunities and Responsibilities in Pharmaceutical Care. *American Journal of Hospital Pharmacy* 1990, 47:533-542.

31. Alsuwaidan, S., Malone, D.C., Billups, S. J., and Carter, B.L. Characteristics of Ambulatory Care Clinics and Pharmacists in Veterans Affairs Medical Centers. *American Journal of Health-Systems Pharmacy* 1998, 55:68-72.

32. Mezey, A.P. and Lawrence, R.S. Ambulatory Care. In A.R. Kovner (ed.), *Jonas's Health Care Delivery in the United States.* New York: Springer Publishing Company, 1995, pp. 122-161.

33. Roemer, M. *Ambulatory Health Services in America.* Rockville, MD: Aspen System Corporation, 1981.

34. Scott, D.M. Ambulatory Care. In R.L. McCarthy and K.W. Schafermeyer (eds.), *Introduction to Health Care Delivery.* Gaithersburg, MD: Aspen Publishers, Inc., 2001, pp. 229-254.

35. Ibid.

36. Clinton, W.J. *The President's Health Security Plan.* Washington, DC: The White House Domestic Policy Council Times Book. New York: Random House, 1993.

37. Ibid.

38. Banta and Jonas, Health and Health Care.

39. Emanuel, E.J. and Emanuel, L.L. The Economics of Dying: The Illusion of Cost Savings at the End of Life. *New England Journal of Medicine* 1994, 330:540-544.

40. Brook, R. and Lohr, K. Will We Need to Ration Effective Health Care? *Issues in Science and Technology,* 1986, 3:1-10.

41. Freymann, J.G. The Public's Health Care Paradigm Is Shifting: Medicine Must Swing with It. *Journal of General Internal Medicine,* 1989, 313-319.

Chapter 2

Financing Health Care in the United States

Lon N. Larson

INTRODUCTION AND PURPOSE

Today health insurance in a variety of forms—private and public programs, conventional insurance and managed care—is commonplace. (In this chapter, the term *insurance* is used to include all public and private prepayment plans.) Given the potential financial consequences of illness, health insurance coverage is perceived as a virtual necessity. In 2001, personal health expenditures averaged just over $4,850 per person or $19,400 for a family of four.[1] Little wonder that health insurance is often a divisive issue in labor contract negotiations, or that persons in entry-level positions highly value a "job with benefits." About 85 percent of the U.S. population has health insurance coverage through private or public programs; the remaining 15 percent or 41 million persons are without coverage and represent a major concern in health care financing.[2]

In addition to patients or potential patients, other groups are concerned about health insurance. These include employers, governments, and providers. Through a historical "accident," health insurance has become intertwined with employment in the United States. Employment-based insurance covered about 63 percent of the population in 2000.[3] Employer-sponsored insurance is a dominant feature of the U.S. health care system. Although it has been proposed as a foundation for health care reform, employer-based insurance has also been criticized as an impediment to reform.[4]

Health care financing is a major issue within federal and state governments. Federal and state governments paid over 43 percent of the nation's personal health expenditures in 2001.[5] Most of the spending was in Medicare and Medicaid, the two largest public sector programs for financing health care services, which covered nearly one-quarter of the population in 2001.[6] Further, the increasing costs of health care are causing problems for government budgeting. Medicaid and Medicare cost over $466 billion in 2000, compared to $13 billion in 1970.[7]

The proliferation and growth of health insurance are also important to providers. In 2001, private or public third-party programs paid over 83 percent of personal health care expenses (i.e., provider revenues).[8] Insurance has affected the way that services are delivered. Its incentives have helped fuel the rapid increases in health care expenditures by reducing the importance of cost as a consideration in decision making by patients and providers. Further, by assuring payment for hospital capital expenditures, insurance has promoted the adoption and diffusion of new technologies.

Through a confluence of factors—organizing social insurance to protect against catastrophic health expenses, accidents of history, and efforts to help the elderly and the indigent—the United States has built a unique health care financing system. This system, with a heavy reliance on the private sector and employment-based insurance, has financed the most technologically sophisticated health care system in the world. However, it has failed to reduce financial barriers to care for a sizable number of persons, and it has fueled a cost escalation trend that has wreaked havoc with government budgets and employee wages.

The purpose of this chapter is to describe, explain, and critique this financing system. The chapter comprises three major sections. The first is an overview of health care financing, including descriptions of private and public programs, their historical development, and definitions of terms. This is followed by an explanation of the flow of funds into the health care system, focusing on the methods of obtaining funds to pay for health insurance, the methods of pricing health insurance policies, and issues that confront policy makers with respect to how we finance health care services. The final section is an explanation of the methods used for paying providers—hospitals, physicians, and pharmacies—and their influence or incentives for provider behavior.

The objectives of this chapter are to enable the reader to

1. develop and critique suggestions for pooling resources to pay for health services,
2. develop and critique suggestions for paying providers, and
3. understand the terms and concepts frequently used in discussions of health care financing.

These terms and concepts include moral hazard; community-rated versus experience-rated premiums; conventional or indemnity insurance versus managed care; problems with employer-based insurance; Medicare and Medicaid; characteristics of a desirable provider payment method; three general methods of paying providers; cost-based reimbursement versus prospective payment; the acronyms of DRGs, UCR, RBRVS; and drug product cost plus professional fee.

HISTORY AND ORGANIZATIONS

A vivid portrait of the evolution of health care financing in the United States can be seen in the trends in personal health expenditures. (Personal health expenditures are spending for services received by individuals, thus excluding spending for activities such as research and construction.) Table 2.1 lists expenditures by source of payment for selected years between 1950 and 2001. Despite its current prevalence and financial import, health insurance is a relatively recent phenomenon in the U.S. health care system. In 1950, the proportion of national health expenditures covered by private health insurance was less than 10 percent. It currently accounts for 35 percent of health spending.[9] The role of governments changed in 1965 with the passage of Medicare and Medicaid. In 1960, federal and state governments represented slightly over 20 percent of health care expenditures, compared to 43 percent in 2001.[10]

In keeping with the underlying philosophies of laissez-faire economics and individualism, the United States has historically relied on the private sector to finance medical care services. Until the Great Depression of the 1930s, paying for medical care was assumed to be the responsibility of

TABLE 2.1. Percent of Personal Expenditures by Source of Payment

Year	Out-of-pocket	Private insurance	Other private	Medicare	Medicaid	Other gov't.
1950	68	9	3	na	na	20
1960	55	21	2	na	na	22
1970	39	23	3	11	8	16
1980	28	29	3	17	11	12
1990	24	33	3	18	12	10
1995	21	32	2	21	15	9
2001	17	35	5	19	17	7

Sources: Rice, D.P. and Cooper, B.S. National health expenditures, 1929-71. *Social Security Bulletin,* January, 1972, (SSA) 72-11700; Levit, K.R., Lazenby, H.C., Braden, B.R., et al. National health expenditures, 1995. *Health Care Financing Review* 1996, 18(1):175-214; Levit, K.R., Smith, C., Cowan, C., et al. Trends in health spending, 2001. *Health Affairs* 2003, 22(1):154-165. na: Not available.

the individual. Insurance or prepayment plans, whether public or private, were nonexistent. Religious and philanthropic organizations supported charity care for the very poor. Furthermore, until the development of relatively expensive modern hospital care, the need to insure against financial risk was minimal. In the 1920s, the Committee on the Costs of Medical Care demonstrated the magnitude and unequal distribution of health care expenses; specifically, a relatively small proportion of persons incurred a relatively large proportion of expenses. The idea of pooling resources to protect against unpredictable, but significant, health care expenses became relevant.[11]

The Depression led to two fundamental changes in health care financing. First were the formulation and beginning of insurance or prepayment plans in the private sector, specifically, Blue Cross and Blue Shield plans. Second, the role of the federal government in social and welfare issues was dramatically changed with the enactment of the Social Security System. Although it failed to pass, federal health insurance was also proposed as a policy option.

Private Plans

Private health insurance began with the formation of Blue Cross plans by hospitals. In 1929, schoolteachers in Dallas contracted with Baylor University to provide specified hospital services for a predetermined monthly payment; thus began Blue Cross. Blue Cross plans were organized as nonprofit organizations to serve a dual mission: to protect individuals from the financial consequences of hospital care and to ensure payment to the hospitals for services rendered. The prepayment concept was endorsed by the American Hospital Association (AHA), which owned the Blue Cross symbol and set the criteria for organizations using it until 1972. The history of Blue Shield is similar to that of Blue Cross, except that it deals with physicians and surgical-medical benefits. There are several Blues plans across the nation; each is an independent corporate entity serving a specific geographic area. In addition to the Blues, commercial (i.e., for-profit) insurance companies such as Prudential, Aetna, Equitable, and many others entered the health insurance business. Over time, the differences between the Blues and the commercials have lessened, so that now it is difficult to see significant differences in their behavior. (Some Blue plans have dropped their non-profit status and become for-profit companies.)

Health insurance policies may be classified as group or nongroup. Nongroup insurance, as its name implies, covers one person or one family. Group insurance, in contrast, is underwritten for a specified group, usually the employees of an organization. In 2001, about 70 percent of the U.S. population was covered by private insurance; 88 percent of these persons were covered by employer-sponsored plans.[12]

With group insurance, the employer typically pays most or all the premium. In 2002, employers on average paid 85 percent of the single premium and 74 percent of the family premium; the monthly premiums were $255 and $663, respectively.[13] As discussed later, the employer's contribution represents tax-free income for the employee. An employer may offer one health plan, and all employees who want insurance coverage must enroll in it. However, many employers (at least the larger ones) offer several health insurance options to their employees, and each employee is able to select the one best suited for him or her.

Health insurance grew rapidly during the 1940s and 1950s. The proportion of persons with some form of health insurance had increased from 20 percent before World War II to over 70 percent in the early 1960s.[14] With wages controlled during the war, insurance was a mechanism to increase compensation in collective bargaining. This quirk in timing led to a key role for employers in financing health care services. The scope of services covered by health insurance was also expanding. Initially, coverage was limited to inpatient hospital care; then it expanded to include coverage for surgical-medical services received during hospitalization. These were referred to as basic hospital and basic surgical-medical benefits. (They are reflected in Parts A and B of Medicare, respectively.) To these benefits, major medical was added. This covers virtually all services, including outpatient services and prescription drugs. Typically, an annual deductible must be met before the insurer pays a specified proportion of expenses (commonly, 80 percent up to a stop-loss or out-of-pocket maximum, after which 100 percent is paid). In addition, special benefits or supplemental coverages emerged for services such as vision, dental, and prescription drugs.

The increasing prevalence and scope of coverage was fueled, in part, by the tax treatment of employer-paid health insurance premiums. The premiums are a deduction for the employer, and they are not considered taxable income for the employee in determining income or payroll taxes. For 2002, this represented about $2,600 in untaxed income for employees with single coverage and nearly $6,000 for family policies.[15] This subsidy is significant. The federal tax subsidy in 1999 was estimated to be over $95 billion; for perspective, this sum approaches the amount spent that year by the federal government for health care for the poor through Medicaid ($108 billion).[16]

For many employees (especially those with higher take-home pay), tax-free insurance coverage of routine medical expenses (e.g., regular, low-cost items such as prescriptions) is preferred to higher taxable wages. Although health insurance may have begun as insurance (that is, a means to protect against financial loss), it has expanded into a prepayment scheme. In other words, it has evolved from protection against catastrophic expenses to prepayment of ordinary medical expenses.

Until the 1970s, the predominant health insurance plans were what are now termed conventional insurance or indemnity plans. (In some contexts, indemnity benefits are differentiated from the service benefits. With the former, a loss is indemnified at a specified amount. The latter, common with Blues plans and prescription drug programs, expresses benefits in terms of services covered, and payment is worked out in participation agreements between insurer and providers. In this chapter, indemnity refers to all conventional plans.) With conventional insurance or indemnity plans, the insurance company and providers are separate and distinct entities. Typically, a conventional policy pays for covered services (within the scope of benefits) that are medically necessary for the treatment of an illness or condition, and which are provided by a licensed, covered provider. Providers are paid on a fee-for-service basis, i.e., a fee is paid for each service performed. The more providers do, the more money they get. Commonly, hospital payment is based on their billed charges, and physician payment is based on a usual and customary (U&C) fee schedule.

Insurance coverage removed much, if not all, of the cost-consciousness of patients and providers. At the time of service, cost was removed as a consideration in treatment choices because "insurance will pay for it." This effect of insurance increasing utilization is referred to as the moral hazard. Ideally, an insured event should be undesired and outside the control of the insured person; neither of these characteristics necessarily describes health care services. In the absence of these characteristics, the insured person may find the presence of the insured event more advantageous than its absence. In other words, insurance may cause the occurrence of the event that it is intended to protect against. Given that the presence of health insurance may affect the use of health services, a moral hazard is present.[17]

The moral hazard is compounded by employer-paid premiums. With the employer paying much of the premium, health care appears to be a "free lunch."[18] The individual employee often does not associate his or her claims with premium increases because the company pays for most or all of it. Using the figures cited earlier for 2002, employees paid $38 per month for single coverage, which was worth $255, and $174 for family coverage worth $663.[19] The situation is analogous to having a credit card—but without monthly statements. However, appearances are deceptive: the employee actually does pay much of the employer's contribution through lower wages.

In response to the demand for cost containment, managed care has proliferated. Since 1973, when the federal government passed the Health

Maintenance Organization (HMO) Act and especially since the early 1980s, many managed care firms entered the health care financing market. As the market matured in the 1990s, some of these firms consolidated or left the market. Managed care organizations (MCOs) may be for-profit or non-profit. Some are owned or operated by the Blues and commercial insurance companies; others are independent. Managed care plans include HMOs, preferred provider organizations (PPOs), and point-of-service (POS) plans.

The key difference between traditional health insurance (i.e., indemnity insurance) and managed care is that the latter integrates the financing or insurance function with health service delivery. An insurer is responsible for paying for services, but is not involved in delivering them. By assuming both activities, the managed care organization has incentives for providing services as efficiently as possible.

Managed care has grown rapidly in the employee benefits market. In 2002, 95 percent of employees were enrolled in some form of managed care plan;[20] this compares to 29 percent in 1988.[21] In recent years, enrollment growth has been greatest in the less-restrictive forms of managed care, PPOs and POS plans. In 2002, these plans enrolled 61 percent of covered workers compared to 42 percent in 1996; during the same time period, enrollment in HMOs declined from 31 to 26 percent of covered workers.[22] This movement to less-restrictive managed care is one reason given for the large increase (8.7 percent) in health expenditures in 2001.[23]

A new form of employee health benefit is emerging. It is in its infancy, and whether it survives and prospers or is merely a short-lived fad remains to be seen. It has been labeled as "defined contribution" or "consumer-driven" insurance, although the terminology is still evolving and terms have different meanings in different contexts.[24] In one variation of defined contribution, an employer contributes to the premium of a catastrophic insurance policy (e.g., a deductible of $5,000) and to a personal health spending account (e.g., $2.000) the employee can use to help pay for routine services. A second variation is that the employer gives each employee a specified amount of money, which the employee then uses to shop in the marketplace, with the aid of Internet technology, for the health plan of his or her choice.[25] Essentially, in this arrangement the role of the employer changes from being a purchaser of health benefits (from one or several insurers and managed care organizations) to giving each employee purchasing power to buy his or her own health insurance.

This new form of defined contribution differs from another arrangement commonly used by large employers.[26] Many employers offer their employees multiple health plans with varying premiums; the employer pays a set amount, regardless of choice, and the employee pays the remainder of the premium. The Federal Employee Health Program is an example of this.

Both the employer and employee were involved in purchasing health benefits; the employer chooses the alternatives that are on the menu, and the employee selects one. In the new arrangement, the employer is no longer involved in purchasing plans; in other words, the employer no longer sets the menu.

Public Programs

Medicare, Title 18 of the Social Security Act, was enacted in 1965. At the same time, a federal-state program for insuring the indigent or poor was enacted. This was Medicaid, or Title 19 of the Social Security Act. In 2001, nearly 14 percent of the U.S. population was covered by Medicare, and over 11 percent was covered by Medicaid.[27]

From a public policy standpoint, the two programs represent different approaches to social welfare policy: Medicare is a social insurance program, and Medicaid exemplifies the welfare approach.[28] These two approaches differ with respect to beneficiaries, benefits, financing, and administration. Briefly, social insurance programs, such as Medicare, are characterized as follows: eligibility is independent of means tests, benefits are earned, the scope of benefits is narrow, financing is through special taxes, and programs are administered centrally with uniform rules. Essentially, welfare programs such as Medicaid are the opposite: eligibility is based on means tests, benefits are broader in scope and are given to the recipients, financing is through general revenues, and administration is decentralized with some variability in the rules.

Medicare employs the social insurance approach to financing health services for the elderly. It is available to all Social Security beneficiaries, regardless of their financial means. Medicare consists of two parts—Part A and Part B—that initially resembled basic hospital and basic surgical-medical insurance, respectively. Part A, the hospital insurance, is mandatory. In addition to hospital services, Part A covers nursing home services, home health services, and hospice services. These coverages do not provide complete protection from the financial costs of care. They have limits to their benefits and include cost-sharing provisions. Part B is optional and covers medical and surgical services. This coverage entails an annual deductible and coinsurance. Unlike Part A, in which Medicare payment is payment in full, physicians who elect to not participate in Medicare can bill the patient for fees above those allowed by Medicare, although the amount that can be "balance billed" is restricted.

Medicaid, in contrast, is a joint federal-state welfare program. The beneficiaries are the poor and medically indigent. Within federal guidelines, each state administers its own program. For instance, the categorically needy (i.e., those eligible for public assistance) must be covered, but the state can also include the medically indigent (i.e., those unable to afford medical care). Medicaid benefits are more comprehensive than Medicare benefits. Some services are mandated, and the state must cover them. These include: inpatient and outpatient hospital services, physician services, independent lab and X-ray services, skilled nursing facility services, family planning services, home health care, transportation, rural health clinics, nurse-midwife services, and EPSDT (early and periodic screening, diagnosis, and treatment). Other services are optional, and a state may or may not cover them. Some of the commonly covered optional services are: prescription drugs, intermediate care facilities, and dental services.

THE FLOW OF FUNDS: POOLING RESOURCES

Health insurance and public financing programs involve two flows of money: first, the pooling of resources, and second, the disbursement of money for services received.[29] This section explores how funds are obtained or pooled; how providers are paid is discussed in a later section. It is important to remember, someone must pay for insurance and other health plans; these plans do not just magically appear with bottomless bank accounts. However, as we will see, our financing systems can make health care look like a free lunch. It is not. Ultimately, individuals—as taxpayers and as purchasers of goods and services—pay for everyone's health care.

We begin with a brief description of the component parts of the health insurance premium, which is the price of insurance. The following equations illustrate the ingredients of a premium:

Premium = Benefit Payments + Administrative Costs
Benefit Payments = Quantities of Services × Unit Prices
Administrative Costs = Administration + Risk + Profit

As indicated in the first equation, a premium can be divided into two parts. One is benefit payments or expenditures; that is, the amount paid for health services. Benefit payments, in turn, are influenced by the quantities of services consumed and their prices (the second equation). The other part of a premium is administrative costs, which are also referred to as the loading charge. Administrative costs include the insurer's costs to administer the policy (marketing, issuing identification cards, processing claims), the fees charged for underwriting or assuming the risk, the cost of conducting cost-containment activities (utilization review), and the profit or reserves of the insurance company (the third equation). In private-sector plans, benefit payments compose about 88 percent of the premium, and all administrative costs the remaining 12 percent.[30]

Benefit payments are payments for the covered medical services received by policyholders or enrollees. With conventional insurance, this is also referred to as the claims experience. The total amount spent for benefit payments reflects two factors: the number of services received and the price paid for each service. Several factors influence the quantity of services used: the health status of the insured person(s); the incidence of disease (e.g., an epidemic); the availability of new services; and, as mentioned previously, the presence of insurance can increase utilization. The price paid by an insurer depends on the prices it has negotiated with providers and the amount of cost-sharing required of the patient.

Cost-containment programs may be directed at either quantity used or per-unit prices. Utilization review, for instance, focuses on the quantity of services. Acquiring price discounts from providers through preferred provider arrangements is a way of lowering the prices paid for services. Patient cost-sharing affects both; it reduces the price paid by the insurance plan and, in addition, it reduces the quantity of services used.[31]

Health insurance premiums can be determined in one of two general ways: community rating or experience rating. In a community-rated premium, the claims experience of all members of the community is used to project per capita benefit payments. The premium is based on the claims experience of everyone—whether young or old, healthy or disabled. Experience-rated premiums are based on the claims experience of a particular group. For instance, groups of young and healthy persons would have lower per capita benefit payments and hence lower premiums than groups comprised of older and less healthy persons. Which is fairer, as we shall see later, depends on one's values.

During the post–World War II time period, competition among insurers intensified. In a competitive market for employee groups, experience rating is preferred over community rating. Any group of employed persons (aged less than sixty-five, not poverty-stricken) is likely to use fewer services than the overall community. Consequently, experience-based rates for employee groups were less than community-based premiums. Given the competition among insurers, experience rating became the usual practice. Although experience underwriting was advantageous for employers and employees, it was not so good for the elderly and others who were unemployed. Without spreading the risks over younger, healthier persons, the experience rates for the elderly (and other high-use persons) became very expensive. Ultimately, the solution for insuring the elderly and the indigent was government intervention in the form of Medicare and Medicaid.

In public programs, tax dollars are used to pay the costs of the programs. The cost of these programs consist of the same elements as private plans, except certain administrative costs (e.g., marketing), risk-related fees, and profit are not applicable. Medicaid is financed jointly by the federal and state government, with the dollars coming largely from federal and state income taxes. The income tax is theoretically a progressive tax: one in which persons with higher incomes pay a larger proportion of their income as taxes. In contrast, Medicare Part A (the hospital insurance) is financed exclusively through a payroll tax, in which a flat amount is paid up to a maximum level of income; income above that amount is not taxed. This payroll tax is regressive, in that persons with high incomes are paying a smaller proportion of their incomes into the Medicare fund than are persons with lower incomes. Medicare Part B is financed by federal income taxes for about three-fourths of total program costs and by beneficiary premiums for the remaining quarter.

Regardless of employer contributions to health premiums or tax coffers, the ultimate payer is the individual. The expense incurred by employers in paying for health benefits is ultimately paid primarily by employees in the form of lower wages, and secondarily by customers in the form of higher prices. Similarly, corporate taxes used to fund public programs are also ultimately passed onto employees or customers.

Issues in Pooling Funds

As a society, we face several important and difficult issues related to the pooling of funds to pay for health insurance. What is the appropriate role of employers in financing health care? How can those who most need coverage become or remain insured at reasonable rates (e.g., persons with high risks or history of health problems)? Is insurance the appropriate model for financing health services? What is the basis for determining fairness and equity in paying for health care? Underlying these questions is the fundamental issue of whether health insurance is a social good that should be purchased collectively, or a private good that can be distributed through the marketplace.

The current system of employment-based insurance results in dramatic disparities in health benefits. Not all employers offer health insurance, and not all persons are working. Generally, smaller firms with lower-wage workforces are less likely to offer insurance. In 2002, 62 percent of firms employing 3 to 199 employees offered health benefits compared to nearly all of the companies with 2,000 or more employees. Only about 55 percent of very small firms (three to nine workers) offered coverage.[32]

The result is that many persons are without health coverage. In 2001, the figure was about 15 percent of those younger than sixty-five.[33] They are simply not included in the pool. Further, poor people are more likely to be without insurance. In 2001, about 30 percent of the poor were without health insurance (or Medicaid)—twice the proportion in the overall population—and nearly half of the workers classified as poor were uninsured, compared to 17 percent of all workers.

The fundamental dilemma with employment-based health insurance is this: should services that are often essential to improving the quality of life, or maintaining life, be distributed on the basis of one's employment status? Although people without insurance may have access to emergency services (and even that is not assured), the situation with respect to more routine services is quite problematic. Imagine a person with diabetes. Like many chronic conditions, successful treatment depends upon effective patient self-management, which requires ongoing monitoring, education, and medication therapy. Continuity in relationships with providers is important. Yet continuous and coordinated care is not readily accessible to a person without insurance. Many uninsured patients, who may need the most assistance in managing their condition, do not receive primary care. They enter the system as patients when the damage is done and complications of diabetes appear.

A comparison of health services and education is instructive. When a person is laid off or becomes unemployed, his or her health insurance benefits are stopped (unless the person pays the employer's full premium). In contrast, education is not tied to employment. The person's children can attend public elementary or secondary schools without paying for the services out-of-pocket. Although employment plays a big role in gaining access to health care services, it is irrelevant in public education. Should these two services, both necessary to realize one's full human potential, be handled so differently?

A second issue (highlighted by the previous diabetes example) is whether the insurance model itself is appropriate for health services. Health benefits may be viewed as insurance or as prepaid services. As mentioned earlier in discussing moral hazard, insurance is intended to protect against the risk of rare, undesired, and unpredictable events. Yet health care services are not necessarily undesirable, nor are they rarely received. This is especially true of primary care services used in the diagnosis and treatment of chronic and minor acute conditions. From an insurance perspective, health coverage should be limited to very serious conditions associated with very large medical expenses; routine services should not be covered. An example is catastrophic coverage, in which patients face large deductibles before benefits begin. In essence, they are covered for health "catastrophes," but they pay for routine, primary care services directly out-of-pocket. Yet discouraging the use of preventive and primary care services—as is done with catastrophic coverage—may be medically and economically unwise. The treatment of diabetes and other degenerative chronic illnesses illustrates this point.

Commonly, persons with the largest health problems have the most difficulty with health insurance. They may be faced with ever-increasing health premiums, or they may be unable to get coverage at all. If they are members of a small employee group, the rates may have become so high that the employer has to drop coverage for the entire group. How can this happen? The insurance model is built upon the idea of protecting against risk; the higher the risk, the higher the premium. For instance, automobile insurance is more costly for bad drivers than good ones because the first is a riskier venture. Similarly, with experience-rated health insurance premiums, one can expect lower premiums with lower utilization; taking it a step further, healthy persons will have lower health insurance premiums than ill persons.

The insurance model in health care is reasonable if utilization of health services is within one's control, just as driving behavior is within our control. But such is not the case. Genetic makeup and social conditions—factors outside the control of individuals—are major determinants of health status. It is difficult to make the case that a person should be penalized with higher health insurance premiums (or being denied insurance at all) because of these uncontrollable factors. The appropriateness of the insurance model in health care depends largely on one's views of the determinants of health status. For those who view illness and subsequent health-services utilization as within the individual's control, the insurance model makes sense. For those who see health as luck—through good genes and a healthy environment—the insurance model is problematic.

A fourth issue is finding a method of pooling resources that is fair and equitable. How should the financing of health services be shared? What is fair? One alternative is for everyone to pay the same amount, regardless of health needs (i.e., use of services) or income. This is illustrated by community rating (discussed earlier). All persons in a community—healthy or ill, young or old, rich or poor—pay the same premium to support the purchase of services. Those who do not use many services (the healthy, the young) subsidize the care of those who do, regardless of their incomes. A second approach is to contribute to the system according to the use of services. This is represented by experience rating for employee groups, in which the premium for a group is based on its utilization and claims experience. Groups with the greater health needs and who use more health services have higher premiums. Historically, all members of a group have paid the same premium. In essence, the employee group is a community that shares the health expenses of its members.

As described, "defined contribution" or "consumer choice" plans are emerging in the marketplace, in which employers no longer purchase health benefits directly, but rather give employees purchasing power to buy their own health benefits. This arrangement reinforces the view that contributions to the health insurance pool should be assessed according to services used. In essence, individuals within a group pay according to the services that each uses. In other words, the healthy pay less, while the unhealthy pay more. A consequence of this approach is the demise of employee health benefits as a form of social insurance, in which all members of a group or community purchase insurance together, and the healthy help pay the expenses of the unhealthy.[34]

A final approach to pooling funds for financing health services is to do so according to one's income or ability to pay. Premiums—community-rated or experience-rated—are a "head tax"; in other words, the same amount is assessed each person in the community or group. Using figures cited earlier for 2002, the average employee paid $174 per month for family coverage (total monthly premium was $660 per month) or an annual assessment just shy of $2,100. The low-wage employee and the chief executive officer each contribute $2,100 to fund the group's health services. Is this fair?

Ethically, financing health services according to one's ability to pay may be the preferred approach. Buchanan argues that one element of a right to health care is that the contributions to pay for services are based on one's ability to pay.[35] In addition, one of the traditional objectives of government health policy is to redistribute resources to those least able to afford care (the other objective is to improve efficiency).[36] Based on this rationale, the financing of health services should be based on ability to pay, so that those with more financial resources contribute more to the community's health care delivery system. An example of this is Medicaid, which is funded primarily by revenues generated through the progressive income taxes of the federal and state government.

With Medicare, the issue of equity also arises. While virtually all individuals pay into the Medicare system when they are working, the benefits received by retirees far exceed the amount they contributed. For instance, the person who retired in 1991 was expected to receive more than five dollars in hospital services for every dollar he or she contributed to Medicare Part A when working.[37] In other words, the young subsidize the care of elderly. Is that equitable, especially since not all elderly are poor and not all young are wealthy? Further, Medicare Part A is financed through a regressive payroll tax; thus lower-paid employees pay a higher proportion of income into Medicare Part A than do higher-paid employees.

In addition, the same Medicare benefits—or the same subsidy—are potentially available to all Medicare recipients, even though their incomes can vary dramatically. Medicare does not pay for all health services (prescription drugs are a noted example). Out-of-pocket medical expenses account for over 20 percent of the income of low-income seniors, but less than 6 percent for high-income elderly.[38] One option for Medicare is to make benefits proportional to income, so that the elderly who are financially needy receive health services at very low cost, while those with financial means pay more. However, this may reduce the social solidarity promoted by a program like Medicare that treats all recipients equally. In short, how to finance—or pay for—Medicare in a fair and equitable fashion is a very complex policy issue.

In sum, should the accessibility of a service such as health care services be based on a person's employment status? What are the determinants of health status? Are they or are they not within the control of the individual? Whose responsibility is it to pay for health care services? What is a fair way to distribute the responsibility across individuals? These questions are at the heart of financing health services.

THE FLOW OF FUNDS: PAYING PROVIDERS

As background, generally in the U.S. economy prices are set by the forces of supply and demand in the marketplace or by government regulation (e.g., utilities). However, in some segments of the health care sector, prices are established in the absence of both; most notably, physicians and hospitals (outside of a few states that regulate hospital rates). The entire health care system is not void of competition, as evidenced by the retail pharmacy and health insurance markets. The lack of pricing controls (market or government) has been a major issue for insurers. What is an appropriate payment rate that is fair to the provider (i.e., covers costs of production, including a fair return on investment) and fair to the payer (i.e., promotes and rewards efficiency, reflective of value)?

The distinction between two types of efficiency is important. These are efficiency in production and efficiency in utilization. The former refers to the resources needed to produce a unit of service (e.g., a hospital inpatient day). Efficiency in utilization is the number and types of services consumed in treating an illness or condition. Both are important to the insurer because both affect health expenditures. As mentioned earlier, health expenditures are the product of the unit price multiplied by the number of units. The per-unit price or cost is largely a reflection of management—be it management of a hospital, pharmacy, clinic, or other provider; the number of units, however, is largely a reflection of medical practice.

Three general categories of payment methods are relevant. One consists of cost-based or charge-based methods. These are fee-for-service, and they involve no risks for the providers. With these methods, there are no incentives to be efficient in production or in utilization. In fact, the incentive is to use more services. In the following section, cost-based hospital reimbursement, physician U&C prices, and product-cost-plus-fee for pharmacies are discussed.

A second category consists of prospective payment. Examples are prospective payment using diagnosis-related groups (DRGs) for hospitals and capitation, in which the provider gets a set amount per member per time period. Here the fees are set ahead of time for episodes of care (e.g., a hospital admission, a patient-year), and the provider is responsible for providing all necessary for that episode. The provider is at financial risk; using too many services on a particular patient may cause the provider to lose money. The incentive facing the provider is to treat the episode of care as inexpensively as possible.

Capitation addresses both efficient production and efficient utilization. For a set dollar amount per person per time period, the provider assumes responsibility for delivering needed services during that time. In other words, the provider assumes financial risk, and therefore has incentives to be efficient in production and in utilization. One problem with capitation of nonphysician providers (e.g., hospitals, pharmacies) is that these providers can control their production efficiency (and per-unit prices) but may have little control over the physicians' utilization decisions. For example, a hospital may operate at peak production efficiency and have a reasonable cost per unit of service, but if unnecessary services are ordered, the average cost per stay in the hospital may be comparatively high. Similarly, a pharmacy can produce services and prescriptions very efficiently, but if physicians prescribe many and/or expensive products, the pharmacy may still lose financially.

A third category consists of salaries for professionals and global budgets for hospitals. Some health maintenance organizations pay their physicians on a salary basis, but generally these methods are not widely used in this country and are not discussed further here.

Hospitals and Facilities

Historically, insurers have paid hospitals on the basis of costs or charges. As insurance with charge- and cost-based reimbursement proliferated, incentives for efficiency in hospital management and utilization were lessened as the risk of loss diminished. Whether routine operating expenses or capital investments, costs could be passed along to the insurance purchaser with impunity. This fostered a competition among hospitals—not to be lower priced, but to be more technologically advanced. With financing provided by insurance reimbursement, hospital services became increasingly sophisticated. Likewise, the presence of insurance removed financial considerations from the decision making of physicians and patients. Because insurance was covering the bill, additional services or procedures could be ordered and used without financially harming the patient (e.g., an admission for observation and testing, extending a hospital stay by an extra day, or one more diagnostic test).

A major change in hospital payment occurred in 1983 when Medicare's Prospective Payment System (PPS) was enacted. Using DRGs as the basis of payment, this system changed the incentives that guide hospital behavior. The system may be viewed as a risk-adjusted payment for each stay or admission. The DRG system is a classification scheme by which hospital admissions or stays are classified not only according to clinical factors, but also according to resource consumption (i.e., economic or cost factors). Factors used to classify a stay include primary diagnosis, comorbidities or complications, and surgical procedure(s) performed, among others.

Each DRG is assigned a weight indicative of its resource consumption. The higher the weight, the greater the resources consumed (e.g., length of stay, intensity of care). A dollar rate is established which, when multiplied by the weight, gives the payment amount for an admission falling in that DRG. (The federal government sets rates for rural and urban hospitals in various regions.) The hospital is paid that rate, regardless of the actual expenses incurred during the stay. For instance, if the costs of treatment are less than payment, a surplus is generated. If costs exceed payment, the hospital suffers the financial loss.

Two elements of the PPS/DRG system made it especially innovative. First, it brought financial risk into hospital management. Second, it redefined the unit of production or output of hospitals to encompass clinical decisions by physicians as well as operational decisions by administrators. Much of the cost of a hospital stay depends on decisions made by physicians. Other than routine room-and-board services, they order all the services (and costs) during a stay, such as lab tests, X-rays, and medications. With prospective payment, these decisions affect the financial health of the hospital. Thus, hospitals are more interested in monitoring and reviewing patient-care decisions.

Prospective payment also has implications for hospital pharmacy. Cost-based reimbursement helped spur the development of innovative pharmacy services and promoted the adoption of new drugs because the costs associated with these endeavors could be passed on to the insurer. In contrast, with prospective payment, the pharmacy becomes a cost center whose expenses must be carefully monitored. For instance, the costs of new, expensive medications must be covered by the prospectively determined payment for that DRG. In this environment, formularies and prescribing protocols are very important. In addition, with prospective payment, innovative pharmacist services are more likely to be implemented if they can reduce the use of medications or other services. Prospective payment also generates demand for cost-saving or cost-effective pharmacist services.

Physicians and Other Professionals

Like hospital services, physician services have not historically been priced in a competitive market. Traditionally, the amount charged has been the professional prerogative of the physician. Advertising and price competition were considered unprofessional. Two methods have been used by insurers to reimburse physicians on a fee-for-service basis: (1) fee schedules and (2) usual and customary (U&C) charges. The latter method is sometimes referred to as usual, customary, and reasonable (UCR). Usual and customary pricing is based on actual charges; profiles of charges for each procedure are established by specialty and by geographic area. The usual charge is defined as the amount typically charged by the physician for that procedure. The customary charge is the prevailing amount charged among all physicians in the area. Often, this is a set percentile (e.g., 75th or 80th) of charges within the area for that procedure. The maximum allowable amount is the lower of these two charges.

The other method of physician reimbursement—the fee schedule—involves a relative value scale (RVS), a dollar conversion factor, and possibly geographic and/or specialty multipliers. A relative value scale compares procedures with respect to their length and complexity. A scale developed recently that has received a great deal of publicity as a possible reform agent in Medicare focused on the resources consumed by each procedure: the resource-based relative value scale (RBRVS). Relative values were based on time and intensity of work, differences in practice costs among specialties, and the opportunity cost of specialized training.[39] The relative values are multiplied by the dollar conversion factor to determine the fee or maximum allowable charge. The conversion factor reflects economic considerations, such as inflation. In addition, adjustments can be made to reflect other relevant variations in the costs of doing business, such as regional variations in wage rates.

Each of these methods has its advantages and disadvantages. U&C profiles require a great deal of maintenance; potentially, a profile for each physician is needed, as well as profiles by specialty and/or area. From an economic standpoint, the U&C system has a couple of deficiencies. Without market or government regulation, physician charges may have little economic rationale, either in relation to costs of production or the value of procedure. Further, if future fees are based on current charges, the incentive is to increase the amount charged. The fee schedule is easier to maintain once the relative values have been determined or assigned. Resource-based relative values are more reflective of input costs than uncontrolled charges. It may be easier to control overall expenditures with the fee schedule because only one value—the dollar conversion factor—must be adjusted. Whether this is an advantage or disadvantage depends on one's perspective. A potential disadvantage for the insurer arises if the relative values deviate significantly from actual charges: patients may have to bear a large portion of the bill.

Pharmacy Third-Party Programs

Direct coverage of outpatient prescription drugs is a relatively recent phenomenon. As mentioned earlier, prescription drugs were initially covered by major medical insurance, in which the subscriber submits claims and receives reimbursement; the provider is not directly involved. The first successful prepaid prescription plan was Prescription Service, begun in 1958 in Windsor, Ontario. In 1964, the California Pharmaceutical Association initiated a prepayment plan, PAID Prescriptions, which was later spun off from the association.[40] In the public sector, outpatient prescription drugs are an optional service under Medicaid. Each state decides whether or not to cover drugs. All fifty states (as well as the District of Columbia) have vendor drug programs. These programs paid $20.6 billion for prescription drugs in 2000; this represented 10.5 percent of all Medicaid expenditures.[41] Medicare does not cover outpatient prescription drugs. Drug coverage was part of the Medicare Catastrophic Coverage Act in 1988, but it was repealed before implementation.

Third-party drug programs often involve two administrative entities. One is the insurance company (or underwriter). The insurer is responsible for assuming the financial risk associated with the coverage. The insurer also determines the level and scope of benefits: which drugs are covered and which are not, the amount of patient cost-sharing, and the level of pharmacy payment. The second entity is a third-party administrator (TPA) or pharmacy benefits manager (PBM). The PBM is responsible for administering the contract: working with pharmacies, enrollees, and prescribers; processing claims; monitoring utilization and cost; and undertaking cost-containment activities.

The most common method of paying pharmacies is to reimburse the (1) acquisition cost of the product dispensed plus (2) a dispensing or professional fee. The acquisition cost is usually estimated; for example, average wholesale price (AWP) less a specified percentage. The professional fee is set; it applies to all prescriptions, regardless of the services actually rendered. It can be varied to promote "desired" behaviors; for instance, a higher fee may be applied to prescriptions filled with generic products.

This reimbursement method has the advantages of being easy to understand and easy to administer. It focuses on the product portion of the prescription, which is more tangible and quantifiable than the service portion. The method simply assumes that the professional service is the same for each prescription, without regard to whether it is new or a refill, the risks of the drug dispensed, or other diseases and medications of the patient. The acquisition cost of the product (the cost of goods sold) is a significant portion of the total cost of a prescription and this method keeps reimbursement rates current with changes in the prices of drug products; prices from manufacturers and wholesalers can be updated daily.

This method of reimbursing pharmacies also has problems. As with any fee-for-service system, the financial incentive is to produce more services. Further, as alluded to previously, this payment formula does not account for differing levels of service associated with different medications and clinical situations. Hence, the financial incentive is to dispense as many prescriptions as possible with the least possible time spent providing services. Further, this method ties pharmacist services to the dispensing of a product— no product, no fee. This runs counter with pharmacists' desire to provide more patient-centered services.

This method also makes it difficult to control the prices paid for drug products themselves. The prices charged by a manufacturer for its products (i.e., wholesale prices) become the basis for reimbursement. This is a given; it is outside the control or influence of the insurer or payer. This would be acceptable if the pharmaceutical manufacturers operated in a competitive market; however, with patent protection and other means of restricting competition, this may not be the case. Without controls on the product portion of the reimbursement, efforts to control the prices paid for prescriptions are limited to the professional fee.

Issues in Paying Providers

Reimbursement methods affect provider behavior; each reimbursement method is accompanied with incentives and disincentives. A "good" method rewards efficiency in production; that is, it has incentives for a provider to produce its services as inexpensively as possible. It also simultaneously rewards efficiency in utilization and promotes quality of care, so that all needed and cost-effective services are provided and unnecessary services are avoided. A good method of reimbursing providers is easily administered and assures accountability; payments reflect the services actually received by the patient. It enhances accessibility by encouraging providers to participate. Finally, a desirable reimbursement method is equitable or fair for both the buyer and seller.

SUMMARY

This chapter has described and explained how health services are financed in the United States. Many thorny issues remain unresolved: How should we pool our resources to pay for health insurance (and thereby, health services)? How should we distribute the burden of paying for health care services? Should it be by a "head tax" via premiums or based on one's ability to pay? How should we pay providers so that both buyer and seller are treated equitably? Can we devise payment methods that simultaneously promote efficiency and quality of care?

NOTES

1. Levit, K., Smith, C., Cowan, C., Lazenby, H., Sensenig, A., and Catlin, A. Trends in U.S. health care spending, 2001. *Health Affairs* 2003; 22(1): 154-164.
2. Mills, R.J. Current Population Reports, Health Insurance Coverage: 2001. Census Bureau, U.S. Department of Commerce, September 2002.
3. Ibid.
4. Budetti, P. Universal health care coverage—Pitfalls and promise of an employment-based approach. *Journal of Medicine and Philosophy* 1992; 17: 21-32; Fuchs, V.R. The Clinton plan: A researcher examines reform. *Health Affairs* 1994; 13(1): 108-114.
5. Levit et al., Trends in U.S. health care spending.
6. Mills, Current Population Reports, Health Insurance Coverage: 2001.
7. Levit et al., Trends in U.S. health care spending.
8. Ibid.
9. Ibid.
10. Ibid.
11. Madison, D.L. Paying for medical care in America. In Henderson, G.E., King, N.M.P., Strauss, R.P., Estroff, S.E., and Churchill, L.R. (eds.), *Social Medicine Reader.* Durham, NC: Duke University Press, 1997.
12. Mills, Current Population Reports, Health Insurance Coverage: 2001.
13. Gabel, J., Levitt, L., Holve, E., et al. Job-based health benefits in 2002: Some important trends. *Health Affairs* 2002; 21(5): 143-151.

14. Chollet, D. Employer-based health insurance in a changing work force. *Health Affairs* 1994; 13(1): 315.
15. Gabel et al., Job-based health benefits in 2002.
16. Woolhandler, S. and Himmelstein, D.U. Paying for national health insurance—And not getting it. *Health Affairs* 2002; 21(4): 88-98.
17. Felstein, P.J. *Health Policy Issues: An Economic Perspective,* Second Edition. Chicago: Health Administration Press, 1999, pp. 50-52.
18. Reinhardt, U.E. Reorganizing the financial flows in U.S. health care. *Health Affairs* 1993; 12(Suppl.): 172-193.
19. Gabel et al., Job-based health benefits in 2002.
20. Ibid.
21. Gabel, J., Liston, D., Jensen, G., and Marsteller, J. The health insurance picture in 1993: Some rare good news. *Health Affairs* 1994; 13(1): 330-334.
22. Gabel et al., Job-based health benefits in 2002.
23. Levit et al., Trends in U.S. health care spending, 2001.
24. Iglehart, J.K. Changing health insurance trends. *New England Journal of Medicine* 2002; 347: 956-962.
25. Gabel et al., Job-based health benefits in 2002.
26. Christianson, J.B., Parente, S.T., and Taylor, R. Defined-contribution health insurance products: Development and prospects. *Health Affairs* 2002; 21(1): 49-64.
27. Mills, Current Population Reports, Health Insurance Coverage: 2001.
28. Felstein, *Health Policy Issues: An Economic Perspective,* pp. 75-102.
29. Reinhardt, Reorganizing the financial flows in U.S. health care.
30. Levit et al., Trends in U.S. health care spending, 2001.
31. Lohr, K.N., Brook, R.H., Kamberg, C.J., et al. Use of medical care in the Rand health insurance experiment: Diagnosis- and service-specific analyses in a randomized clinical trial. *Medical Care* 1986; 24(Suppl.): S39-S50.
32. Gabel et al., Job-based health benefits in 2002.
33. Mills, Current Population Reports, Health Insurance Coverage: 2001.
34. Fuchs, V.R. What's ahead for health insurance in the United States? *N Engl J Med* 2002; 346: 1822-1824; Taylor, H. How and why the health insurance system will collapse. *Health Affairs* 2002; 21(6): 195-197.
35. Buchanan, A. Philosophic perspectives on access to health care: Distributive justice in health care. *Mt. Sinai Journal of Medicine* 1997; 64: 90-95.
36. Felstein, *Health Policy Issues: An Economic Perspective,* pp. 263-272.
37. Ibid., p. 81.
38. Ibid., p. 80.
39. Hsiao, W.C., Braun, P., Dunn, D., and Becker, E.R. Resource-based relative values. *JAMA* 1988; 260: 2347-2360.
40. Gagnon, J.P. Third party reimbursement: How did we get where we are today? *American Pharmacy* 1980; NS20: 703-710.
41. National Pharmaceutical Council. *Pharmaceutical Benefits Under State Medical Assistance Programs, 2001.* Reston, VA: National Pharmaceutical Council, 2002.

Chapter 3

Managed Care and Pharmacy Services

Kenneth W. Schafermeyer

BACKGROUND AND RATIONALE
FOR MANAGED HEALTH CARE

In the United States we have witnessed dramatic changes in the way health care is *provided,* as well as the way it is *financed.* Access to health care services and the cost of these services has been in large part a function of the growth of health insurance. The growth of health insurance during the past half century has helped preserve financial security and improve access to health care for millions of Americans. Health insurance has also ensured payment for health care providers, fueled the growth of hospitals, and stimulated the development of new health services.

Employers view labor costs, including employee benefits such as health insurance, much the same way as other raw materials are used in production. To remain competitive in the global marketplace, employers feel that they have to minimize their costs. The scope of this issue can easily be understood when one considers that U.S. auto manufacturers spend more on health care benefits for their employees than they do for the steel used in their cars. Since health benefits in other industrialized nations are paid by the government—rather than employers—increased health care costs can put U.S. companies at a competitive disadvantage. Employers consider rising health care costs to be a serious problem, and the area that is growing the fastest—and drawing the most attention now—is the prescription drug benefit.

Traditionally, health care providers were always reimbursed on a fee-for-service basis; in other words, they received a fee for each service performed. Because providing additional services means additional revenue, fee-for-services systems offer little financial incentive to control utilization, reduce costs, or enhance the quality of care. As health care costs increased rapidly during the 1970s and 1980s, employer groups sponsoring health benefit plans demanded that health insurance programs control costs. Health insurance companies responded by restricting reimbursement to providers and by controlling the use of health care services.

The federal government influenced far-reaching changes in the health insurance industry when President Nixon signed the Health Maintenance Organization (HMO) Act of 1973. This legislation provided financial assistance for the development of HMOs and required employers with more than twenty-four employees to offer their workers the option of joining an HMO as an alternative to conventional insurance. HMOs created a reimbursement system that gave providers incentives to focus on prevention and wellness instead of the traditional "sick care" encouraged by fee-for-service reimbursement.

Until recently, health care services were *financed* but not *managed*. Historically, government and private employers sponsoring health insurance programs demanded cost controls but showed relatively little interest in improving quality or ensuring positive outcomes—ordinary management functions for most businesses. More attention is now being devoted to analyzing claims databases to assess and improve the quality of health care services in an effort to control costs and enhance patient outcomes. This new focus on managing the health insurance benefit is referred to as managed health care.

STRUCTURE OF THE MANAGED CARE INDUSTRY

Although managed care plans are often referred to as "third parties," there are actually many different individuals or companies involved in addition to the patient, the health care provider, and the payer. Each participant has its own specific function. Following is a list of the most important participants in employer-sponsored group health insurance programs.

Patients

The patient may be

1. an employee of a company that sponsors a health insurance plan,
2. a dependent of the covered employee,
3. a retiree receiving health insurance as a retirement benefit, or
4. a beneficiary of a government program such as Medicare or Medicaid.

Sometimes employees are represented by labor unions that negotiate benefits on behalf of employees. In this case, labor contracts may specify the types of health care and prescription coverage that employees and their dependents receive. Patients often have to pay a portion of the cost for health services received. This patient cost sharing (discussed in more detail later) is designed to control utilization of health services by making patients more cost conscious.

Sponsors

The sponsor of an insurance program—usually an employer or government agency such as Medicare or Medicaid—assumes responsibility for obtaining coverage and pays some or all of the program costs. Since health care costs can be unpredictable, these insurance benefit programs can present a great deal of financial risk for sponsors, especially small groups (i.e., a few hundred people or less). Health benefit plans are also complex to administer. Therefore, most employer groups sponsoring employee health benefits programs enlist the help of insurers and administrators.

Insurers

The process of insuring is known as underwriting. Underwriters assume financial risk for health services in return for premiums paid by employer groups. Because of the unpredictable nature of health insurance coverage, most insurance companies limit their own risk by obtaining reinsurance. In essence, the insurance company buys its own insurance policy to limit its risk. Since it is their business to limit risk, underwriters and reinsurance companies are reluctant to speculate that new health care services (such as reimbursing for pharmacists' cognitive services) will save money unless they can base their predictions on empirical evidence.

Insurance companies have workers who are responsible for conducting statistical analyses to determine the income (premiums) that must be earned to cover their estimated expenses. These individuals, known as actuaries, determine the cost for each type of service provided, the utilization rates for these services, and the administrative expenses for the insurance program. Actuaries can adjust their estimates based on the previous year's expenses for either a specific geographic area (community rating) or for a specific employer group (experience rating). These adjustments affect premiums for the next year, depending on whether the claims expenses were higher or lower than the actuary's estimate.

Sometimes corporations decide that it is unnecessary to use insurance companies to underwrite health benefit programs and decide to self-insure instead. To protect workers, most states require self-insured plans to put a large sum of money aside into a reserve fund to cover any unexpected health benefit claims. Because self-insurance is a risky strategy and ties up a considerable amount of money, most employers use the underwriting services of an insurance company instead.

Administrators

Like underwriting, administration is a complex activity and health insurance program sponsors often contract with specialized companies to administer their health care benefits. The administrative functions include

- developing and maintaining a network of health care providers,
- maintaining eligibility files and identifying eligible beneficiaries,
- providing information about the health benefit program to providers and beneficiaries,
- adjudicating and paying claims,
- auditing providers, and
- reporting on service utilization and costs.

A few companies, such as the various Blue Cross/Blue Shield plans, provide both underwriting and administrative services. Some health care services, such as prescriptions, vision, dental, and mental health are "carved out" of health benefit plans and administered separately. Administrators for carved-out prescription drug programs are known as pharmacy benefit managers (PBMs).

Employer groups and insurers usually have little or no contact with health care providers, but they certainly have a great deal of influence on them. Administrators, however, are much more visible to providers because providers contract directly with health care administrators and are in constant communication with them.

TYPES OF HEALTH INSURANCE PROGRAMS

The way in which a health insurance plan is organized and operates has a major impact on the degree of control it exercises over health care providers and, consequently, provider revenues and services. Following is a description of the three basic types of health insurance programs: (1) traditional indemnity, (2) managed indemnity, and (3) managed care.

Traditional Indemnity

These plans do not contract with health care providers and have little or no control over the utilization and cost of health care services. Patients pay the provider for each service received and submit their own claims to the insurance company for reimbursement. These plans were popular from the 1950s to the 1970s but, because they did little to control costs, they are not used much today.

Managed Indemnity

These types of health insurance plans allow all providers to participate and receive reimbursement on a discounted fee-for-service basis. Costs are also controlled through patient cost sharing and some basic controls on utilization. Since the provider group is not restricted, these plans have limited ability to extract large volume discounts from providers.

Managed Care

The defining feature of these plans is the use of provider networks.[1] These plans include or exclude providers based on their compatibility with the plan's objectives. There are several types of managed care organizations (MCOs) that are usually categorized according to their relationship with physicians. The three major types of MCOs are HMOs, preferred provider organizations (PPOs), and point-of-service (POS) plans.

HMOs

HMOs place physicians at financial risk either directly or indirectly and generally restrict patients from using providers that are not part of the network. These risk arrangements can take several different forms. In the most common form, capitation, MCOs pay the physician a flat amount each month for each person (i.e., per head or per capita) and the physician is responsible for providing any needed care. The physician is taking the risk that the capitation fees, plus copayments paid by patients at the time of service, will be adequate to cover the costs for care provided to enrolled patients.[2] Since physicians get paid the capitation fee for each patient whether or not they provide any services to them, the incentive is to keep patients healthy and prevent wasteful or unnecessary expenses. Consequently, these programs tend to promote preventive care and wellness.

Another form of financial risk assumed by providers is the creation of a withhold or reserve fund in which a percentage of fees (usually 10 to 25 percent) are withheld and distributed at the end of the year.[3] Physicians who perform poorly lose their portion of their withhold, which is then redistributed to those physicians who do the best jobs of controlling costs and utilization.

Referrals are controlled through the use of "gatekeepers." Gatekeepers are usually primary care physicians who must coordinate and authorize the use of all specialty or ancillary services, such as laboratory services, referrals to specialists, and hospital admissions. The rationale is to avoid unnecessary and expensive use of specialists and other health services. Gatekeepers are often put at risk for the services that they provide as well as for other services that they authorize.[4]

There are four basic types of HMOs:

1. *Staff-model HMOs* directly employ physcans and other health care professionals. As employees of the HMO, they see only HMO patients and are generally paid a salary without directly taking risk.
2. *Group-model HMOs* consist of large, multispecialty group practices that are capitated. Providers in group-model HMOs generally see only HMO members.
3. *Network-model HMOs* consist of smaller group practices that receive capitation but are not exclusively dedicated to one HMO.
4. An *independent practice association* (IPA) is an organization that contracts with individual physicians to provide medical services. Although the IPA itself is capitated, it may reimburse physicians on a modified fee-for-service basis, often with incentives such as withholds and bonuses based on performance of the group or the individual physician. IPAs are the least-restrictive type of HMO; they are the most popular with patients and providers because they offer more choices.

HMOs can vary widely in the amount of control they exercise. Because of the dynamic nature of the managed care industry, the distinctions among the various types of HMOs are not always clear.

PPOs

PPOs usually reimburse providers on a discounted fee-for-service basis but do cover some expenses for "nonparticipating providers" who are not part of the network. Patients pay a smaller percentage of the cost when they use a network—or "preferred"—provider. For example, a patient may pay a $10 copayment when visiting a network physician and $25 when visiting a nonpreferred provider. Patients are required to select their primary care physician from among an approved list. Since physicians participating in PPO plans do not assume financial risk, the managed care organization controls costs by emphasizing fee reductions and utilization controls (discussed later). PPOs are much less restrictive than HMOs and, consequently, are much more popular today.

POS Plans

POS plans are a type of hybrid and often require physicians to assume risk but allow patients to select their providers at the time of service rather than selecting a primary care physician at the time of enrollment. Like PPOs, POS plans allow out-of-network services at a higher cost to the patient.

PRESCRIPTION DRUG BENEFITS

The increasing cost of prescription drugs is a major concern for employers who sponsor health insurance benefits for employees (and often their dependents). Expenditures for prescription drugs have been rising faster than any other health care cost—over twice the rate of inflation for other goods and services.[5]

Employers and government agencies that pay for prescription drugs are looking to managed care organizations to help control increases in prescription drug expenditures. They are also shifting some of the burden to the insured individuals by expecting them to pay a larger portion of health care expenses out of their own pockets.

Pharmacies generally are not put at risk because they do not have as much control over the types and amounts of drugs that are prescribed and dispensed. Instead, most pharmacies are reimbursed on a discounted fee-for-service basis with varying degrees of control over the types and amounts of medications that can be dispensed. These controls are discussed in more detail later in this chapter

Functions of Pharmacy Benefit Managers

PBMs provide two basic functions: (1) they serve as brokers for prescription benefits by arranging services between payers and providers and (2) they use databases and various tools to influence the cost and quality of health care services. As brokers, PBMs combine existing pharmacies into large networks, process claims, identify eligible beneficiaries, and reimburse network pharmacies. These are PBMs' core services and, because they have become standardized through the National Council for Prescription Drug Programs (NCPDP), they are virtually the same for every PBM.

In their second role (as managers of data, costs, and quality) PBMs offer various value-added services. These services include maintaining formulary systems, conducting drug utilization review, educating providers, educating patients, and performing disease-management programs, among others. Descriptions of each of these functions follow.

Maintaining Pharmacy Networks

PBMs contract with community pharmacies to create a network of pharmacies from which patients can receive prescriptions. The network may be an "open panel," in which all pharmacies are invited to participate or a "closed panel," in which only selected or "preferred" pharmacies are included. In selecting a network, PBMs consider factors such as location, cost, and ability to perform services as specified in the contract—known as the "participating pharmacy agreement." PBMs can reduce administrative expenses and negotiate lower fees by contracting with fewer pharmacies. The selected pharmacies, in turn, expect to receive an increase in prescription volume.

Some networks are so restrictive that they may include a very limited number of pharmacies or a single pharmacy chain. Although these exclusive networks offer more limited access, they also have lower pharmacy reimbursement rates.

Some managed care organizations prefer to provide prescription services from their own pharmacies, which are located in centralized clinics along with the MCO's other health care providers. These "in-house" pharmacies are closely managed to reduce inventory and prescription costs.

Pharmacy Reimbursement for Prescription Claims

Prescription reimbursement consists of three components: the PBM's cost for the drug ingredients, plus the dispensing fee, minus the amount paid by the patient in the form of copayments, coinsurance, or deductibles. These factors are shown in Equation 3.1.

$$\text{Rx Payment} = \text{Ingredient Cost} + \text{Dispensing Fee} \quad (3.1)$$
$$- \text{Patient Cost Sharing}$$

Ingredient costs. Ingredient costs (also known as the cost of goods sold) represent between 75 and 80 percent of the cost of the average prescription.[6] Pharmacy reimbursement for drug ingredient costs is usually based on the average wholesale price (AWP). AWP is the list price established by the manufacturer. AWP is higher than the actual acquisition cost (AAC) that pharmacies pay for drug products. As shown in Equation 3.2, the difference between the average wholesale price and the pharmacy's actual acquisition cost is known as the earned discount.

$$AWP - AAC = Earned\ Discount \qquad (3.2)$$

The amount of the pharmacy's earned discount varies depending on the purchasing volume of the pharmacy (volume discount), the pharmacy's ability to pay early (cash discount), and special deals and promotions the pharmacy is able to obtain (trade discounts) (see Equation 3.3).

$$Earned\ Discount = Volume\ Discount + Cash\ Discount \qquad (3.3)$$
$$+ Trade\ Discount$$

These discounts are very important because they decrease the pharmacy's acquisition cost (see Equation 3.4). This, of course, results in a higher gross margin (GM) (i.e., the difference between the selling price and the cost to the pharmacy for the product that was sold) (see Equation 3.5). By supplementing low dispensing fees, earned discounts have allowed pharmacies to participate in managed care plans that would otherwise have been unprofitable.

$$AWP - Earned\ Discounts = AAC \qquad (3.4)$$

$$Reimbursement - AAC = GM \qquad (3.5)$$

Because the earned discounts vary among pharmacies and even for the same pharmacy from time to time, managed care plans usually do not reimburse pharmacies for their actual acquisition cost. Instead, the participating pharmacy agreements usually specify that reimbursement for drug ingredient costs will be based on an estimated acquisition cost (EAC) calculated as a percentage of the average wholesale price (see Equation 3.6).

$$(AWP - (x\%\ of\ AWP)) = EAC \qquad (3.6)$$

When a drug product has generic equivalents, managed care plans usually limit reimbursement to the generic price, referred to as the maximum allowable cost (MAC). Each managed care plan creates its own MAC list. On those occasions when a physician requires the brand-name product, some managed care plans allow full reimbursement for the higher-cost product if the pharmacist indicates that the prescription was a "dispense as written" (DAW) order.

Dispensing fees. The second part of the reimbursement for a managed care prescription is the dispensing fee paid to the pharmacy. This is a fixed amount paid to the pharmacy for each prescription dispensed. PBMs, of course, try to keep total reimbursement for ingredient costs and dispensing fees as low as possible while still maintaining an adequate provider network.

Patient cost sharing. The third component of Equation 3.1 is patient cost sharing. Patient cost sharing can take one of three forms: a copayment, a deductible, or coinsurance. A copayment requires patients to pay a specified dollar amount every time a service is received (for example, $50 per hospital admission or $5 per prescription). Copayments are the most common form of patient cost sharing for prescription benefits. A deductible requires patients to pay their health care expenses until a specified dollar amount has been paid out-of-pocket during a given period of time, usually a year. (For example, the insurance company begins paying health expenses once a patient has incurred $200 of health care expenses during the policy year.) Because patients can receive health services from several different providers, it has been difficult to determine exactly when the deductible requirement has been met. The expansion of online computerized claims processing makes it easier to keep track of expenses; therefore, more plans are using deductibles in their programs. The third form of patient cost sharing, coinsurance, requires the patient to pay a specified percentage (usually 20 percent) of the cost of the service; the plan pays the remainder.

Plans without any patient cost sharing have "first-dollar coverage." Although first-dollar coverage was once common, most plans use patient cost sharing as a financial incentive to avoid using unnecessary health care services. To be effective, however, patient cost sharing provisions should not be so high as to discourage use of necessary health services.

Cost-sharing provisions may also include out-of-pocket limits (i.e., a stop-loss provision) and/or maximum benefits. Patient cost sharing, usually in the form of a copayment, effectively decreases MCOs' prescription costs by shifting some responsibility for payment directly to the patient. This not only decreases prescription costs but may also decrease the utilization rate. Although copayments are the most common type of patient cost sharing, the use of coinsurance has been increasing.[7] Copayment levels have been increasing significantly since the mid-1990s; coinsurance levels, however, have not changed because the actual dollar amount paid by patients increases as the price of prescriptions increases.

To encourage patients to ask for generic prescriptions, many managed care plans require patients to pay a tiered copayment—a relatively low copayment for generic drugs, a higher copayment for preferred brand-name drugs, and an even higher copayment for nonpreferred brand-name products. Some plans have created a fourth tier for certain "lifestyle" drugs—such as Viagra—with a copayment of $50 or more or a 50 percent coinsurance. A fifth tier is sometimes reserved for nonformulary products and has what is euphemistically referred to as a "100 percent copayment." Multitiered cost-sharing levels are being coordinated with formulary systems to encourage patients to request their physicians to prescribe less expensive medications.

Payment

To be adequate, the total reimbursement should cover the cost of drug ingredients dispensed (i.e., the costs of goods sold (COGS) or AAC) plus the overhead cost incurred by the pharmacy in dispensing the prescription (i.e., cost of dispensing or COD) and a reasonable return on the pharmacy's investment (i.e., net profit or NP). If reimbursement covers only the pharmacy's cost without any profit, then it pays at the break-even point (BEP). That portion of the reimbursement that exceeds the pharmacy's AAC for drug ingredients is know as the gross margin (GM). (See Equation 3.7.)

$$\text{Reimbursement} = \text{AAC} + \overset{\overbrace{\qquad\text{BEP}\qquad}}{\underset{\underbrace{\qquad\quad\text{GM}\quad\qquad}}{\text{COD}}} + \text{NP} \qquad (3.7)$$

For most plans, total reimbursement for a managed care prescription will not exceed the pharmacy's usual and customary (U&C) price (i.e., the price most commonly charged to private-pay patients). Therefore, pharmacy reimbursement is usually the lower of

1. the specified EAC plus the dispensing fee,
2. the specified MAC plus the dispensing fee, or
3. the pharmacy's U&C charge.

Some plans are shifting from paying an estimated acquisition cost for drug ingredients based on a percentage of the AWP to a wholesale acquisition cost (WAC). WAC is based on surveys of wholesale pricing data rather than manufacturer's list prices. Sometimes reimbursement is specified as WAC plus "x" percent, with "x" being somewhere between 0 and 2 or 3 percent (see Equation 3.8).

$$AAC = WAC + x\% \qquad (3.8)$$

Mail Service

Most PBMs offer mail-service pharmacies as part of their service—either through their own mail-order facility or by contracting with one. With huge prescription volumes, these mail-service pharmacies negotiate discounts on product costs and try to achieve economies of scale to reduce dispensing costs.

PBMs may require members to use only a mail-service pharmacy for certain prescriptions—usually maintenance medications for chronic conditions—or they may give incentives, such as discounted copayments, to encourage members to use the mail-service pharmacy. Although PBMs serve as brokers for pharmacy services, they are in the unique position of actually competing with their network pharmacies by channeling patients away from their contractual partners to their own mail-order pharmacies. When a prescription benefit plan makes the mail-service program optional, community pharmacies are wise to make their patients aware of their advantages regarding accessibility and the value of face-to-face interaction between pharmacist and patient.

CONTROLLING COSTS AND ENCOURAGING COMPLIANCE

Controlling Costs

As shown in Equation 3.9, managed care prescription costs consist of three major components: unit costs, the utilization rate, and program administration costs. To control costs, a PBM may address any or all of these components.

$$\text{Rx Program Costs} = (\text{Prescription Costs} \times \text{Utilization Rate}) \qquad (3.9)$$
$$+ \text{Administrative Costs}$$

Prescription Costs

Limitations and Restrictions. One way to decrease prescription expenditures is to restrict the quantity of prescription medications that are covered.

These restrictions prevent patients from getting unnecessarily large quantities of medications. A typical restriction is no more than a one-month supply (which is defined as thirty days in some plans or as much as thirty-four days in others). Some plans that limit most prescriptions to a one-month supply will allow larger quantities for specified "maintenance medications" that are taken on a long-term basis for chronic conditions (e.g., high blood pressure medications). For example, if the patient is taking 2 tablets per day, a maximum of 100 tablets may be dispensed at one time, even though this is actually a 50-day supply. Allowing oral contraceptives to be dispensed as a three-month supply would be another example. Typically, mail-service pharmacies offer reduced copayments as an incentive for patients to use their mail program rather than a community pharmacy.

Formularies

Another common way for PBMs to decrease prescription costs is to establish formularies—lists of drugs identified as the preferred treatment for specific diseases and conditions—that often give preference to generics and low-cost brand-name products. Physicians and pharmacies are required—or at least strongly encouraged—to use products that are approved by the formulary. These formularies may exclude certain therapeutic classes of drugs, such as products used for cosmetic purposes, appetite suppressants, smoking-cessation products, medications for erectile dysfunction, experimental medications, parenteral medications (other than insulin), and certain compounded medications. Formularies may cover certain drugs within a therapeutic class while excluding others.

Formularies can be categorized as either open or closed. Open formularies have few restrictions. Cost-control efforts are aimed at encouraging use of preferred products—through newsletters and online messaging, for example—or creating incentives for physicians, pharmacies, or patients to comply with formulary guidelines.

Closed formularies consist of a limited list of approved products—usually generics plus about 300 to 1,000 brand-name drugs. Although only drugs on the closed formulary list are covered, sometimes more than one drug product is available within a therapeutic category if there is a significant demand on the part of prescribers. Closed formularies always have a process that allows the use of nonformulary drugs under certain circumstances without making these drugs readily available to all patients. This process, known as prior authorization (PA), requires the managed care plan to review each case to determine whether patients meet certain predetermined criteria.

Open formularies are relatively easy to maintain and are more widely accepted by patients, physicians, and pharmacists. Because managed care organizations and managed care plans want to increase satisfaction and do not want to be seen as questioning physicians' judgment, open formularies are much more popular than closed formularies.

As a part of formulary development, PBMs negotiate discounts on selected drugs directly with pharmaceutical manufacturers. These discounts take the form of rebates that are paid by manufacturers to the PBMs for each dosage unit dispensed. Manufacturers are willing to give these rebates if their drugs are given preferred status by the PBM and they see an increase in the use of their products.

Utilization Rate

It can be seen from Equation 3.9 that the biggest factor affecting prescription costs is the utilization rate, because it is a multiplicative, rather than additive function. For example, a patient who is having an ulcer treated with a prescription for a proton pump inhibitor (PPI) could incur some significant and unnecessary costs if he or she takes the medication beyond the time recommended for acute ulcer treatment. By limiting use of the PPI to the recommended dosage and duration of therapy, the plan can save as much as $100 a month or more. Therefore, it is to the plan's advantage to make sure that expensive medications are not overutilized.

One of the primary tools used by PBMs to control utilization is drug utilization review (DUR).* DUR is a very important tool that has a significant impact on community pharmacy practice. Traditional DUR programs have attempted to control unnecessary utilization by avoiding duplication of therapy and reducing drug abuse and misuse. Today, PBMs are using drug-specific therapeutic guidelines to detect potential drug-therapy problems such as drug interactions, contraindications, improper dosage or duration of therapy, unusual refill patterns, and overusage.

DUR programs can be prospective or retrospective. Prospective DUR is conducted at the time prescription claims are processed and result in alert messages sent to the pharmacy's computer while the prescription is being dispensed. These messages are designed to prevent potential problems. Retrospective DUR is conducted *after* the prescription is dispensed. Since this type of DUR program looks at prescribing, dispensing, and utilization trends over time, its focus is on provider education. By detecting problems

---

*Although some professionals differentiate between the terms *drug utilization review* and *drug use evaluation,* the distinction is not important for this discussion.

and alerting providers, retrospective DUR programs attempt to improve future prescribing. In most cases these educational efforts consist of newsletters and, when necessary, direct letters to individual physicians and/or pharmacies alerting them to potential problems and suggesting possible solutions.

DUR programs and DUR on-screen messages can require substantial time on the part of pharmacy personnel. DUR messages can be helpful in managing utilization, complying with program design, and improving patient safety. It is easy to see that avoiding unnecessary prescriptions, therefore, can result in savings that are much more significant than simply obtaining a discount on unit costs. Nevertheless, unit costs are very important and PBMs apply a significant amount of effort in trying to minimize them.

Administrative Costs

The third component of PBMs' prescription costs shown in Equation 3.9 is administrative costs. Managed care organizations incur costs in contracting with pharmacies, communicating with patients and providers, maintaining pricing files, processing claims, making payments, maintaining formularies, operating DUR programs, and performing the other functions listed in this chapter.

To reduce costs, PBMs can look at any of the items listed here or in Equation 3.9. Since dispensing fees are less than 25 percent of unit costs, the additional amount of savings that can be achieved by further decreasing fees is limited. Greater savings can be earned by increasing patient cost sharing or by decreasing drug ingredient costs through the use of generics and formularies. Encouraging proper utilization is also an important strategy.

Prescriber Education

Physician profiling is an extension of retrospective DUR and is used to report prescribing patterns. Two measures that are commonly reported are number of prescriptions per-member, per-month (PMPM) and prescription costs PMPM. Typically these reports (often referred to as "report cards") are provided to individual physicians, showing not only their practice patterns but also the average practice patterns of their physician counterparts, thereby providing a benchmark for comparison.

Counterdetailing (also known as academic detailing) is an extension of physician profiling used by some health plans. Those physicians identified by the report cards as having high costs or unusual prescribing patterns are visited by a health plan representative and encouraged to prescribe in ways that will reduce overall costs while maintaining program quality.[8]

Patient Education and Disease Management

Almost all PBMs offer one or more patient education programs. The goal of these programs is to produce voluntary changes in patients' behavior that will improve health. Such efforts take a variety of forms, from passive educational mailings to disease-management programs.

Disease-management programs are designed to improve drug and related health care utilization for patients with certain common, high-cost diseases in which prescription drug therapy plays a central role. Disease management programs often focus on disease states such as diabetes, asthma, hyperlipidemia, and specialized drug therapy such as anticoagulation therapy. The most common intervention method is mailing educational materials directly to the patient.

IMPACT OF MANAGED CARE ON PHARMACY

Professionally and economically, managed health care has profoundly affected pharmacy practice. Managed care controls on reimbursement have resulted in declining gross margins for pharmacies. Successful pharmacies, however, responded by controlling their ingredient costs and becoming more efficient through computerization and increased use of pharmacy technicians. In addition to lower reimbursement, managed care has resulted in extra work for pharmacy personnel that is required for prior authorization, online prospective DUR, formulary restrictions, and answering patients' questions about their prescription benefit plan.

Although most community pharmacists recognize the downside, there are also potential advantages. It is not coincidental that growth of pharmaceutical care occurred simultaneously with the growth of managed care. In theory, both concepts are consistent and pharmacy education has changed dramatically to help new pharmacists learn to manage care and affect positive patient outcomes. The hope and expectation is that pharmaceutical care services will be recognized as a valuable part of managed care and not just a cost to be controlled. In the broader perspective, greater focus on patient outcomes and cost-effectiveness will encourage pharmacists, physicians, and other health care providers to collaborate for the benefit of the patient in order to realize the goal of optimally managed health care.

NOTES

1. Miller, R.H. and Luft, H.S. Managed Care Plans: Characteristics, Growth, and Premium Performance. *Annual Review of Public Health* (1994): 15, 437-459.

2. Rognehaugh, R. *The Managed Health Care Dictionary.* (Gaithersburg, MD: Aspen Publishers. 1996).

3. Mack, J.M. Managed Care Relationships from the Physician's Perspective. *Topics in Health Care Financing* (1993): 20(2), 38-52.

4. Medicome International, A thru Z. Managed care terms, *Medical Interface.* (n.d.): Bronxville, NY: Author.

5. United States Department of Labor, Bureau of Labor Statistics. Available at <http://data.bls.gov/cgi-bin/surveymost?cu>.

6. West, D.S. (ed.). *NCPA-Pharmacia Digest* (Alexandria, VA: National Community Pharmacists Association, 2002).

7. *The Takeda and Lilly Prescription Drug Benefit Cost and Plan Design Survey Report, 2001.* (Indianapolis, IN: Eli Lilly and Company, Inc., 2001).

8. Graden, S.E. and Schafermeyer, K.W. Performance Reporting for Managed Care Prescription Programs. *Journal of Managed Care Pharmacy* 1998; 4:160-166, 170.

Chapter 4

The Health Professions

Albert I. Wertheimer

INTRODUCTION

The U.S. health care industry consumes more than 15 percent of the value of all of the goods and services produced in the United States, and functions through the efforts of millions of men and women employed in the health field. In fact, the health care industry is usually considered the third largest industry in the United States today. Defense and agriculture are the other industries at the top of such lists. The workers in the health care industry are categorized into several hundred different occupations. Some of these occupations are considered professions. There are various definitions that discern professions from occupations. Most definitions, though, agree that at least several characteristic activities must be present for an occupation to receive the status of a profession. Some of these characteristic activities include

- exercising self-regulation and policing;
- putting the interests of the patients first (altruism);
- exercising judgment in the routine conduct of one's work; and
- becoming the exclusive keeper of a body of knowledge.

Generally, there is a trade-off in contemporary societies where the controlled access to the professions is granted, yielding a monopolistic situation. However, in exchange, members of that professional body agree to be accountable to the society, to pass required licensure examinations, and to maintain their competence. So, pharmacists or physicians have wide latitude in their professional practices based upon their professional judgment and, in exchange, they agree to pass rigid licensing examinations after qualification from specified, approved educational institutions of mandated course content and length. In addition to continuing their education through attendance at mandatory continuing education programs. Regulatory boards routinely inspect pharmacists' and physicians' practice sites and receive any complaints from consumers.

PRESCRIBING AUTHORITY

When considering specific personnel roles and responsibilities, pharmacists are interested in the controls placed on the prescribing of drugs. Those who are permitted to write prescriptions for prescription-legend drugs are listed in Table 4.1. These tabular data require a little further explanation. The conventional physician (MD) may practice, including the writing of prescriptions, within the state or states in which he or she is licensed. No major difference exists between the education of physicians in the United Kingdom and the United States, but in the United States, medical study follows a four-year undergraduate education. In the United Kingdom, medical

TABLE 4.1. Professions with Drug-Prescribing Authority

Title	Abbreviations	Authority	Notes
Medical doctor (allopathic)	MD	Independent	
Dentist	DDS or DMD	Independent	For appropriate use—dental related
Podiatrist	DSC, PodD, DPM	Independent	As appropriate—for extremities (hands, feet)
Osteopathic physician	DO	Independent	
Optometrist	OD	Independent	Most for ophthalmic products in a number of states (usually office-based diagnostics only)
Veterinarian	DVM	Independent	For animals only
Nurse Practitioner	NP	Dependent	Protocols, prescriptions need to be cosigned (varies in scope)
Physician assistant	PA	Dependent	Protocols, prescriptions need to be cosigned (varies in scope)
Chiropractor	DC	None	No prescribing authority whatsoever
Certified nurse midwife	CMW	Dependent	May prescribe only medication specified by a practice agreement in collaboration with a supervising physician

education usually begins immediately after completion of secondary school; therefore, in England, the physician earns a bachelor of medicine degree (MB). This certification is accepted in the United States as equivalent to MD when the physician successfully completes the several U.S. licensing examinations.

In dentistry, the DMD and DDS are also interchangeable and equal, but one's academic degree is based upon the traditions at one's professional school. The podiatrist (previously called the chiropodist) is legally entitled to prescribe drugs as related to his or her practice requirements. The pharmacist should not be surprised to see antibiotics, analgesics, and dermatological products ordered by a podiatrist, but must use professional judgment if a prescription is for a drug used for hypertension, arrhythmias, contraception, and so on, is presented, as these, in most cases, would be considered beyond the practice scope of podiatry.[1]

Osteopathic physicians (DOs) have, for all intents and purposes, the same education as medical doctors (MDs), but are educated in a different system with different origins. Practice laws in most states permit MDs and DOs to undertake the same spectrum of activities. The osteopath, to be sure, must not be confused with the optometrist (OD). The doctor of optometry attends a four-year curriculum following undergraduate study. These persons examine eyes and fit spectacles and contact lenses. Optometrists are allowed to prescribe topical prescription medications in all 50 states. A total of 38 states and the District of Columbia allow optometrists to prescribe oral and systemic drugs. Please see individual state board of pharmacy Web sites to determine the range of prescriptive authority for optometrists in a particular state.

Doctors of chiropractic (DC) are educated in a four-year curriculum. Chiropractors have no prescribing authority; however, many recommend natural vitamins as therapies for many conditions. Chiropractors, for the most part, consider prescription drug medications as substances foreign to the body and thus do not consider drugs appropriate interventions.

Veterinarians diagnose and treat animals. They are not permitted to write prescriptions for humans for any reason. As an added word of caution, when one sees DVM on the top of prescriptions, one should be aware that doses may well not be similar to those usually encountered in treating adult humans.

Numerous other categories of paraprofessionals exist that have dependent prescription-writing authority in concert with protocols or supervisor requirements. Some of the many different names for persons who screen, examine, and diagnose for physicians or treat under their direct or indirect supervision are physician assistants (PAs), nurse practitioners (NPs), and medex (MX). Most have written instructions that enable them to prescribe a specified range of drugs under certain conditions dealing with patient status and the results of their physical assessment of the patient. In fact, at many clinics and health maintenance organizations (HMOs), the patient first meets a nurse practitioner. If the problem appears to be trivial or simple, the nurse practitioner may send the patient for tests, bed rest at home, or out with a prescription for an over-the-counter or prescription drug. Where written protocols are not employed, some practices use a prescription pad on which the physician cosigns or initials the order, indicating that he or she has reviewed the case and approves or endorses the decisions of the paraprofessional. However, greater latitude for independent prescriptive authority is clearly gaining support.

Pharmacist Prescribing

The pharmacist's role in prescribing medication has greatly expanded over the past few decades. The majority of the public is unaware of the role pharmacists play in healthcare delivery in addition to dispensing drugs. Drug utilization review (DUR), administration of vaccines, patient counseling, drug-level lab test monitoring and consultation, prescription of emergency contraception, equivalent drug selection, and direct drug prescribing are among the expanded roles of pharmacists. Due to the state regulation of pharmacy licenses, the roles of pharmacists vary from state to state.

One of the first pieces of legislation to expand the role of pharmacists was passed in 1986 in Florida. This legislation granted pharmacists the ability to prescribe drugs that are listed on a strict formulary. This formulary has been expanded since it was originally passed in 1986.

Pharmacists have also been granted prescriptive authority of vaccinations. State legislation depicts the rules and regulations of this practice in addition to the formulary of vaccinations. New Mexico and many other states allow pharmacists to administer vaccinations according to state statutes. Please see Appendix A for a listing of vaccines and associated injectable drugs that can be prescribed by pharmacists under protocol arrangements in New Mexico. Appendix B lists the various states with some sort of prescriptive authority under protocol for pharmacists.

Recently, pharmacists have obtained the capability of prescribing emergency contraception to patients. Pharmacists must have a physician to partner them, but they do not need to be partnered with that patient's physician. This legislation has been enacted in California, Oregon, New Mexico, and Washington, to name a few.

HEALTH MANPOWER

A listing of the overall numbers of the major health professions in the United States can be found in Table 4.2. This listing is the latest available; however, it may be dated, since it was published in 2001.

Health Care Professions: Terms and Procedures

In 2001, more than 7 million persons were employed in the health arena in the United States. At that time, an astounding 800 primary and alternate job titles had been identified.[2] Before delving into this massive list, it is important to understand a few terms and procedures, including accreditation, certification, registration, and licensing.

Essentially, two types of credentialing are used. One recognizes the competence of educational programs to prepare personnel. This is generally referred to as accreditation. The second recognizes the competence of individuals to deliver services. This includes the practices of certification, registration or association membership, and licensure.

Accreditation

Accreditation may be defined as the process by which an agency or organization evaluates and recognizes a program of study or an institution as meeting certain predetermined qualifications or standards. It applies only to institutions and their programs of study or their services. Accreditation of a training program implies that the educational institution meets the standards that have been established by the accrediting agency in collaboration with professional groups.

The two types of accreditation are institutional and specialized. Institutional accreditation means that the total institution has met the standards established by the accrediting agency. Specialized or program accreditation means that a part or parts of an educational institution have met certain criteria, usually relating to a single profession. Thus, accreditation of the whole educational institution may not be the equivalent of specialized accreditation for each one of its several parts or programs. This is chiefly due to the fact that different accrediting agencies are responsible for the various programs and, as a result, variations occur in their criteria for accreditation, definitions of eligibility, and the procedures they use for establishing standards.[3]

TABLE 4.2. Active Principal Health Personnel in the United States in 2001

Category	Number active (in thousands)
	1,993
Doctors of medicine, total	836.2
Professionally active	798
Place of medical education	
U.S. medical graduates	619.9
Foreign medical graduates	204.8
Sex	
Male	630.2
Female	205.9
Nonfederal	811.9
Patient care	652.3
Office-based practice	514
General and family practice	87.1
Cardiovascular diseases	21.2
Dermatology	9.6
Gastroenterology	10.8
Internal medicine	135.9
Pediatrics	64
Pulmonary diseases	8.8
General surgery	36.5
Obstetrics and gynecology	40.4
Opthamology	18.2
Orthopedic surgery	22.4
Otolaryngology	9.4
Plastic surgery	6.4
Urology	10.1
Anesthesiology	36.1
Diagnostic radiology	21.4
Emergency medicine	23.9
Neurology	12.4
Pathology, anatomical, clinical	17.6
Psychiatry	38
Other specialty	5.4
Hospital-based practice	138.3
Residents and fellows	92.9
Full-time hospital staff	45.4
Other professional activity	41
Not classified	38.3

Category	Number active (in thousands)
Federal	20
Patient care	16.6
Office-based practice	0
Hospital-based practice	23.3
Other professional activity	3.406
Inactive/unknown address	84.5
Doctors of osteopathy	44.7
Dentists, number	168
Nurses, number (active registered)	2,696
Podiatrists	18
Optometrists	29.5

Source: American Medical Association, *Physician Characteristics and Distribution,* 2003 Edition, Chicago: AMA 2003.

Certification and Registration

Certification may be defined as the process by which a nongovernment agency or association grants recognition to an individual who has met certain predetermined qualifications specified by that agency or association. Registration is the process by which qualified individuals are listed on an official roster maintained by a government or nongovernment agency.

Within some professions, specialty boards, certification boards, and/or registries are established by the profession itself for the purpose of distinguishing quality. Persons who meet certain requirements of education, experience, and competency and pass an examination given by the board may use a specific professional designation. For example, MT indicates that the medical technologist had been registered by the Board of Registry of the American Society of Clinical Pathology (ASCP). These organizations not only qualify persons who meet their standards but also usually know of persons working toward qualification. They maintain lists of all persons registered to date. The lists may appear in published form, as in the *Directory of Medical Specialists,* which provides information on all physicians who are diplomats of the twenty-two medical specialty boards approved by the American Medical Association.[4]

In December 1977, sixty-five professional health associations formed the National Commission for Health Certifying Agencies as the result of an acknowledged need to develop and encourage high standards of professional conduct among health certifying agencies. The commission has set nationwide standards for the certifying agencies which attest to the competence of the individuals who participate in the health care delivery system.

License or Permit

Licensure may be defined as the process by which an agency of the government grants permission to (1) persons meeting predetermined qualifications to engage in a given occupation and/or use a particular title or (2) institutions to perform specified functions. A license or permit to practice within a state, issued by a state agency, is a means of identifying some health personnel. More than thirty occupations in the health field are licensed in one or more states. All states and the District of Columbia require that the following health personnel be licensed to practice: chiropractors, dental hygienists, dentists, environmental health engineers, nursing home administrators, optometrists, pharmacists, physical therapists, physicians (MDs and DOs), podiatrists, practical nurses, psychologists, registered nurses, and veterinarians. Another eighteen occupations are licensed in at least one state, and one occupation is licensed only in Puerto Rico.[5]

To give the reader a general feeling for the size of this manpower pool and an idea of the types and variety of such personnel, a listing from a 2001 federal government report is presented in Table 4.3. Obviously, the numbers constantly change, but the sheer magnitude and proportions in different areas are worthy of consideration.

Before leaving this topic, note that a 1984 report indicated that about eight million persons were working in the health care industry.[6] Note also that this figure excludes the large but unknown number of housekeeping, kitchen, and maintenance personnel also employed in the health care industry.

In the remaining sections of this chapter, the medical profession will receive a closer look, the pharmacy profession will be scrutinized. Finally, some current issues and trends will be examined.

PHYSICIANS

Physician Specialization

In the 1930s, about 80 percent of physicians were in primary care and general practice, with about 20 percent in specialties. Specialists earning higher incomes received greater respect and had other advantages, includ-

TABLE 4.3. Estimated Persons Employed in Health Occupations, 2000

Health field and occupation	Active workers
Total	11,914,564
Administration of health services	323,913
Health department, public health administrator	7,985
Hospital administrator and assistant	26,065
Nursing home administrator and assistant	24,531
Voluntary health agency administrator and program representative	15,332
Medical and health services managers	250,000
Anthropology and sociology	2,912
Anthropologist (cultural and physical)	1,379
Sociologist (medical)	1,533
Automatic data processing in the health field	7,666
Systems analyst and programmer	7,666
Basic sciences in the health field	136,660
Medical scientist	37,000
Research scientist (other than physician, dentist, veterinarian)	99,660
Biomedical engineering	64,797
Biomedical engineer	7,000
Biomedical engineering technician	12,265
Clinical engineer	1,532
Health and safety engineers	44,000
Chiropractic	50,000
Chiropractor	50,000
Clinical laboratory services	304,276
Clinical laboratory scientist	9,276
Medical and clinical laboratory technologist	148,000
Medical and clinical laboratory technician	147,000
Dentistry and allied services	589,000
Dentist	152,000
Dental hygienist	147,000
Dental assistant	247,000
Dental laboratory technician	43,000
Diagnostic technology	247,000
Cardiovascular technologists and technicians	29,000
Diagnostic medical sonographers	33,000
Nuclear medicine technologists	18,000

TABLE 4.3 *(continued)*

Health field and occupation	Active workers
Radiologic technologists and technicians	167,000
Dietetic and nutritional services	75,000
Dietetic and nutritionist	49,000
Dietetic technician	26,000
Economic research in the health field	770
Economist (health)	770
Environmental sanitation	37,050
Sanitarian	29,130
Technician and aide	7,920
Food and drug protective services	78,340
Inspector (health, food and drug, other)	25,300
Food and drug chemist, microbiologist	1,840
Food technologist	46,000
Food technician	5,200
Funeral directors and embalmers	65,000
Funeral director	32,000
Embalmer	7,000
Funeral attendants	26,000
Health and vital statistics	2,070
Health statistician	1,690
Vital record registrar	230
Demographer	150
Health education	43,000
Health educator	43,000
Health information and communication	16,000
Biomedical photographer	4,600
Health information specialist and science writer	6,100
Medical writer	2,150
Technical writer and editor	2,300
Medical illustrator	850
Library services in the health field	15,800
Medical librarian	4,600
Medical library technician and clerk	11,200
Medical records	235,000
Registered record administrator	9,200
Accredited record technician	13,800

Health field and occupation	Active workers
Other medical record personnel	76,000
Medical records and health information technician	136,000
Medicine	773,000
Physician (MD)	728,000
Physician (DO)	45,000
Medical support occupations	530,300
Medical assistants	329,000
Medical equipment preparer	33,000
Medical transcriptionists	102,000
Medical equipment repairer	28,000
Opthalmic medical assistant	38,300
Midwifery	6,700
Lay-midwife	3,600
Nurse midwife	3,100
Nursing and related services	4,882,000
Registered nurse	2,194,000
Licensed practical nurse and licensed vocational nurse	700,000
Nursing aide, orderly, attendant	1,373,000
Home health aide	615,000
Occupational therapy	104,000
Occupational therapist	78,000
Occupational therapy assistant	17,000
Occupational therapy aide	9,000
Opticianary	68,000
Dispensing optician	68,000
Optometry	40,900
Optometrist	31,000
Optometric assistant	7,700
Optometric technician	2,200
Orthotic and prosthetic technology	5,000
Orthotist and prosthetist	5,000
Pharmacy	464,000
Pharmacist	217,000
Pharmacy technician	190,000
Pharmacy aide	57,000
Physical therapy	212,000
Physical therapist	132,000

TABLE 4.3 (continued)

Health field and occupation	Active workers
Physical therapy assistant	44,000
Physical therapy aide	36,000
Physician extender services	58,000
Physician assistant	58,000
Podiatric medicine	18,000
Podiatrist	18,000
Psychology	182,000
Psychologist	182,000
Respiratory therapy	110,000
Respiratory therapist	83,000
Respiratory therapy technician	27,000
Secretarial and office services in the health field	464,000
Receptionist, assistant, aide	150,000
Medical secretary	314,000
Social work	193,500
Social worker (medical, public health, mental health, and substance abuse)	187,000
Social work assistant and aide	6,500
Specialized rehabilitation services	87,790
Corrective therapist	2,000
Educational therapist	770
Manual arts therapist	1,700
Music therapist	3,400
Recreational therapist	29,000
Home economist in rehabilitation	920
Radiation therapist	16,000
Massage therapist	34,000
Speech pathology and audiology	101,000
Audiologist	13,000
Speech language pathologist	88,000
Veterinary medicine	163,000
Veterinarian	59,000
Veterinary technologist and technician	49,000
Veterinary assistants and laboratory animal caretakers	55,000
Vocational rehabilitation counseling	27,600
Vocational rehabilitation counselor	27,600

Health field and occupation	Active workers
Miscellaneous health services	803,000
Electrocardiograph technician	17,000
Electroencephalograph technician	9,200
Emergency medical technician	440,000
Operating room technician	19,100
Orthoptist	700
Athletic trainers	15,000
Medical appliance technician	13,000
Ophthalmic laboratory technician	32,000
Mental health counselor	67,000
Psychiatric aides	65,000
Psychiatric technician	54,000
Surgical technologist	71,000

Source: Hecker, D. Occupational Employment Projects to 2010, *Monthly Labor Review,* 124(11): 57 (November 2001).

ing control of hours, a more limited body of knowledge in which to remain current, and client control. As a result, by 1970, over 70 percent of physicians (DOs and MDs) in the United States were in practices limited to specialty boundaries. The result of this pendulum swing was an oversupply of specialists and a shortage of primary care physicians. The federal government aided efforts aimed at producing more primary care practitioners, with the outcome that family practice became a specialty area, and the number of family practices grew in the late 1970s and 1980s. A review of MD practice types is presented in Table 4.2.

In the late 1960s and early to mid-1970s, there were physician shortages in numerous areas and within several medical specialty areas. As a result, some of the clinical pharmacy activities were welcomed by some members of the medical community. Since the mid-1980s, the physician shortage has turned into a glut, as paraprofessionals, greater manpower production, and the use of automation have decreased the demand. Some argue that the self-help movement, the continued growth of chiropractic medicine, better public health education, prevention campaigns, improved immunizations, and nutrition have further reduced the demand for physician services. Some clinical pharmacy functions may then be in jeopardy as physicians try to reclaim lost functions and maintain their income levels.

PHARMACY PERSONNEL AND PRACTICE SITE

From 1978 to 1979 the federal government conducted a massive man-power study of pharmacists. The National Center for Health Statistics (NCHS) conducted an inventory of all licensed pharmacists in the United States. The data collection spanned two years in an effort to time each state survey to correspond with the state license renewal period for pharmacists. Results have been updated periodically by the National Association of Boards of Pharmacy (NABP). As the degree structure in pharmacy has changed from a BS-dominated profession to a PharmD-dominated gradua-tion and practice degree, the licensure profile of pharmacy will change ac-cordingly. At present, 74 percent of pharmacists hold BS degrees, and the balance is dominated by PharmD graduates (15 percent). Other pharmacists hold MS and/or PhD degrees. This data is from the National Pharmacists Workforce Survey published in 2000 by the American Association of Colleges of Pharmacy, Pharmacy Manpower Project, Inc.

Specialization

The Board of Pharmaceutical Specialties is composed of representatives from the American pharmaceutical organizations. This organization has prepared guidelines for groups desiring specialty status within the profes-sion. Several groups have petitioned recently. Nuclear pharmacists have succeeded in obtaining this designation, along with pharmacotherapeutics and oncology.

The growth of specialization within the profession is bound to have an impact. It could be in higher salaries, intraprofessional turf battles, the greater use of pharmacist substitutes, the growth of labor-union representa-tion, or perhaps in other areas not even envisioned today. Preparing for the expected growth in the use of pharmacy technicians, the American Society of Health-System Pharmacists created the Task Force on Technical Person-nel in Pharmacy, which prepared proposed guidelines for the use of techni-cians and other information for the use of hospital pharmacy directors.[7] A number of others have considered these personnel questions, but the future direction of the overall health care system will determine the future of phar-macy practice, for the most part, as the tail cannot wag without the dog.

ISSUES AND TRENDS

The issues and trends in pharmacy are essentially similar to those facing all health professions. All health professions worry about the impact of technology and change, keeping current with new discoveries, financial security, and the status and welfare of the profession. In pharmacy, the full impact of the specialization trend has not yet been fully appreciated. Varying components of specialization may be positive or negative, depending on where one is looking. Little to no evidence is available for predicting whether hospitals or extended care facilities or other large employer groups will acknowledge specialty status or whether the specialty group itself will be successful in convincing accreditation organizations to require the use of board-certified specialists.

The use of auxiliary personnel is also in need of rigorous evaluation. Pharmacy technicians are trained in increasing numbers at vocational-technical schools, junior colleges, and on the job. The limitation on their fullest utilization appears to be what some consider arbitrary or baseless limits or ratios. No evidence says that a pharmacist cannot effectively supervise many technicians under the appropriate circumstances.

The pharmacy technician group has organized. It has its own journal, *The Journal of Pharmacy Technology,* and one can expect to hear more from its representatives. It is, essentially, a time bomb, as the profession can be expected to be called upon to define limitations of the use of technical personnel and technician practice. Technicians, on the other hand, may argue that they are equally competent to perform certain functions.

The jury is still out as to whether the concept of pharmaceutical care will be accepted by payers, patients, and other health professions and HMOs.

Technology should have a major impact. Computers are expected to continue their spread into every aspect of health care activity. Artificial intelligence will further fuel this diffusion of computer involvement. Major strides in robotics may affect pharmacy staffing, especially in routine, repetitive tasks such as repackaging, ointment making, and other bulk compounding. Other automation involving counting machines, generation of labels from the spoken word, and changes in dosage forms and delivery systems will surely affect personnel needs and training requirements in the near future.

Politics and economics will also have a significant impact on pharmacy practice. Budget pressures on HMOs and health insurers may catalyze cost-cutting efforts in pharmacy. This may also be the case with services rendered for the government, whether cost-containment activities are continuous or not. How well conventional pharmacy practice fares in defending its turf against physician dispensing, mail-order pharmacy, and other internal and external assaults on the status quo will likewise have a major impact on practice characteristics.

In summary, the needs of health manpower appear to be a complex web of interacting concerns that vibrate in reaction to numerous forces: economic, political, technical, governmental, professional, and historical, among others. These reactions result in decisions and compromises that further result in practice and education changes several or more years later. Pharmacy manpower activities are not insulated from or immune to external forces or unpredictable events. Discussions today about the role of pharmacy in home care might be translated into actual practice changes in a few years.

APPENDIX A

Vaccines and Related Drugs Dispensible by Pharmacists in the State of New Mexico

Authorized Drugs

Diphtheria, tetanus, and pertussis vaccine (DTP)
Diphtheria, tetanus, and acellular pertussis vaccine (DTaP)
Diphenhydramine injection
Epinephrine injections (premeasured syringe)
Haemophilus influenza B vaccine (HIB)
Hepatitis A vaccine
Hepatitis B vaccine
Inactivated polio vaccine (IPV)
Influenza vaccine
Measles, mumps, and rubella vaccine (MMR)
Meningococcal vaccine
Oral polio vaccine
Pneumococcal vaccine
Tetanus toxoid
Tetanus and diphtheria toxoid (Td)
Varicella vaccine
Other vaccines as determined by the Centers for Disease Control and Prevention or the New Mexico Department of Health that may be required to protect the public health and safety in an established emergency

Source: New Mexico Board of Pharmacy Protocol for Pharmacist Prescribing Vaccines. Available online at <http://www.nm-pharmacy.com/body_vaccination_protocl.htm>.

Immunization Fact Sheet: APhA

Currently, the thirty-six states in which pharmacists can provide immunizations are as follows: (This information is based upon a survey of state pharmacy association executives.)

*Alabama	Montana
*Alaska	*Nebraska
*Arkansas	*Nevada
*California	*New Mexico
Colorado	*North Carolina (limited)
*Delaware	*North Dakota
*Georgia	*Ohio
Hawaii	*Oklahoma
Idaho	*Oregon
*Indiana	Pennsylvania
*Iowa	*South Carolina
Kansas	*South Dakota
* Kentucky	*Tennessee
* Massachusetts (pilot)	*Texas
* Michigan	*Utah
* Minnesota	*Virginia
* Mississippi	*Washington State
* Missouri	*Wisconsin

* States known to have pharmacists actively administering immunizations.
Note: The Illinois Department of Professional Regulation legal counsel has interpreted administration to be limited to pharmacokinetic services (personal communication, September 23, 2003).

For more information, contact Mitch Rothholz, AphA vice president, Professional Practice, 202-429-7549 (FAX: 202-628-0443), Lisa Geiger, director, State Government Affairs, 202-429-7575 (FAX: 202-628-0443), or Elizabeth Keye, group director, Strategic Alliances and Industry Relations, 202-429-7597 (FAX: 202-223-7193).

APPENDIX B

American Pharmaceutical Association States with Some Form of Collaborative Drug Therapy Management (CDTM) As of January 2003

Total number of states with some form of CDTM: 40
Total number of states with statutes authorizing some form of CDTM: 35
Total number of states with only regulations authorizing some form of CDTM: 5
Statutory Authority (35 States):

Arizona
Arkansas
California
Connecticut
Delaware[a]
Florida
Georgia
Hawaii
Illinois
Indiana
Iowa
Kansas
Kentucky
Maryland
Michigan
Minnesota
Mississippi
Montana
Nebraska
Nevada
New Mexico
North Carolina
North Dakota
Ohio
Oregon
Pennsylvania
Rhode Island
South Carolina
South Dakota

Texas
Utah
Virginia
Washington
Wisconsin
Wyoming
Board of Pharmacy Regulations (5 States):
Alaska
Idaho
Louisiana
Tennessee
Vermont

Note: In addition to the 40 states listed, the Territory of Guam also has statutory authority for collaborative practice.
ªDelaware authority limited to immunization prescribing under protocol.

NOTES

1. Anonymous, *Health, United States, 2003.* Hyattsville, MD: U.S. Department of HHS, 2003.
2. Bureau of Health Manpower Education. *Certification in Allied Health Progressions. 1971 Conference Proceedings.* Washington, DC: DHEW, 1972.
3. Pennell, M.Y., Profitt, J.R., and Hatch, T.D. *Accreditation and Certification in Relation to Allied Health Manpower.* Washington, DC: DHEW, 1971.
4. Jonas, S. and Kovner, A. *Healthcare Delivery in the United States.* New York: Springer Publishing Company, 2002.
5. Kapantais, G. *Summary Data from the National Inventory of Pharmacists: United States, 1978-79.* NCHS, No. 85, DHHS. Washington, DC: GPO, 1982.
6. Davis, H. *Characteristics of Pharmacists: United States: 1978-79.* Vital and Health Statistics, Series 14. Public Health Services, DHHS, 1984.
7. Ibid; Kapantais, Summary Data.

BIBLIOGRAPHY

American Association of Colleges of Pharmacy, Pharmacy Manpower Project, Inc. Arlington, VA: American Association of Colleges of Pharmacy, 2005. <http://www.aacp.org/site/page.asp?VID=1&CID=1056&DID=6195&TrackID=>.
American Medical Association, Physician Characteristics and Distribution, 2003. Chicago: AMA, 1996.
Anonymous. ASHP Statement on Supportive Personnel in Hospital Pharmacy. *Am J Hosp Pharm* 1971; 28: 516.

Anonymous. Statistical Abstract of the United States Census Bureau. Available on-line at <http:www.census.gov/prod/www/statistical-abstract-04.html>.

Anonymous. Toward a Well-Defined Category of Technical Personnel in Pharmacy. *Am J Hosp Pharm* 1987; 44: 2560.

Bureau of Health Professions, PHS, DHHS, 5600 Fishers Lane, Rockville, MD.

Health Resources Administration, Public Health Service, DHHS. Supply and Characteristics of Selected Health Personnel. HRA81-20. Washington, DC: GPO, 1981.

Hecker, D. Occupational Employment Projections to 2010, *Monthly Labor Review,* 2001; 124(11): 57.

Knapp, K.K. Pharmacy Manpower: The Need for an Improved Database. *Am J Pharm Educ* 1988; 52(summer):15.

Miller, W.A. Further Developing Clinical Pharmacy As a Differentiated Type of Pharmacy Practice. *Am J Pharm Educ* 1984; 48(fall): 332.

1995-96 NABP Survey of Pharmacy LAW. Park Ridge, IL: National Association of Boards of Pharmacy, 1996.

U.S. Department of HHS, Public Health Service, National Center for Health Statistics. *Vital and Health Statistics,* Series 12, 13, and 14. Washington, DC: U.S. GPO, 1979.

Chapter 5

Pharmacists in the U.S. Health Care System

Craig A. Pedersen

INTRODUCTION

The integration of topics between this chapter and others is significant, since pharmacist interaction with the health care system is essential for the appropriate provision of pharmaceutical products and services. This chapter presents a summary of important workforce and education issues in pharmacy today.

WORKFORCE

Pharmacy workforce issues are a great concern of pharmacists today and will continue to be into the future. As the practice of pharmacy shifts more toward the provision of a service and becomes less about the product, and the transition to pharmaceutical care continues, pharmacists have undergone a shift in workforce requirements. Real or perceived shortages of pharmacists can greatly influence pharmacy practice and education. Shortages drive up pharmacist salaries as employers recruit heavily from a dwindling supply of pharmacists. Schools of pharmacy have faced mounting pressure from pharmacist employers to expand enrollments in an increasingly attractive profession. Recently, many new schools of pharmacy have opened in this environment of a perceived shortage of pharmacists. These new schools are depending on a high number of students continuing to apply to pharmacy school and on student's optimism for their future job opportunities.

Equally of concern is an oversupply of pharmacists. Elementary laws of supply and demand in economics predict that an oversupply of pharmacists will decrease wages. New graduates and experienced pharmacists alike would have difficulty finding employment in a market with an oversupply of pharmacists. This can be seen today in cities where schools of pharmacy are located. Recent graduates have more difficulty finding employment in saturated markets, but if graduates are willing to move to an area undersupplied with pharmacists, they frequently receive multiple offers from prospective employers. Furthermore, salaries for pharmacists in cities with pharmacy schools can be lower than in cities without pharmacy schools. Workforce is itself greatly influenced by the areas of education and practice. The supply of pharmacists is directly tied to school enrollments. Periods of proclaimed shortage and surplus routinely follow contraction and expansion of those enrollments. The activities of pharmacists in different settings are influenced by the professionalization and practice expectations acquired during their educational experience. The increasing number of pharmacists functioning in nondistributive roles further confounds workforce assessments and projections.

With the central role of the pharmacy workforce in any consideration of pharmacists in the U.S. health care system established, let us proceed to answer the question, "How did we get where we are today?"

Historical Considerations

In the mid- to late-1960s, the federal government developed a greater interest in health workforce because of a perceived shortage of health care professionals. This interest resulted in a program of federal grants to schools as incentives to increase enrollments. These grants, called capitation grants because they provided monies directly to schools for each student enrolled, were successful in causing enrollments to substantially increase through the 1970s.

The government's interest in health workforce was evident through another program. Through the Bureau of Health Manpower, a series of studies were commissioned to estimate the supply of practitioners in several health professions, including pharmacy. At about that time, Christopher Rodowskas, then a faculty member at the Ohio State University College of Pharmacy, had conducted research in this area and had authored an article detailing an impending crisis in professional productivity, citing a projected gap between the demand for prescriptions and the number of practicing pharmacists available to provide them to the public.[1] In 1974, the American Association of Colleges of Pharmacy (AACP) received a federal contract to conduct a national survey of pharmacists. Drs. Rodowskas and W. Michael Dickson headed this project, termed the Pharmacy Manpower Information Project (PMIP). It was conducted with assistance from the National Association of Boards of Pharmacy (NABP) and took three years to complete. In addition to assisting the Pharmacy Manpower Information Project, the National Association of Boards of Pharmacy had collected and reported information on the supply of pharmacists in the United States in 1968, 1972, and

1978. Unfortunately, neither the PMIP nor the NABP databases were maintained or updated.

The failure to maintain or update these valuable data sources has created problems for all parties involved in the pharmacy workforce. The Bureau of Health Professions (BHP) of the Health Resources and Services Administration (HRSA), which has responsibility for reporting on the status of the health professional workforce to Congress, used the 1978 database to adjust for estimated deaths, retirements, and other separations to project future workforce supply. The accuracy of these projects naturally decreased as one moved further from the base year of 1978, making any projections of future workforce supply or demand uncertain at best.

To address this problem, a Pharmacy Manpower Database Project Steering Committee was formed in 1987. The committee, composed of representatives from all major national pharmacy organizations, was charged with collecting and maintaining a database of all pharmacists licensed to practice in the United States. State boards of pharmacy assist in the collection of information during their regularly scheduled relicensure periods. Both AACP and NABP have management responsibilities for the project. Follow-up · surveys through the state boards of pharmacy are to be conducted every three or four years, roughly in accordance with the relicensure schedule of each state. In 1991, the Pharmacy Manpower Steering Committee completed a national survey of licensed pharmacists, the first since 1978, led by Dr. Stephen Schondelmeyer and Dr. Holly Mason at Purdue University.

As with previous data on the pharmacy workforce, the survey was not kept current and the pharmacy profession again found itself without any understanding of the demographic and practice characteristics of the pharmacy workforce. Furthermore, the demand for pharmacists appeared high in the late 1990s. Therefore, in 1999, with the background of an apparent pharmacist shortage and the paucity of data regarding demand for pharmacists, the Pharmacy Manpower Project (PMP) sponsored a project to quantify pharmacist demand. Katherine Knapp was the lead investigator on the project.

In early 2000, PMP also contracted with members of the Midwest Pharmacy Workforce Research Consortium to obtain reliable information on demographic and practice characteristics of the pharmacist workforce in the United States during 2000. The objectives of this investigation were to (1) describe the pharmacist workforce in the United States in terms of demographic and practice characteristics, (2) examine factors influencing hours annually worked by pharmacists, and (3) describe work patterns in terms of setting and hours worked. The research team included Dr. William R. Doucette, University of Iowa; Dr. Caroline A. Gaither, University of Michigan; Dr. David A. Mott, University of Wisconsin–Madison; Dr. Craig

A. Pedersen (project director), The Ohio State University; and Dr. Jon C. Schommer, University of Minnesota.

Perhaps at no other time in the history of pharmacy in the United States was the state of the workforce of such interest as it was in 2000. The Bureau of Health Professions (BHP) (via PL 106-129) had an extremely high level of interest in the supply of pharmacy, given the congressional mandate to examine the issue. What made this issue so timely was the apparent imbalance in the supply and demand of pharmacists. Demand for pharmacists greatly outstripped the supply and, coupled with the implementation of entry-level doctor of pharmacy programs, the imbalance was likely to persist into the near future. This imbalance led to drastic increases in wages, as companies competed for workers using salary and sign-on bonuses as recruitment incentives.

Released in December 2000, the HRSA National Center for Health Workforce Information and Analysis study validated observed issues facing the profession. The report documented (1) the emergence of a shortage of pharmacists, (2) sharp increases in demand for pharmacy services, and (3) declines in pharmacy school applications. The HRSA study also suggested that factors causing the shortage were not likely to abate without fundamental changes in pharmacy practice and education, and that the results of shortage included less time for pharmacists to counsel patients, greater potential for fatigue-related pharmacist errors, and fewer pharmacy school faculty.[2]

In 2004, to track changes occurring since 2000, the PMP again contracted with the Midwest Pharmacy Workforce Research Consortium to collect similar demographic and practice characteristics of pharmacists. Dr. Dave Mott at the University of Wisconsin–Madison leads this investigation. It is important to note that PMP is the only organization supporting extensive examination of the profession, in particular the importance of maintaining current demographic and practice characteristics of the pharmacy workforce. It is these data that help define the direction of pharmacy practice, and they can be used to understand the issues pharmacists face in practice.

SUPPLY

Although pharmacists comprise the third largest health profession, the exact supply of pharmacists is not well documented.[3] Unfortunately for the pharmacy profession, no consistent national effort is made to track all pharmacists' careers. Such information would be very powerful and could be used to better predict supply characteristics. The information used to predict supply typically focuses on samples of pharmacists.

The BHP, a federal agency which estimates the number of people in the workforce for the health professions, biennially reports estimates of the number of pharmacists. The pharmacist workforce is reported by sex and age. BHP uses a model to estimate numbers of pharmacists and to draw conclusions about the balance between supply and requirements for the pharmacy workforce.[4] In 1992, the Pharmacy Workforce Steering Committee reported 194,570 licensed pharmacists.[5] Of these, only 171,611 (88.2 percent) were actively practicing pharmacy. These figures coincide with figures released by the BHP.[6] In 2000, the HRSA National Center for Health Workforce Information and Analysis study on the pharmacist workforce reported the active number of pharmacists to be 196,011.[7,8] In 2005, it is estimated that there will be 210,321 active pharmacists.[9]

Current estimates of demographic and practice characteristics of the pharmacy workforce come from two main sources: The National Pharmacists Workforce Survey in 2000, and the Study of Supply and Demand for Pharmacists by the BHP in 2000.[10]

Factors Related to Supply

Female Pharmacists

The number of females in pharmacy school and in practice has seen dramatic growth over the past thirty-five years. The proportion of females in the pharmacist workforce dramatically increased from 13 percent in 1970 to 18 percent in 1980, 32 percent in 1990, and women pharmacists represented 46 percent of the workforce in 2000.[11] It is estimated that women will predominate the pharmacist workforce beginning in 2004 or 2005. These increases occurred primarily because of large proportions of female pharmacy graduates.

With this change in the pharmacist workforce, there is growing concern over how demographics will impact the pharmacist workforce. Several research studies have addressed female labor force participation relative to male participation. In a 1982 study LoPachin and Dickson reported that women worked approximately 67 percent of the hours worked by men.[12] Also in 1982, Shepherd and Kirk reported the figure to be approximately 77 percent.[13] Knapp reported that female pharmacists in California worked approximately 88 percent of the hours males worked.[14] In 1992, it was observed that female pharmacists in their child-rearing years prefer to practice pharmacy part-time rather than full-time.[15] Mott and colleagues compared data from the workforce surveys in 1990 and 2000. In this investigation it was found that the proportion of females practicing full-time increased (from 61.7 percent in 1990 to 69.9 percent in 2000) and the proportion of females working outside of pharmacy and not working decreased (9.1 percent in 1990 versus 6.6 percent in 2000).[16] The studies over time suggest that as the number of female pharmacists increases in the pharmacy workforce, the impact on the supply of pharmacists of part-time workers remains an issue and must be followed.

Length of Education

With the recent movement toward adoption of the doctor of pharmacy as the sole entry-level degree in the profession of pharmacy two factors can influence the supply of pharmacists: (1) When the program switches to a PharmD curriculum, a year will exist when the program will graduate no pharmacists; and (2) The real potential for schools to decrease class size in order to accommodate the increased length of curriculum.[17] In 1993, Knapp reported the degree conversion will continue to cause a reduction in pharmacy graduates, and the magnitude will be less than 20 percent.[18] These conclusions were borne out as pharmacy schools have now converted to all-PharmD programs. The supply of pharmacy graduates has been increasing recently; as schools have increased class sizes enrollments increased 9 percent from 2002 to 2003.[19] Coupled with additional pharmacy schools opening, the number of graduates should increase in the near term.

Advanced Training

As the practice of pharmacy becomes more sophisticated, the need for more highly trained practitioners increases. Many students and practitioners will demand that programs be made available to prepare them for this new work environment. In response to the perceived need, schools will continue to develop these programs. Currently, many schools are offering nontraditional doctor of pharmacy degree programs as a direct result of the move toward an all-PharmD level of education. While enrolled either full-time or part-time in advanced training programs, many students will remove themselves from the workforce to some degree. In this case, advanced training beyond the bachelor of science level, therefore, serves to lower the actual number of pharmacists available to practice at any one time.

Enrollment

The projections of pharmacist supply are partially based on expected pharmacy school enrollments. Enrollment is neither easily predicted nor consistent over time. Schools of pharmacy experienced remarkable growth in the early to mid-1970s, no growth in the late 1970s, decline in the early to mid-1980s, renewed growth in the late 1980s, no growth or decline in the early 1990s, and now renewed growth in the 2000s. These fluctuations are due to changes in composition, qualifications, and size of the target enrollment group, and also to various uncontrollable and unpredictable factors such as job attractiveness (salary, working conditions, security) of the profession relative to other professions (nursing, medicine, allied health, dentistry, education, etc.); market conditions for people in related fields (health, biology, chemistry); affordability of a pharmacy education (tuition, loans), and other alternative careers (high tech, computers, biotechnology). Because of the many factors which influence enrollment, perhaps the best statement that can be made about them, and thus about the supply of pharmacists, is that no projection can be made with absolute certainty. Nonetheless, estimates could more closely approximate enrollments of pharmacy students and supply of pharmacists if these factors are addressed.

Decreased Interest

The real possibility certainly exists of decreased interest in pharmacy education. Current pharmacist job satisfaction, salary, and placement could impact potential students' interest in pharmacy education. This did not appear to be a problem in the late 1980s as both enrollments and applications were on the rise.[20] During the mid- to late-1990s applications to pharmacy schools began to wane as other careers became more attractive. However, in the early 2000s when the dot-com bubble burst and the economy suffered, pharmacy again became more popular. Downturns in the economy usually stimulate interest in stable careers such as pharmacy and health care in general. In 2005, pharmacy schools were again seeing high interest in their programs.

Pharmacist Work Patterns

Employee pharmacists tend to work fewer hours than owner pharmacists (thirty-six to forty hours versus forty-eight to fifty-four hours, respectively).[21] The reductions in independent pharmacy ownership throughout the 1990s resulted in the number of employee pharmacists increasing.[22]

Knapp proposed a loss of 1,457 full-time equivalents (FTEs) as a result of fewer independent pharmacy owners.[23] Furthermore, the work patterns of male pharmacists over their careers has been shown to be different than female pharmacists, with male pharmacists working on average 6 more hours per week than female pharmacists.[24] Contributions of pharmacists to the workforce in the form of FTEs is an important adjustment that models of pharmacy supply must account for to ensure that they are as accurate as possible. For example, if all pharmacists were willing to work only half the hours they currently work, the demand for pharmacists would double overnight.

Pharmacists Leaving the Profession

Supply of pharmacists is influenced by the number of pharmacists leaving the profession. As pharmacists leave their positions for other fields, there are fewer pharmacists to maintain the existing level of service for the public. Currently, pharmacists leaving the profession to pursue other career interests does not appear to be a significant problem.[25] A study of more than 1,000 pharmacists showed that recent graduates are staying with pharmacy as a career to a greater extent than earlier graduates.[26] Furthermore, in 2000, it was estimated that only 3 percent of licensed pharmacists were working in a profession other than pharmacy.[27]

Foreign Pharmacy Graduates

The impact of foreign pharmacy graduates is largely ignored as a potential impact on supply of pharmacists. To date, no good information or data source is available on foreign pharmacy graduates. Nevertheless, the potential for increases in the supply of pharmacists cannot be ignored. This is especially true now that the Accreditation Council for Pharmacy Education (ACPE—formerly American Council on Pharmaceutical Education) has accredited the Lebanese American University and recognized the accreditation decisions of the Canadian Council for Accreditation of Pharmacy Programs. These decisions will have an impact on the supply of pharmacists in the United States.

DEMAND

Demand for pharmacists has been a hotly debated issue. Traditionally, estimates of demand have relied on historical trends. Current information on demand for pharmacists can be found in a number of sources: The BHP's

(HRSA report) examination of the pharmacist market in 2000; the aggregate demand index; a consensus report of a conference on need for pharmacy services in 2020, facilitated and reported by David Knapp; and reports from professional and trade organizations.[28,29,30] Each provides important data on demand for pharmacist services.

The HRSA report cited increasing numbers of outpatient prescriptions, increasing age of the population, third-party share of prescription volumes, automation, use of technicians, work setting and activities, salaries, and expanding professional roles as important factors in determining demand. These factors will be discussed later in this chapter.

The support of PMP led to the development of the Aggregate Demand Index (ADI) by Katherine Knapp. Data for the ADI are collected from month surveys of individuals who are involved in the hiring of pharmacists across the United States. The survey panel represents a broad spectrum of pharmacy practice and geographical areas. In December 1999, the ADI average was 4.4, where 5 = high demand: difficult to fill open positions; 3 = demand in balance with supply; and 1 = demand is much less than the pharmacist supply available. This backdrop led Congress, in December 1999, to direct the Department of Health and Human Services and HRSA to conduct a study that documented the extent of the shortage.[31] Since the release of the HRSA report in 2000, the ADI average has declined. In March 2005, data on the ADI Web site show that two states were classified as having "high demand," 37 states had "moderate demand," 10 states were "balanced," one state had a "moderate surplus," and one state had a "high surplus" of pharmacists. In March 2005, the ADI average was 3.93. These data suggest that the hyperdemand for pharmacists had certainly moderated. Current data may be viewed at <http://www.pharmacymanpower.com>.

In 2002, PMP sponsored a conference for the purpose of establishing a professionally determined need for pharmacist services in 2020. Working with the current use estimate of 196,700 pharmacists in 2001, the conference projected a shortfall of 157,000 pharmacists in 2020, based on a need for 417,000 pharmacists and an estimated supply of 260,000 pharmacists. They emphasized the need for pharmacists to move even more rapidly to redeploy from order fulfillment to patient care. It was suggested that by using technology, automation, robotics, and supportive personnel to their fullest, order-fulfillment efficiency could be improved by a factor of five. Furthermore, conference participants suggested that even if these improvements in efficiency were accomplished, many more pharmacists would need to come from new graduates, foreign pharmacists, and improvements in productivity in patient care. Finally, emphasis was placed on the importance of pharmacists rapidly meeting professionally determined needs for pharmaceutical care; otherwise, it was suggested, either the care would not be provided to patients or care would be provided by others. These suggestions certainly identify the challenges ahead for pharmacists.

Professional and trade organizations such as the National Association of Chain Drug Stores, National Community Pharmacists Association, American Society of Health-System Pharmacists, and the American Pharmacists Association each issue periodic information on the demand for pharmacist services. Each group brings an important perspective to different segments of the pharmacy industry. For example, it has been reported that the number of vacancies in hospital pharmacy declined from an estimated 3,000 in 2002, to 2,000 in 2003.[32,33] These data help shape policy decision for hospital pharmacists.

Factors Related to Demand

Knapp has contended that there is less agreement over the factors associated with demand for pharmacists than supply.[34] Given the variability in the determinants of supply cited previously, and rapidly changing demand projections, demand for pharmacists should also be viewed cautiously.

Aging Population

People sixty-five years of age and older represent an ever-increasing percentage of the population and consume a greater percentage of prescription medication. It is predicted that people sixty-five years of age and older will represent 20 percent of the population and will consume 40 to 50 percent of medicines in the year 2030.[35] Furthermore, this population group often requires a greater percentage of pharmacist's time per prescription, because of increased likelihood of drug interactions due to multiple therapies and the special communication needs of the elderly.[36] For estimates of pharmacist demand to be more accurate, consideration must be given to the nature of the population the pharmacists will serve. Without this clarification of the population, projections of pharmacist demand will underestimate the true need.

New Service Roles

Demand estimates by the BHP do not include the changing role of pharmacists in society. Greater emphasis on clinical practice and the cost justification of services provided has increased the demand for pharmacists to provide nondistributive services. The growth of nursing home consulting, home health care pharmacy, managed care pharmacy, and inpatient clinical pharmacy are examples of this increased demand. As these areas continue to grow, traditional demand estimates for pharmacists will increasingly underestimate the actual demand.

Augmenting demand estimation is the recent movement toward pharmacists providing medication therapy management services (also sometimes referred to as pharmaceutical care, disease management, population management, or cognitive services) in the community practice setting. Evidence from Washington State and North Carolina suggest that targeted medication therapy management services in ambulatory settings can reduce costs and improve care.[37-43] The pharmacists who are practicing in the pharmaceutical care model of the future are working to firmly establish the future of pharmacy practice. Other pharmacists are providing cognitive services, outside of traditional patient counseling, within a community pharmacy.

Now that pharmacist-provided medication therapy management services has evidence to support lower costs and improved patient outcomes, pharmacy has been successful in lobbying for inclusion of such a benefit in the expansion of Medicare prescription drug coverage. In December 2003, Congress passed and President Bush signed the Medicare Prescription Drug Improvement and Modernization Act of 2003. This major policy change to include prescription drugs in the Medicare benefit will have a dramatic effect on demand for pharmacists. Models should be constructed that account for these changes in practice roles.

New Jobs

The traditional models of community and hospital practice are changing rapidly. Included in this change is the expansion of employment opportunities in pharmacy. This chapter is not the appropriate place to comprehensively present the varied roles and spectrum of pharmacy practice. Rather, a limited discussion can be found toward the end of the chapter. Katherine Knapp has reviewed the evidence for the impact of new types of jobs on demand for pharmacists and concludes that, "the overall impact of pharmacy workforce of the 'niches' that are being created for pharmacists remains to be determined."[44]

New Technology/Technicians

These two factors are combined because they share a common purpose. Improved technologies and the expanded role of technicians serve to increase the efficiency of the practicing pharmacist. Computers have become more of a necessity than a luxury in nearly all pharmacy practice settings.

Improved speed, ease, and accuracy of data retrieval and prescription processing have resulted in higher productivity levels per pharmacist. Automated dispensing machines further improve efficiency and reduce the demand for additional pharmacists.

Supportive personnel, or pharmacy technicians, have traditionally functioned in all pharmacy practice settings. The profession is finally attempting to deal with such important issues as the formalization of the education and training of technicians and the roles and number of technicians in the workplace. Both proponents and opponents of these issues have expressed themselves with passion, suggesting that these issues concerning technicians have far-reaching consequences for the pharmacy profession.

Expanded use of technicians and further development of their role will influence the nature of the pharmacist's work. Whether it will affect demand for pharmacists depends on which scenario will unfold. One scenario has technicians assuming a greater share of the distributive functions, thereby allowing pharmacists to meet the current demand for advanced clinical services in all practice settings. Given this development, expanded use of technicians will have little or no effect on demand for pharmacists. The second scenario has an ever-increasing technician-to-pharmacist ratio occurring in all practice settings. Technicians replace pharmacists, thereby reducing the demand for pharmacists.

Population Density

Demand for pharmacists varies by geographic area. Currently the distribution of pharmacists between urban and rural areas is not optimal. Employers in urban areas often have very little difficulty filling pharmacist positions. Conversely, employers in rural areas often have difficulty finding pharmacists to fill open positions. This phenomenon is not unique to pharmacy, but also can be seen in other health professions such as medicine, nursing, dentistry, and allied health. The impact that shifting patient populations have on demand for pharmacy services is not well quantified and should be considered when demand for pharmacy services is estimated.

SURPLUS OR SHORTAGE?

Over time, compelling evidence has been presented supporting the proposition that we are or will soon be experiencing a pharmacist shortage.[45-48] At the same time, an oversupply of pharmacists has been observed in certain areas of the country.[49] At best, one can conclude that the workforce is a complicated issue that becomes more complex as one examines it more fully. However, several statements can be made with confidence:

1. Pharmacist surplus or shortage is the practical expression of pharmacist workforce. Workforce assessments are made from component supply and demand determinations. We have only recently begun to understand the current estimate of supply through efforts of the PMP. However, no agreed-upon method for determining demand has been found.
2. The PMP has greatly improved the accuracy of pharmacy supply estimates and projections by considering the previously mentioned factors affecting pharmacist demand.
3. Although workforce is a national issue, pharmacist surplus or shortage is a regional or local issue. Workforce and surplus or shortage determinations can be in disagreement but correct in their own right, given the geographical location of interest.
4. Most factors affecting supply that have not been routinely considered in supply estimates will lower the actual and projected supply of pharmacists available to practice.
5. Most factors affecting demand that have not been routinely considered in demand estimates will raise the actual and projected demand for pharmacists.

PEW HEALTH PROFESSIONS COMMISSION REPORT

In 1995, the Pew Health Professions Commission released its third report, *Critical Challenges: Revitalizing the Health Professions for the Twenty-First Century.* The report sparked substantial interest primarily due to its provocative suggestions regarding workforce downsizing in medicine, nursing, and pharmacy. These recommendations were viewed as controversial by many in the health professions and in the public.

Specifically, the commission made the following recommendations for pharmacy:[50]

1. Reduce the number of pharmacy schools 20 to 25 percent by the year 2005.
2. Evenly distribute these closings to avoid creating underserved areas.
3. Increase focus of professional pharmacy education on issues of clinical pharmacy, system management, and teamwork and collaboration with other health care providers.

The basis underlying these recommendations was the direction of the dramatic transformations of the American health care system occurring today. The focus has been on the transformation of the organization and financing of health care. It is thought that these systems of care will soon realize the role of all health care professionals in delivering care that improves quality, lowers cost, and enhances patient satisfaction and quality of life. In deriving its recommendations for pharmacy, the commission focused on the increasingly clinical nature of the pharmacy profession and the pharmaceutical care paradigm. It was established that purely distributive pharmacy's time had come and gone. In the future, pharmacists would move away from the product to provide a service.

In many ways the commission's report is consistent with curricular changes occurring in schools of pharmacy. What is not consistent is the recommendation to decrease the number of graduates by 20 to 25 percent. At this time, the pharmacy profession is involved in a major transformation of professional tasks. Schools of pharmacy are continually updating their curriculums to keep pace with the changes requiring additional clinical pharmacy training and knowledge of the pharmaceutical care process. It is impossible to predict how these changes will affect the profession. If Johnson and Bootman are correct in their estimation of the number of drug-related problems it seems plausible that the demand for pharmacist-provided clinical services to prevent these drug misadventures will only increase as the baby boomer generation enters retirement age.[51] The reality today remains that pharmacy school graduates and pharmacists continue to be in strong demand with no change expected in the foreseeable future.

EDUCATION

The previous sections addressed the question of pharmacist supply and demand. This section examines the education that prepares an individual for practice.

Pharmacy education is similar to education in other professional areas. It is constantly changing to assure pharmacists practicing in the future meet the needs of the health care system. This change, however, is best described as slow. One must have a good understanding of past historical events in pharmacy to gain an appreciation for how pharmacy education has evolved and where pharmacy education is going.

Historical Considerations

Kremers and Urdang state that wherever civilization arises pharmacy is found because it fulfills one of humanity's basic needs.[52] Efforts to discover or to create means of protecting or curing humans from illness can be traced to the beginning of the historical period, about 3000 B.C. At that time, the Sumerians developed a system of cuneiform writing. A relatively recent translation of those writings indicates the presence of materia medica of about 400 drugs of vegetable or mineral origin. It is reasonable to assume that these tablets were the basis of what was passed to succeeding generations of persons skilled in the art of medicine preparation. Thus it can be argued that education in the area we currently consider pharmacy be traced back 5,000 years.

It is beyond the scope of this chapter to detail the contributions of various cultures to the evolving nature of pharmacy education. The most recent edition of Kremers and Urdang's *History of Pharmacy,* revised by Sonnedecker, is an excellent resource for this purpose.[53] However, picking up the trail of pharmacy education in Renaissance Europe is instructive because this was the model upon which pharmacy in the United States was based.

Apprenticeship was the only acceptable means by which an individual became a pharmacist in early Renaissance Europe, and apprenticeships generally lasted five or six years. A student was then required to complete a three- to seven-year clerkship, depending on the country. At the end of this training with a practicing pharmacist, the student had to pass what was considered a rigorous examination testing knowledge and skill in making medicinal preparations. The requirement of formal education, usually at universities, was adopted at different times in different countries, largely owing to the organizational strength of practicing pharmacists. By the early nineteenth century, however, all countries required pharmacy apprentices to complete coursework prior to taking the examination.

The development of pharmacy education in the United States is best understood against this backdrop. In colonial times, pharmacy was considered an art that was best learned under the tutelage of a practitioner. The reasons for this belief and practice were twofold. First, this method of learning how to prepare medicines was the existing model in the countries from which the settlers had recently emigrated. Second, the nature of settling a new land necessitated a more practical, rather than theoretical, approach to passing knowledge and skill from one generation of practitioners to the next.

In the larger cities, pharmacists' organizations developed to protect the public from bad or adulterated drugs and to foster their own interests and those of the profession. One such association of practicing pharmacists, the

Philadelphia College of Pharmacy (associations called themselves colleges, patterned after English custom), initiated course offerings in 1821 to individuals wishing to obtain knowledge that would supplement their practical experiences. The courses were taught at night by groups of pharmacists and were not required for eligibility to practice. However, from this humble beginning sprang the system of pharmaceutical education as we know it today.

Over the next forty to fifty years, didactic pharmaceutical education remained in the hands of pharmacists' associations. Not until after the Civil War did state land-grant universities offer pharmaceutical education. Today, most pharmacy schools are affiliated with either a university or college. In 1905, New York became the first state to require a diploma of any kind as a prerequisite for the licensing examination. The transition that occurred in the United States from strictly experiential preparation for pharmacy practice to a combination of formal coursework at universities and practical experiences mirrored the transition that had taken place in Europe.

Three trends characterize pharmaceutical education in the United States during the twentieth century: (1) progressive lengthening of the pharmacy curriculum, (2) standardization of the educational experience, and (3) the development of clinical pharmacy.[54,55]

Increased Length of Curriculum

The pharmacy curriculum has increased in length throughout this century for many reasons. The rapidly expanding scientific knowledge base required for practice necessitated additional coursework for practitioners to remain competent. Pharmacy also suffered from being perceived as a technical occupation. The expanded curriculums led to clarification of pharmacy's place as a profession, rather than as a technical occupation, in modern medicine.

The American Association of Colleges of Pharmacy, previously known as the American Conference of Pharmaceutical Faculties, established guidelines concerning curriculum length for member schools to follow to remain in good standing. The guidelines and year of implementation are as follows:

Year	Curriculum length
1907	2 years
1925	3 years
1932	4 years
1960	5 years
1992	6 years

In 1992, the AACP adopted policies that support a single professional educational program in the doctoral level (PharmD). The debate that surrounded the movement to an all-PharmD curriculum raged for nearly forty years. The movement to make the PharmD the profession's sole entry-level degree can be traced back to 1948, when a national survey led to the recommendation that a six-year degree should be mandatory. It was this proposal that led to an AACP requirement in 1960 that colleges and schools of pharmacy adopt a five-year BS program. By this time, however, California schools had embraced the six-year model, offering the six-year PharmD exclusively.

As pharmacokinetics and clinical pharmacy rose in prominence in the 1970s, the American Pharmaceutical Association (now the American Pharmacists Association) endorsed the PharmD as the entry-level degree. The American Society of Health-System Pharmacists (previously the American Society of Hospital Pharmacists) followed this lead a few years later. The debate within the profession continued until 1989, when the American Council of Pharmaceutical Education proposed new educational standards that included the call for the entry-level PharmD. In 1992, the American Pharmaceutical Association, the American Society of Health-System Pharmacists, and NARD (now National Community Pharmacists Association) issued a joint statement in support of an entry-level doctor of pharmacy degree.

Controversy surrounded the ACPE proposal and the joint statement. McLeod summarized the main reasons both in favor and against the all-PharmD degree.[56] Reasons in favor of an all-PharmD degree include

1. adding dignity and status to the pharmacy profession,
2. more than five years is needed to train contemporary pharmacy practitioners,
3. providing all students with equal opportunities to advance in the profession,
4. placing pharmacists on more equal footing with physicians,
5. all pharmacists should possess significant clinical and therapeutic skill, which are not attainable in the five-year degree program, and
6. the PharmD degree will transform the profession.

Reasons cited against an all-PharmD degree include

1. educational costs will increase,
2. costs to consumers will increase,

3. most pharmacists with five-year degrees are currently underused with respect to their clinical and therapeutic competence,
4. most pharmacists are predominantly involved in technical dispensing functions,
5. not enough clinical faculty and facilities to train all students at the PharmD level, and
6. graduates produced will not be equal in caliber to post-BS trained PharmD graduates, and thus the gains made by previous PharmD graduates will be diluted.

The debate over moving to an all-PharmD curriculum has waned as the six-year PharmD is implemented across the country, but the controversy still exists in the profession.

Standardization of the Curriculum

The content of educational offerings in schools and colleges of pharmacy across the country varied prior to the turn of the twentieth century, primarily because little thought had been given to the need for consistency. No detailed agreement existed either between schools or between schools and state boards of pharmacy. The need for consistency of curriculum became apparent as states began requiring graduation from a school or college of pharmacy as a prerequisite for examination. When New York, the first state to require a diploma, tried to decide what pharmacist training should encompass, the national scope of the problem became apparent.

A committee composed of representatives of the American Conference of Pharmaceutical Faculties, the National Association of Boards of Pharmacy, and the American Pharmaceutical Association convened in 1906 to address this problem. *The Pharmaceutical Syllabus* set forth a curriculum outline that member schools could use as a guide. This publication and subsequent editions served as the first successful effort to create some consistency in pharmacy curricula.

The Pharmaceutical Syllabus met its demise in 1946 due to concern over the restrictiveness of its guidelines and influence over the schools. The intent of the National Syllabus Committee lives on through the formation, in 1932, of the American Council of Pharmaceutical Education. The council, composed of representatives of the National Association of Boards of Pharmacy, the American Pharmaceutical Association, the American Association of Colleges of Pharmacy, and the American Council on Education, continues to develop standards for pharmaceutical education. The ACPE has avoided charges of dictating specifics by emphasizing more general requirements for admission and graduation, such as years of study, hours of instruction, amount of laboratory work, and amount of experiential training. In addition, the council periodically visits schools to assess compliance with published standards. The reports of the council carry a considerable amount of importance for schools and their respective universities because school strengths and weaknesses are identified by this external accrediting body. The improved standard of pharmaceutical education in schools across the country can be directly attributed to the profession's acceptance of the Council and its growth over the past 73 years.

Clinical Pharmacy

Clinical pharmacy has been a relatively recent development in pharmacy practice and education. Practitioners and researchers have offered various definitions of the term. Barker, in a letter to the editor of the *American Journal of Hospital Pharmacy*, stated that such a variety is confusing. He offered the following framework for clarification:

> As a method of teaching, clinical pharmacy involves: (1) the teaching of basic pharmaceutical sciences by demonstration, using patients instead of laboratory animals, and (2) the teaching of how to select and apply basic pharmaceutical sciences to the healing of patients via case study. As a pattern of practice, clinical pharmacy involves: (1) hospital pharmacy practice at the bedside, and (2) community pharmacy practice emphasizing patient contact.[57]

This definition of clinical pharmacy was important for several reasons. First, patients are viewed as an integral part of every aspect of clinical pharmacy. This was a marked divergence from the generally accepted social role of pharmacy up to that time; namely, solely to make medicines available to patients. Thus, clinical pharmacy is the vehicle by which pharmacy practice and education shifted from a product orientation to a patient orientation. This shift necessitated the reevaluation of existing pharmacy education and fueled the development of patient-oriented courses in pharmacy schools, such as communications, therapeutics, pharmacokinetics, patient assessment, and ethics.

Second, Barker views clinical pharmacy practice as behaviorally defined, not setting defined. The definition clearly allows for clinical pharmacy to exist wherever a pharmacist embraces its philosophy. Unfortunately, as clinical pharmacy developed, it has been most often associated with hospital pharmacy practice only, where it has found its greatest success. Structural opportunities and barriers of the hospital and community practice settings are part of the reason for this dichotomy. Pharmacy education has also played a part: clinical pharmacy courses are separate entities in the curriculum, apart from other pharmacy practice courses, and instructors of clinical pharmacy are primarily hospital based. The recent development of team teaching by clinical and basic science faculty and of clinical residencies in community practice suggests that efforts to rectify this situation are being made.

Increasingly more clinical pharmacy faculty are shifting emphasis from a hospital-based environment to an ambulatory care environment. This shift out of the hospital and away from rounding with physicians is a move that will incorporate Barker's second pattern of practice of clinical pharmacy: which emphasizing patient contact in the community. Practitioners are becoming involved in clinics on subjects such as anticoagulation, breathing problems, diabetes, lipids, and high blood pressure. These pharmacists are practicing clinical pharmacy in clinic settings without dispensing a prescription product. Other pharmacists are practicing clinical pharmacy in their retail stores by conducting detailed patient interviews and designing patient-specific care plans to better manage their patients' diseases.

A Profile of Pharmacy Education

Schools, Programs, and Students

As of 2003, there were 89 schools and colleges of pharmacy.[58] This represents an increase of 10 schools since 1996.[59] Of these, 56 were in state-supported universities and 33 were in private institutions. The 89 schools operate with a complement of 3,918 full-time faculty and 833 part-time faculty, increases of nearly 800 full-time faculty and 400 part-time faculty since 1996.

In 2003, all 89 schools offered only the PharmD as the sole entry-level professional degree. This is a marked changed from the 13 schools that offered the PharmD as the entry-level degree in 1990 and the 27 schools that offered the PharmD as the sole entry-level degree in 1996. Thirty-one schools offer the PharmD as a post-BS degree.

Programs are generally six years in length. Most programs have a clearly delineated preprofessional component of two years, with the remainder of the program dedicated to professional education. These programs are commonly called 2-4 programs. Some programs incorporate more of the general education requirements into the professional program, hence they have fewer preprofessional years. These programs would be considered 1-5 or 0-6 programs.

In the 2003-2004 academic year, 43,047 students were enrolled full-time in a professional pharmacy degree program. Over 67 percent of all pharmacy students were female. The number of students already holding BS degrees has been steadily increasing and totaled 3,603 in 2003. One school, Ohio State University, has taken a leadership role in elevating the PharmD degree on their campus to a postgraduate professional degree, much like medical school education. In this model, students must generally complete a bachelor's degree prior to enrolling in the PharmD program. This trend toward more students having bachelor's degrees has led some to suggest that all programs will adopt this postgraduate professional model of pharmacy education.

Sixty-seven schools have graduate programs in pharmacy at the MS level or at the PhD level. In the 2003-2004 academic year, 3,331 students were enrolled full-time in graduate programs offered at schools of pharmacy, 2,597 in PhD programs, and 734 in MS programs. Fifty percent of all full-time graduate students were female.[60]

Areas of Study

The education a pharmacy student receives today encompasses three major areas: (1) general education required by the degree-granting institution; (2) didactic pharmaceutical education, composed of basic pharmaceutical sciences, applied managerial and behavioral sciences, and pharmacy practice; and (3) experiential education.

General education requirements are established by the degree-granting institution. For example, anyone receiving a bachelor of science degree, regardless of major, might have to successfully complete courses in English, mathematics, social science, humanities, language, and in physical, chemical, and biological sciences. Frequently, the student takes these courses before enrolling in the pharmacy degree program; however, some schools incorporate these general education courses into the professional program.

Didactic pharmaceutical education is the coursework completed while enrolled in pharmacy school. The basic biomedical sciences—anatomy, physiology, biochemistry, and medical microbiology—are foundation courses. Study in the basic pharmaceutical sciences is a major component of a pharmacist's education.

Basic pharmaceutical sciences consist of a variety of content areas. Pharmaceutics is the study of the basic physiochemical principles applicable to the understanding of drugs and the development and evaluation of different pharmaceutical dosage forms and drug delivery systems. Pharmacokinetics is the study of the mathematical time course of drug absorption, distribution, metabolism, and excretion. Pharmacology is the study of the therapeutic effect of drugs. Toxicology is a specialized branch of pharmacology that deals with the mechanism and effect of poisonous or toxic chemicals of various origins. Immunopharmacology emphasizes immunology and pharmacology as they relate to the modulation of the immune response. Pharmacognosy, the study of drugs of natural origin (focusing on isolation and purification of the biologically active component of the natural product), has reemerged as a discipline of interest as more natural products are being investigated for use in various disease states. Medicinal chemistry is the branch of chemistry that examines the relationship of the chemical properties of compounds to their biologic activities, with emphasis on modification of molecular structure to enhance pharmaceutical utility.

Applied managerial and behavioral sciences have become an increasingly important component of the pharmacy curriculum. Pharmacists must have a good understanding of the legal, structural, economic, administrative, and behavioral aspects of pharmacy practice to function in the pharmaceutical marketplace, regardless of practice setting. Courses in this area generally include pharmacy law, ethics, financial and human resource management, health care systems, communications, pharmacoeconomics, and medication use systems. Typically, these courses attempt to apply the theories of more basic social and administrative sciences to pharmacy practice.

Pharmacy practice courses are applied in their approach. These courses cover specific aspects of pharmacy practice, such as over-the-counter medicines, home medical equipment, parenteral drug delivery systems, dispensing laboratories, and others.

The experiential component of pharmacy education is designed as a transition from purely didactic material to actual practice. The roots of the experiential component are found in the system of apprenticeship prevalent in the United States prior to 1900. The experiential component, regardless of length or structure, has remained a vital part of a pharmacist's education. It has three parts: internship, externship, and clerkship. Internship refers to the experience gained through work in a pharmacy practice setting. The student has the responsibility of securing employment and acquiring internship experience before taking the licensing board exam. Externship refers to the school-directed practical pharmacy experience students acquire before graduation from school. The pharmacist supervisors, who are approved by the schools, are called preceptors. Students work with preceptors in pharmacy practice settings and gain academic credit for the experience by completing the structured externship program, and the student's participation and performance is verified and graded by the preceptor. Clerkship refers to the structured experiences a student acquires in a patient care area. Like the externship, the clerkship is directed by the school and academic credit is given to the student, whose performance is graded by approved preceptors. The primary difference between the two is that the clerkship experience is much more clinically oriented, with direct patient care activities emphasized over distributive or managerial activities.

Boards of pharmacy of each state determine the experiential requirements of candidates for the licensing exam. Although there is great variation across states, an example of a common requirement is that the students must have 1,500 hours of pharmacy practice experience, 640 hours of which can be acquired in conjunction with academic credit, meaning externship and clerkship.[61] Students should consult their respective boards of pharmacy for state-specific requirements.

Clinical pharmacy as a development in pharmaceutical education has been discussed. However, it is difficult to define clinical pharmacy as an area of study. Clinical pharmacy involves the direct patient care activities of pharmacists. As such, clinical pharmacy was considered the domain of pharmacy faculty who had direct patient contact. As pharmacy practice and education have embraced a greater patient care orientation, clinical pharmacy education has become a part of all aspects of a pharmacy student's educational experience. Practically speaking, this means that clinical pharmacy faculty and basic pharmaceutical sciences faculty collaborate in areas of clinical pharmacokinetics, clinical toxicology, patient assessment, clinical anatomy and physiology, and clinical biochemistry. Clinical pharmacy faculty and pharmacy administration faculty collaborate on courses in communications, patient compliance, health care systems, and both dispensing and parenteral drug product laboratories. The conditions that separate clinical pharmacy from other areas of study have changed. As pharmacy education becomes more oriented toward patient care, clinical pharmacy is being incorporated into the different areas of the curriculum. While clinical pharmacy remains an area of expertise and the knowledge base of practitioners and educators becomes increasingly complex and sophisticated, clinical pharmacy is becoming the type of practice expected of practitioners exposed to the current program of study in schools of pharmacy.

Continuing Education

The Report of the Study Commission on Pharmacy listed three intellectual skills necessary for the practice of any health profession. These skills are problem identification, problem solving, and the skills and habits of continual learning.[62] In a time when scientific knowledge is increasing so rapidly, continuing education is a necessary defense against professional obsolescence. Continuing education is society's safeguard against professional incompetence, and the debate over whether it should be mandatory has become moot. As of 2003, only Hawaii's board of pharmacy did not require pharmacists to participate in continuing education activities as a prerequisite for relicensure.[63] Although the requirements vary between states, fifteen hours of continuing education per year is common.

The American Council for Pharmacy Education approves providers of continuing education. Among these providers are schools of pharmacy, national and state pharmacy associations, pharmaceutical companies, large retail pharmacies, publishers, and others.

Practice Setting

This chapter is not the appropriate place to comprehensively present the varied roles and spectrum of pharmacy practice opportunities. Rather, a brief discussion of practice settings will follow. The reader is encouraged to explore pharmacy career opportunities through networking with pharmacy practitioners and accessing publications, such as *The Pfizer Guide* to pharmacy career opportunities.[64]

The historical roots of pharmacy practice can be traced to independent community pharmacy. Today, community pharmacy still predominates as a practice setting and includes independent and chain-pharmacy settings. A chain pharmacy is defined as a pharmacy organization with four or more units under the same management. Chain pharmacy has experienced significant growth and consolidation through the 1980s and 1990s.

Pharmacy students today continue to enter chain-pharmacy practice settings in large numbers upon graduation. Several factors may account for this finding. Growth and expansion have provided many opportunities for employment in the chain setting. Employment in this setting offers ease of geographic mobility. A pharmacist can relocate and still remain with the same employer, avoiding searching for a new position and losing accrued benefits. Prospective employees are usually offered highly competitive and attractive salary and benefit packages, compared to other pharmacy practice settings. Also, chains offer a diversity of corporate advancement opportunities unavailable in many other settings.

An area where chain pharmacy has enjoyed particular success is in its association with prepaid group insurance plans. Benefit managers of large corporations have the responsibility of assuring access to quality pharmacy services at affordable prices for their employees. Chain pharmacy is viewed by benefit managers as a viable provider of these services and therefore has captured a sizable share of the prepaid group insurance plan business. The association appears to be an area of continued growth for chain pharmacy.

Hospital pharmacy has always served as a distinct alternative to pharmacists who want to practice in a setting other than the community. With its growth and the opportunities it provides its practitioners, hospital pharmacy has become a preferred setting for many, as opposed to an alternative setting. Hospital pharmacy has restructured itself to meet the need of improved drug use and control in the institutional setting. A national survey of hospital pharmacy services confirms this trend.[65-71] Hospital pharmacy is providing increased opportunity for pharmacy practitioners.

Each of these practice settings can offer something unique to the prospective pharmacy employee. The strengths of each practice setting, as seen by pharmacists in those settings, were reported by Schulz.[72] Independent pharmacy was viewed by its pharmacists as challenging, interesting, allowing the pharmacist to use knowledge, providing good working conditions, and providing opportunities for patient interaction. Chain pharmacy's strengths were seen by the responding pharmacists as offering financial rewards for one's work, security, and providing the opportunity for patient contact. Hospital pharmacists saw their positions as interesting, providing a setting in which they could use their knowledge.

In the section on workforce earlier in this chapter, it was stated that alternative opportunities for pharmacists must be considered in any discussion of workforce; specifically, the supply of pharmacists. The growth of nontraditional, alternative practice sites warrants further examination. Some of these practice opportunities have arisen due to consumer demand. Others have been successful because of changing reimbursement mechanisms and the demand for alternative service voiced by third-party payers. Still others may be different in philosophy and scope of activity but continue to operate under the more traditional physical structure of community or institutional pharmacy.

Supermarket pharmacy has enjoyed rapid growth in recent years. Much of the success of supermarket pharmacy may be attributed to the convenience of one-stop shopping it offers to customers. Another key may be that the typical supermarket may generate tens of thousands of customers each week without the pharmacy. As the pharmacy begins operations, it already has the traffic necessary to be successful.

Deep-discount pharmacy is a relatively recent player in the pharmacy market. Its strategy has been to offer lower prices through lower gross margins and to succeed on high volume and inventory turnover. This practice site has seen varied levels of success. The early 1990s saw some contraction in the numbers of these pharmacies due to poor or fraudulent business practices. Recently, this practice site has successfully positioned itself in the market as a low-price alternative for consumers.

Franchise pharmacy may be considered a partnership between franchiser and franchisee. The franchiser provides managerial and administrative assistance, including cooperative buying, advertising, marketing, and accounting. In return, the pharmacist pays an origination or licensing fee and a royalty, usually a percentage of gross sales to the franchiser. Although typically a franchise pharmacy is considered a small, apothecary-type shop, franchise opportunities exist for pharmacies of all sizes.

Mail-order pharmacy provides another opportunity for pharmacists. Although we may consider mail-order pharmacy a recently developed practice site, it has been around for over fifty years. The Veterans Administration, established in 1946, is the country's largest mail-order pharmacy operation. The VA fills mail-order prescriptions through 172 medical centers and 226 outpatient clinics throughout the country. Pharmacists employed by the VA are considered federal pharmacists and must be licensed in one state to be eligible for practice at the VA in any state. Retired Persons Services, which administers the mail-order business for the American Association of Retired Persons, is a private, nonprofit mail-order business established in 1959. It is the second-largest mail-order pharmacy in the country and offers practice opportunities for pharmacists in 11 states and the District of Columbia. Although the VA and AARP mail-order pharmacies are nonprofit, most of the other mail-order businesses are either private or public for-profit operations. Mail-order pharmacy prescription volume has grown approximately 50 percent annually since 1981. This growth has been fueled by increased demands for cost containment by third-party payers and the preference for additional convenience by consumers.[73]

It is estimated that over 6,500 pharmacists work in the pharmaceutical industry.[74] Sales positions are usually the entry-level position for pharmacists. Companies hire pharmacists for sales positions because of pharmacists' knowledge of pharmacology and the marketplace in general. More than 60 percent of all pharmacists in industry work in sales or marketing. Sales responsibility can be either general or specific, depending on the structure of the sales force or particular company. Some sales positions may give the pharmacist responsibility for detailing many products to all professionals who use the product. Other positions may focus on only a few products within certain therapeutic categories or promote the products to certain specialty professions. The remaining pharmacists in industry work in a variety of areas: research and development, quality control, manufacturing, policy development, and public relations. Although entry-level positions in these areas are available to the pharmacist with an entry-level pharmacy degree, advancement usually requires a graduate degree.

Pharmacy positions in government can be classified as military or civil service.[75] Pharmacists working in armed services facilities function much the same as pharmacists in other institutional practice settings. Pharmacists have responsibility for the daily operation of the pharmacy, where they have instituted unit-dose distribution systems, clinical pharmacy services, and technician training programs. Armed service pharmacy offers other opportunities as well, including opportunity for international service, fully sponsored advanced education, and a well-defined career advancement ladder. As commissioned officers, pharmacists enjoy the benefits the position affords.

Numerous practice opportunities exist for pharmacists in the government besides those in the armed services. These include the Public Health Service, with the following practice sites: Centers for Disease Control and Prevention, Food and Drug Administration, National Institutes of Health, and Veterans Administration. Each offers unique opportunities not found in traditional pharmacy practice settings, ranging from extensive primary care practice opportunities in rural settings to participation in advanced experimental drug therapies.

Space prohibits further listing of alternative practice sites where pharmacists work. Two types of practice though, should be mentioned, although they do not always constitute a physically distinct practice site. Consultant pharmacy is an example. A consultant pharmacist is one who provides consultant pharmaceutical services to long-term care facilities or other related institutions or organizations. Consultant pharmacy began as a distinct type of practice in the 1960s, encouraged by federal legislation that sought to protect long-term care residents from poorly controlled drug therapy. The consultant pharmacist provides three basic services to the institution: administrative, operational, and clinical.[76] These services include developing policy-and-procedures manuals, cost-containment programs, documentation of drug-related problems, in-service education, and drug regimen review. A review of pharmacist-conducted drug regimen reviews indicates a significant net benefit to the institution from this one consultant pharmacist service alone.[77]

Managed care provides another practice opportunity. Some managed care organizations provide their own in-house pharmacy. This type of practice setting may be considered a hybrid of institutional and community practice. In these cases pharmacists have access to patient medical information and may practice in the same facility with other health care practitioners, similar to an institutional environment, yet they interact with ambulatory patients in a manner that is similar to community practice. Other opportunities for pharmacists include involvement in contracting, practice evaluation, design and implementation of studies that assess cost-effectiveness, formulary development, education of patients and/or providers, reimbursement methods, drug utilization review, consulting, and other activities.[78] With the growth of managed care, unique practice opportunities for pharmacists have been created.

CONCLUSION

The dimension of a pharmacist's job and the role the profession plays in the future will be determined by how well pharmacy manages the interrelationships among the topics covered in this chapter. Precise estimates of pharmacist workforce are needed to ensure that sufficient numbers of pharmacists are available to serve society. Sophisticated means of assessing demand are necessary to guarantee that pharmacy has practitioners who themselves have evolved with the needs of the public they serve. Concerns over the impact of pharmaceutical care, health care reform, and reports such as that from the Pew Commission must be addressed by the profession. The educational institutions that prepare and provide the workforce must not become anachronisms, clinging to a gloried past while the world, and the practice of pharmacy, reels in change. The settings, depending on the quantity and quality of practitioners developed at the institutions, must seek the frontier of practice where the profession is defined. New settings will be created and traditional ones will change to provide additional opportunities for pharmacists. Pharmacists' activities will continue to be viewed as professional if they serve a societal purpose. Pharmacy's participation in the provision of health care in the United States is tied to its success in addressing these basic issues.

NOTES

1. Rodowskas, C.A. The pending crisis in professional productivity. *Journal of the American Pharmaceutical Association* (1970) NS10: 196-199.

2. U.S. Department of Health and Human Services. *The pharmacist workforce: A study of the supply and demand for pharmacists* (Washington, DC: U.S. Department of Health and Human Services, Health Resources and Services Administration, Bureau of Health Professions, 2000).

3. Gebbie, K., J. Merrill, and H.H. Tilson. The public health workforce. *Health Aff (Millwood)* (2002) 21(6): 57-67.

4. U.S. Department of Health and Human Services (eds.), *Health personnel in the U.S.: Eighth report to Congress, 1991* (Washington, DC: Government Printing Office, 1992).

5. Anonymous. *Pharmacy workforce project* (Park Ridge, IL: Pharmacy Workforce Project, 1993).

6. Knapp, K.K. Pharmacy manpower: Implications for pharmaceutical care and health care reform. *Am J Hosp Pharm* (1994) 51: 1212-1220.

7. U.S. Department of Health and Human Services, *The pharmacist workforce.*

8. Gershon, S.K., J.M. Cultice, and K.K. Knapp. How many pharmacists are in our future? The Bureau of Health Professions Projects Supply to 2020. *J Am Pharm Assoc (Wash.),* (2000) 40(6): 757-764.

9. U.S. Department of Health and Human Services, *The pharmacist workforce;* Gershon, Cultice, and Knapp, How many pharmacists are in our future?

10. U.S. Department of Health and Human Services, *The pharmacist workforce;* Pedersen, C.A. Doucette, W.R, Gaither, C.A., Mott, D.A., et al. *Final report of the National Pharmacist Workforce Survey: 2000* (Alexandria, VA: Pharmacy Manpower Project, Inc., 2000).

11. U.S. Department of Health and Human Services, *The Pharmacist workforce.*

12. LoPachin, M. and W.M. Dickson. A comparison of male and female labor force participation in Wisconsin. *Contemp Pharm Pract* (1982) 5: 183-188.

13. Shepherd, M.D. and K.W. Kirk. Analysis of pharmacy practice patterns of men and women pharmacy school graduates. *Contemp Pharm Pract* (1982) 5: 189-197.

14. Knapp, K.K. Pharmacy manpower: The need for an improved database. *American Journal of Pharmaceutical Education* (1988) 52(2): 152-156.

15. Knapp, K.K., M.J. Koch, L. Norton, and M.A. Mergener. Work patterns of male and female pharmacists: A longitudinal analysis 1959-1989. *Eval Health Prof* (1992) 15(2): 231-249.

16. Mott, D.A., Doucette, W.R., Gaither, C.A. et al. A ten-year trend analysis of pharmacist participation in the workforce. *American Journal of Pharmaceutical Education* (2002) 66(3): 223-233.

17. Knapp, K.K. Questions which relate to manpower issues and the entry-level PharmD debate. *Am J Pharm Educ* (1993) 57: 269-275.

18. Ibid.

19. American Association of Colleges of Pharmacy. *Fall 2003 profile of pharmacy students* (Arlington, VA: American Association of Colleges of Pharmacy, 2003).

20. Schering Laboratories. *A profession in transition: The changing face of pharmacy* (Schering Laboratories, 1988).

21. Eli Lilly and Company. *Lily digest 1990* (Indianapolis, IN: Eli Lilly and Company, 1990); NCPA. *2003 NCPA-Pfizer digest* (Alexandria, VA: National Community Pharmacists Association, 2003); Knapp K.K., Questions which relate to manpower; Pedersen, C.A., Doucette, W.R., Gaither, C.A., Mott, D.A. et al., *Final report of the National Pharmacists Workforce Survey: 2000* (Alexandria, VA: Pharmacy Manpower Project, Inc., 2000).

22. Pedersen et al., *Final report of the National Pharmacists Workforce Survey.*

23. Knapp, Questions which relate to manpower.

24. Pedersen et al., *Final report of the National Pharmacists Workforce Survey.*

25. Ibid; Knapp, Questions which relate to manpower.

26. Knapp et al., Work patterns of male and female pharmacists.

27. Pedersen et al., *Final report of the National Pharmacists Workforce Survey.*

28. U.S. Department of Health and Human Services, *The pharmacist workforce.*

29. Knapp, K.K. and J.C. Livesey. *The aggregate demand index: Measuring the balance between pharmacist supply and demand, 1999-2001.* 2002. *J Am Pharm Assn* (2002) 42(3): 391-398.

30. Knapp, D.A., *Professionally determined need for pharmacy services in 2020* (Alexandria, VA: Pharmacy Manpower Project, Inc., 2002).

31. U.S. Department of Health and Human Services, *The pharmacist workforce.*

32. Pedersen, C.A., P.J. Schneider, and D.J. Scheckelhoff. ASHP national survey of pharmacy practice in hospital settings: Dispensing and administration—2002. *Am J Health Syst Pharm* (2003) 60(1): 52-68.

33. Pedersen, C.A., P.J. Schneider, and D.J. Scheckelhoff. ASHP national survey of pharmacy practice in hospital settings: Monitoring and patient education—2003. *Am J Health Syst Pharm* (2004) 61(5): 457-471.

34. Knapp, *Professionally determined need for pharmacy services in 2020* Pharmacy manpower.

35. Bauwens, S.F. Counseling the aging patient. *Patient Couns Comm Pharm* (1985) 3(4); 3-9.

36. Ibid.

37. Christensen, D.B., Holmes, G., Fassett, W.E. et al. Principal findings from the Washington State cognitive services demonstration project. *Manag Care Interface* (1998) 11(7): 60-62,64.

38. Smith, D.H., W.E. Fassett, and D.B. Christensen. Washington State CARE project: Downstream cost changes associated with the provision of cognitive services by pharmacists. *J. Am Pharm Assoc (Wash)* (1999) 39(5): 650-657.

39. Christensen, D.B., Holmes, G., Fassett, W.E. et al. Influence of a financial incentive on cognitive services: CARE project design/implementation. *J Am Pharm Assoc (Wash)* (1999) 39(5): 629-639.

40. Christensen, D.B., Holmes, G., Fassett, W.E. et al. Frequency and characteristics of cognitive services provided in response to a financial incentive. *J Am Pharm Assoc (Wash)* (2000) 40(5): 609-617.

41. Cranor, C.W. and D.B. Christensen. The Asheville project: Short-term outcomes of a community pharmacy diabetes care program. *J Am Pharm Assoc (Wash),* (2003) 43(2): 149-159.

42. Cranor, C.W. and D.B. Christensen. The Asheville project: Factors associated with outcomes of a community pharmacy diabetes care program. *J Am Pharm Assoc (Wash)* (2003) 43(2): 160-172.

43. Cranor, C.W., B.A. Bunting, and D.B. Christensen. The Asheville project: Long-term clinical and economic outcomes of a community pharmacy diabetes care program. *J Am Pharm Assoc (Wash)* (2003) 43(2): 173-184.

44. Knapp, *Questions which relate to manpower.*

45. LoPachin and Dickson, A comparison of male and female labor force participation; Knapp and Livesey, *The aggregate demand index;* Knapp, *Professionally determined need for pharmacy.*

46. Manasse, H.R. Jr. Pharmacy's manpower: Is our future in peril? *Am J Hosp Pharm* (1988) 45(10): 2183-2191.

47. Knapp, K.K. and M.D. Ray. A pharmacy response to the Institute of Medicine's 2001 initiative on quality in health care. *Am J Health Syst Pharm* (2002) 59 (24): 2443-2450.

48. Cooksey, J.A., Knapp, K.K., Walton, S.M. et al. Challenges to the pharmacist profession from escalating pharmaceutical demand. *Health Aff (Millwood)* (2002) 21(5): 182-188.

49. Knapp, *Professionally determined need for pharmacy.*

50. Pew Health Professions Commission. *Critical challenges: Revitalizing the health professions for the twenty-first century* (San Francisco, CA: Pew Health Professions Commission, 1995).

51. Johnson, J.A. and J.L. Bootman. Drug-related morbidity and mortality: A cost-of-illness model. *Arch Intern Med* (1995) 155(18): 1949-1956.

52. Sonnedecker, G.A. (ed.), *Kremers and Urdang's history of pharmacy,* Fourth edition (Philadelphia: J.B. Lippincott Company, 1994).

53. Ibid.

54. Hepler, C.D. The third wave in pharmaceutical education: The clinical movement. *Am J Pharm Educ* (1987) 51(4): 369-385.

55. Mrtek, R.G. Pharmaceutical education in these United States—An interpretive historical essay of the twentieth century. *Am J Pharm Educ* (1976) 40(4): 339-365.

56. McLeod, D.C. All-PharmD degree alone will not significantly alter the pharmacy profession. *Ann Pharmacother* (1992) 26(7-8): 998-1000.

57. Barker, K.N. Defining clinical pharmacy. *Am J Hosp Pharm* (1969) 26: 197.

58. AACP. *Academic pharmacy's vital statistics* (Alexandria, VA: American Association of Colleges of Pharmacy, 2004).

59. AACP. *Academic pharmacy's vital statistics* (Alexandria, VA: American Association of Colleges of Pharmacy, 1995).

60. AACP. *Academic Pharmacy's Vital Statistics,* 2004.

61. NAPB, *2002-2003 National Association of Boards of Pharmacy survey of pharmacy law including all 50 states, D.C., Guam, and Puerto Rico* (Chicago, IL: National Association of Boards of Pharmacy, 2003), pp. 1-100.

62. Study Commission on Pharmacy. *Pharmacists for the future: The report of the Study Commission on Pharmacy* (Ann Arbor, MI: Health Administration Press, 1975), p. 128.

63. NAPB, *2002-2003 National Association of Boards of Pharmacy survey.*

64. Giorgianni, S.J. (Ed.). *The Pfizer guide: Pharmacy career opportunities* (New York: Merritt Communications, Inc., 1994, pp. 1-355.

65. Pedersen, Schneider, and Scheckelhoff, ASHP national survey of pharmacy practice, 2002; Pedersen, Schneider, and Scheckelhoff, ASHP national survey of pharmacy practice, 2003.

66. Santell, J.P. ASHP national survey of hospital-based pharmaceutical services—1994. *Am J Health Syst Pharm* (1995) 52(11): 1179-1198.

67. Reeder, C.E., Dickson, M., Kozma, C. et al. ASHP national survey of pharmacy practice in acute care settings—1996. *Am J Health Syst Pharm* (1997) 54(6): 653-669.

68. Ringold, D.J., Santell, J.P., Schneider, P.J. et al. ASHP national survey of pharmacy practice in acute care settings: Prescribing and transcribing—1998. *Am J Health Syst Pharm* (1999) 56(2): 142-157.

69. Pedersen, C.A. et al. ASHP national survey of pharmacy practice in acute care settings: Monitoring, patient education, and wellness—2000. *Am J Health Syst Pharm* (2000) 57(23): 2171-2187.

70. Ringold, D.J., J.P. Santell, and P.J. Schneider. ASHP national survey of pharmacy practice in acute care settings: Dispensing and administration—1999. *Am J Health Syst Pharm* (2000) 57(19): 1759-1775.

71. Pedersen, C.A., P.J. Schneider, and J.P. Santell. ASHP national survey of pharmacy practice in hospital settings: Prescribing and transcribing—2001. *Am J Health Syst Pharm* (2001) 58(23): 2251-2266.

72. Schulz, R.M. Positive work characteristics of three pharmacy practice settings. In *Final report to the NACDS* (Alexandria, VA: National Association of Chain Drug Stores, 1986).

73. Konnor, D.D. The mail service pharmacy industry: Growing by meeting the needs and managed care. *J. Res Pharm Ecom* (1990) 2(1): 3-14.

74. Wade, D.A. Opportunities in the pharmaceutical industry. In *The Pfizer guide: Pharmacy career opportunities* (New York: Merritt Communications, Inc., 1994), pp. 294-299.

75. Skolaut, M. Pharmacists government. In A. Oslo (ed.), *Remington's pharmaceutical services* (Easton, PA: Mack Publishing Company, 1980), pp. 42-48.

76. Tertes, E., P. Wilson, G. Greenberg, and S. Nicholson. The role of the consultant pharmacist. *Am Drug* (1986) 2: 83-98.

77. Kidder, S.W. Cost-benefit of pharmacist-conducted drug-regimen reviews. *Consult Pharm* (1987) 9/10: 394-398.

78. Tindall, W.N. New career opportunities in managed care pharmacy. In Giorgianni, S.J. (Ed.) *The Pfizer guide: Pharmacy career opportunities* (New York: Merritt Communications, Inc., 1994), pp. 204-208.

Chapter 6

Pharmacy Organizations

Joseph Thomas III

INTRODUCTION

Much of what happens in health care is influenced by the activities of the many organizations that represent various health care occupations or corporations involved in health care. These organizations have such impact on the various professions' roles in the health care system that the nature of an occupation's organizations and the role played by those organizations have been used by sociologists as criteria in determining whether an occupation is considered a profession. In fact, coming together to create formal organizations or associations has been described as essential for the existence of a profession.[1] Saunders and Wilson summarized that view by stating that a number of people performing the same function does not constitute a profession. They asserted that a "profession can only be said to exist when there are bonds between the practitioners, and these bonds can take but one shape—that of formal association."[2] This chapter examines the nature of the varied organizations that represent pharmacy-related groups. The functions performed by the organizations, the ways those organizations influence pharmacists' roles in the health care system, and the delivery of pharmaceutical services will be explored.

ROLE OF PHARMACY ORGANIZATIONS

The activities performed by professional organizations, and pharmacy organizations in particular, are of interest to individual practitioners—and future practitioners—because the activities of the organizations help to define the profession. Society, including patients, other health care professions, and health care insurers are affected by the organizations' influence on the nature of health services provided, the cost of those services, and where those services are provided. This section examines the range of functions performed by pharmacy organizations. We will first examine the role

113

that organizations play for individual practitioners and the profession the organizations represent.

Profession and Individual Practitioners

The formation of an organization normally is initiated by a group of individuals sharing common interests that motivate development of some formal structure (i.e., organization), to work toward those common interests. It seems reasonable to begin by examining the services that organizations provide to individuals and/or the profession in which those individuals practice. We will investigate what motivates individuals to invest their time, dollars, and other resources in forming or in serving as members of professional organizations.

Networking and Professional Identity

Individuals join pharmacy organizations as well as other professional organizations to associate and network with individuals who share like interests and activities. The interaction with members of the same occupation helps individuals to develop awareness of the position of the group's occupation in society. Sharing of work accomplishments, work challenges, and professional contributions through meetings, written materials, and other communications helps individuals to develop a view of pharmacy's collective role in society. The resulting sense of shared responsibility and accomplishment is so valued that it motivates individuals to join and support the formal organization.[3]

Educational Services, Publications, and Meetings

The meetings sponsored by pharmacy organizations are an attraction for many individuals who join pharmacy organizations. As described previously, the meetings provide an opportunity for member pharmacists to network and interact with other individuals in the same profession. The meetings attract individuals to organizations for reasons other than just socializing with peers. Most organizations' meetings also include educational sessions on topics of primary interest to organization members. The opportunity to obtain information on new therapies, approaches to managing therapy of patients with a specific diseases, or on management techniques that can be applied in practice are all incentives that motivate individuals to join and maintain membership in pharmacy organizations. Members may possess a strong motivation to learn and enhance their skills or, at mini-

mum, may need to complete mandatory continuing education requirements. Some individuals may prefer to obtain their continuing education in
a live, interactive format rather than by other means. Regardless, the annual
meetings are perceived by some individuals as an important benefit that
leads to establishing and maintaining membership in an organization. Most
organizations hold series of regular meetings and ad hoc meetings in addition to their main annual meetings. The additional meetings may range
from educational sessions on topics of interest to meetings devoted to
planning action in advocating for policy decisions. The meetings also may
serve as forums for organization subgroups with special practice interests.

Most pharmacy organizations offer members a variety of publications
and programs that are either available only to members or available to members of the organization at lower cost than to nonmembers. The range of materials provided by pharmacy organizations is very broad. Many organizations publish a journal or magazine that is provided as part of the package of
services included in the membership fee. The journals often include reports
on the organization's business meeting, summaries of issues facing pharmacy, and lobbying activities of the organization. Many of the journals include continuing education articles and mechanisms by which official continuing education credits can be obtained for reading and completing exams
on the articles. The journals provide members with a means of maintaining
contact with actions of paid staff and elected officers of the organization on
behalf of the organization's membership.

Many organizations publish monographs on specific topics. For example, community-practice-based organizations may sponsor publication of
monographs on management of the community practice or on management
of therapy of patients with a specific disease. Such publications bring together information on a specific topic and structure it in a format to make it
more easily accessible to members. Such publications are often available to
the publishing organizations' members at discounts.

Promoting the Profession

Pharmacy organizations continue to play a very active role in defining
and advancing the role of the profession in the health care system. Pharmacy organizations were often founded in response to a perceived threat to
the profession, a desire to advance the profession, or a desire to promote
greater development of a special area of pharmacy practice. Many individuals support various organizations because of the organizations' roles as advocates for the profession. The organization acts as a collective voice for
members on issues that affect pharmacy and public health. The organiza-

tions are often involved in communicating with legislators and regulatory agencies on laws and regulations that affect pharmacy. The organizations help members to develop a common viewpoint that can be consistently communicated to policymakers and which may carry more weight than many discordant voices speaking on an issue. Many pharmacists perceive a personal obligation or responsibility to support efforts toward advancing the profession that motivates them to support pharmacy organizations.

Pharmacy organizations not only work as advocates with legislators and regulators on policy issues but they also provide an avenue for defining the profession's role vis-à-vis other health professions, as well as engaging those professions in dialogue on such issues. In doing so, pharmacy organizations sometimes serve as the collective voice for a group of pharmacists in interacting with organizations representing other health professionals such as physicians.

Goal Setting

If a profession is to avoid stagnation, there must be active examination of societal changes and setting of goals. Pharmacy organizations provide opportunities for individuals involved in the profession to review health care trends and to discuss their relevance for the future of the profession. Such dialogue provides a means for identification of goals related to the future of the profession. The issues addressed may vary, from whether pharmacists should be involved in administration of drugs used in capital punishment to whether pharmacists should seek the right to independently initiate drug therapy for patients.

Forum for Policymaking for the Profession

Most pharmacy organizations operate on the basis of some form of representative decision making. As a result, the organizations provide a forum for representative policymaking within the profession. Individual members of the organization are provided a structured means of affecting the direction of the profession. That process helps each organization to provide a collective voice for its members. It also allows members to influence policy positions of the organization as well as health policy in general.[4]

Society

Pharmacy organizations play an important role in protecting the social welfare through setting standards for the profession. These functions can be realized through a variety of approaches. In its most informal form, organizations provide members with a common concept of the roles and responsibilities of members of the profession. The socialization of individuals that takes place through involvement in an organization can be quite influential in the development of individuals' personal practice philosophies, personal practice standards, and a professional ethos that guides their practices. However, pharmacy organizations also play formal roles in setting standards. Based on their specialized knowledge, professions are granted a certain amount of autonomy and given authority and responsibility for self-regulation. Through their interaction with legislative bodies, organizations provide information needed to define the realm of practice for the profession.

We have examined the many services that pharmacy organizations provide members and their contributions to society. Before discussing some of the many pharmacy organizations that exist, it would be useful to explore the historical development of pharmacy organizations within the United States.

HISTORICAL DEVELOPMENT
OF PHARMACY ORGANIZATIONS

Prior to the Revolutionary War, dispensing medications to patients was an activity normally performed by physicians. Although nonphysicians specializing in drugs (druggists) existed, their main activity was to supply physicians with drugs and chemicals. Initially, the druggists primarily imported drugs and chemicals. Over time, they changed their focus from importation to the manufacture of drugs and chemicals. The focus on chemistry and preparation of prescription orders served as the beginnings of the U.S. chemical and pharmaceutical industries.[5] It also furthered the separation of pharmacy activities from those of physicians and speeded development of a separate professional identity for pharmacists.

Prior to the 1850s, pharmacy was not organized in any formal way to promote education of pharmacists or to regulate the practice of pharmacy. Pharmacy associations first formed in response to activities undertaken by physicians to regulate the sale of drugs. The first pharmacy organizations formed were local associations. One of the earliest and most notable groups was the Philadelphia College of Pharmacy. The use of the term "college" was based on English custom; only later did the term *college* come to refer primarily to the schools teaching pharmaceutical subjects. However, the first local associations did establish schools for the training of individuals interested in taking up the occupation of pharmacy. The organizations also set up legal controls, established processes for licensing individuals wishing to enter the occupation, and generally sought to maintain practice at a level that would elevate the occupation.[6]

Ironically, development of pharmacy organizations did not proceed from the local associations to the next larger geographical levels, such as states and regions. Instead, formation of a national organization, the American Pharmaceutical Association, was spurred by several local associations from multiple states. The national organization later encouraged and supported the founding of state associations to assist in enacting state legislation and regulations that promoted the goals of the association.[7]

SPECIFIC PHARMACY ORGANIZATIONS

Existing pharmacy organizations are examined in this section. The organizations have been grouped in the following categories: national practitioner organizations; state practitioner organizations; local practitioner organizations; national trade organizations; and educational, regulatory, or foundation organizations. National practitioner organizations are those national organizations which primarily have pharmacists as members. State and local practitioner organizations are the state- and local-level counterparts of the national practitioner organizations. National trade organizations are those organizations which normally have corporations as members and represent those corporate interests.*

National Practitioner Organizations

American Pharmacists Association (APhA)

The American Pharmacists Association is considered the oldest national pharmacy association. It was founded in 1852 and was known as the American Pharmaceutical Association until 2003, when it changed its name to better reflect the makeup of its membership. The impetus for its formation was the perceived need for an organization that could represent the opinions of all pharmacists, not just a local group, in working with the American Medical Association on efforts to control the quality of imported drugs.[8] The organization has espoused a view of representing the whole of phar-

---

*The content in this section was influenced by and includes material adapted from Lucinda Maine, "Pharmacy Organizations," pp. 288-306 in *Pharmacy and the U.S. Health Care System*, ed. Jack E. Fincham and Albert I. Wertheimer. Binghamton, NY: Pharmaceutical Products Press, 1991.

macy since its founding and has over 50,000 members. The organization has three academies, the Academy of Pharmacy Practice and Management, the Academy of Pharmaceutical Research and Science, and the Academy of Students of Pharmacy. The academies contain smaller sections based on more specialized interests. Several other national associations began as special subgroups within the APhA and later went on to become separate organizations.

The association publishes a refereed journal, newsletters, books, continuing education pieces, and a variety of other publications. The association lobbies on pharmacy issues and works with other pharmacy associations and organizations outside of pharmacy on pharmacy and health-related issues.

National Community Pharmacists Association (NCPA)

The National Community Pharmacists Association was most recently known as the NARD. When the organization was formed in 1898, it was known as the National Association of Retail Druggists. The organization's name was shortened to NARD in 1987 and then changed to the National Community Pharmacists Association in 1996. The group first developed to address the commercial interests of independent pharmacy owners, and still works to represent the interests of independent community pharmacy owners. It lobbies on issues related to pharmacy practice and other legislative issues that affect community pharmacies. The organization publishes a journal and several specialty publications, such as one for pharmacies providing home intravenous infusion services. The organization offers a student membership category and works to encourage development of new independent community pharmacies.

American College of Apothecaries (ACA)

The American College of Apothecaries was founded in 1940. It is an organization of pharmacists interested in maintaining progressive professional practice and prescription compounding services. The association describes its purpose as translation and dissemination of knowledge, research data, and recent professional pharmacy practice developments for the benefit of pharmacists, pharmacy students, and the public. The organization publishes several periodicals. The members of ACA are designated "fellows." The organization has several membership categories. Full fellows must be owners, partners, stockholders, or managers who make policy decisions in a professional pharmacy practice. Associate fellows are member pharmacists employed by full fellows or recommended by three full fellows. A student membership category, student fellow, also exists for students who have completed at least two years of prepharmacy curricula. In addition to information dissemination, the organization takes positions on policy issues related to pharmacy practice and promotes professional pharmacy practice.

American Society of Health-System Pharmacists (ASHP)

The American Society of Health-System Pharmacists had its origin in a subsection on hospital pharmacy that was created within the American Pharmaceutical Association in 1932. The group became a separate association in 1942. When the group was founded in 1942, it was known as the American Society of Hospital Pharmacists. For an eight-year period, from 1986 to 1994, the organization was officially known as the ASHP. Its name was changed in 1994 to the American Society of Health-System Pharmacists.

The ASHP's membership consists primarily of pharmacy practitioners, pharmacy students, and pharmacy residents with an interest in hospital pharmacy. The organization represents their interest in lobbying and provides a variety of services to its members. The organization sponsors the Mid-Year Clinical Meeting, perhaps the largest annual pharmacy-related meeting. Just as the American Pharmacists Association, the American Society of Health-System Pharmacists publishes a wide variety of materials including books, continuing education pieces, journals, and references texts.

National Pharmaceutical Association (NPhA)

The National Pharmaceutical Association was founded by African-American pharmacists in 1949 to work toward improvement of the position of such pharmacists within the profession. The association works as an advocate for improvement of pharmaceutical services and health care in general for minority and indigent populations and serves as a vehicle for minority pharmacists to engage in collective dialogue with other pharmacy organizations and other health care organizations. The NPhA sponsors an annual national convention of its members with continuing education programming and organization business meetings. The association has provided scholarships for pharmacy students and works toward recruitment of African-American and other underrepresented ethnic groups to the study of pharmacy and to careers in pharmacy. Student chapters of the organization exist in many schools of pharmacy, and these have been active in assisting with student recruitment and retention efforts.

American Society of Consultant Pharmacists (ASCP)

Founded in 1969, the American Society of Consultant Pharmacists grew out of the desire of a group of pharmacists to improve the use of pharmaceuticals in extended care facilities. ASCP members "manage and improve drug therapy and improve the quality of life of geriatric patients and other individuals residing in a variety of environments, including nursing facilities, subacute care and assisted living facilities, psychiatric hospitals, hospice programs, and home and community-based care" (http://www.ascp.com/about/). The organization and its members were given a major boost in 1974, when regulations for nursing home participation in Medicare and Medicaid required pharmacist review of patients' drug regimens. Membership has grown from just over 1,000 in 1976 to over 6,500. The organization sponsors an annual meeting and a mid-year clinical meeting.

American College of Clinical Pharmacy (ACCP)

The American College of Clinical Pharmacy is a practitioner organization that works toward providing "leadership, education, advocacy, and resources enabling clinical pharmacists to achieve excellence in practice and research" (http://www.accp.com/about.php). Founded in 1979, the organization is young relative to others. Its mission includes fostering growth of clinical services, promoting the value of clinical pharmacy services, facilitating pharmaceutical and biomedical research, dissemination and application of research findings, and promoting excellence in clinical pharmacy education. The organization offers three classes of membership, full member, associate member, and affiliate member. Students, residents, and fellows may also join under a special member category with reduced membership fees.

American Association of Pharmaceutical Scientists (AAPS)

Founded in 1986, the American Association of Pharmaceutical Scientists consists primarily of pharmaceutical scientists from varied segments of the profession, including the pharmaceutical industry and academia. The organization has over 7,000 members. Its mission has been described as serving the pharmaceutical sciences, the health professions, and the public interest by providing a forum for free interchange and dissemination of scientific knowledge, influencing the formation of public policy relevant to health sciences, collectively promoting pharmaceutical sciences, and fostering career growth and development of members.[9]

The organization sponsors an annual meeting and provides members with a variety of publications including several newsletters, several scientific journals, workshops, and short courses. Activities include lobbying on pharmacy and other health-related issues as well as sponsoring scholarships and grants.

Academy of Managed Care Pharmacy (AMCP)

As managed care grew, it was probably inevitable that an organization focusing on the specific interests of that group would develop. Formed in 1989 specifically to address the issues of managed care pharmacy, the Academy of Managed Care Pharmacy is a relatively young national organization. The organization addresses what has been described as the "unique needs and interests" of managed care pharmacists. AMCP publishes a scientific journal, newsletter, and other materials and its membership is said to be more than 4,800.

State Organizations

Many pharmacy organizations have memberships based within a specific state or region within a state. Since the licensing and much of the regulation of pharmacy and other health professions are based on state laws, the state associations play a significant role in the health care system. Some of the organizations have several thousand members and budgets of over a million dollars. For example, in 1995 the California Pharmacists Association had over five thousand members and an annual budget of nearly $2.5 million. Other states such as Florida, North Carolina, and Texas have pharmacy associations with over three thousand members.[10]

Each state pharmacy association generally publishes a journal that is distributed to its members. The journals include continuing education articles and analysis of general trends affecting pharmacy, but they also offer information on legislative and policy issues specific to the association's home state. The state associations tend to be actively involved in lobbying on state legislation or regulations that affect pharmacy. Since government health insurance programs such as Medicaid are operated at the state level, the associations often serve as a collective voice for pharmacists on reimbursement and other issues related to such programs. The associations also have been very active in communicating with state legislatures and regulatory bodies on expansion of the role of pharmacists. For example, the state associations have worked toward passage of laws allowing pharmacists to initiate or modify drug therapy as a means of facilitating a more active role in managing drug therapy.[11] States often have several associations based on members' practice interests, such as hospital pharmacy, community pharmacy, and in some cases long-term care pharmacy. However, some of the state associations have explored mergers and consolidations as one method of dealing with rapid change in the health care system.

Local Organizations

Local pharmacy associations that cover a county or perhaps a city in more metropolitan areas are common. The organizations bring together practitioners serving patients in a geographic area such that the pharmacists often interact with some of the same physicians, nurses, hospitals, and other providers of health care services. Providing a means of networking with individuals serving that common group, the organizations often sponsor local continuing education meetings, provide community service, and may work to encourage individuals to enter pharmacy. Some of the organizations sponsor scholarships for pharmacy students. The local associations also provide a group that can interact with its local counterpart in the medical and other professions.

National Trade Organizations

Consumer Healthcare Products Association (CHPA)

Consumer Healthcare Products Association was founded in 1881 to represent makers of cosmetics, medical supplies, and medications for home use. Originally named the Propriety Association, its name was changed to the Nonprescription Drug Manufacturers Association in 1989. It expanded its scope to include representation of the nutritional supplement industry in 1998 and took on its current name in 1999. The organization publishes a newsletter and other materials for companies that produce nonprescription drugs or nutritional supplements. The organization also takes an advocacy role in representing its members' interests. The organization promotes the role of nonprescription medications and nutritional supplements and promotes responsible use of these medications.

Generic Pharmaceutical Association (GPhA)

The Generic Pharmaceutical Association represents manufacturers and distributors of finished generic pharmaceuticals, manufacturers and distributors of bulk active pharmaceutical chemicals, and suppliers of the generic pharmaceutical industry. It tracks legislative and regulation activities for its members. The organization presents information on behalf of its members in forums considering legislation, regulations, or policy that relate to the pharmaceutical industry. The association also conducts meetings and seminars on topics of interest to its members.

Healthcare Distribution Management Association (HDMA)

The Healthcare Distribution Management Association was formed in 1876 as the Western Wholesale Druggist's Association. Its name was changed to the National Wholesale Druggists' Association in 1882 and later to its current name in 2001. The association represents pharmaceutical and related health care product distributors. It membership includes health care product manufacturers, distributors, and service providers. International companies may hold membership in the organization.

The association works to maintain dialogue between members of the health care distribution chain. The association gathers data on the health care distribution industry and publishes a variety of periodic reports with statistical data on the industry. The association works to educate customers and policymakers about the services provided by health care product distributors and the value added by distributors in the health system. The association is an active advocate for the health care product distribution industry. The organization sponsors meetings and programs to educate association members about issues related to the industry and on methods to increase productivity.

National Association of Chain Drug Stores (NACDS)

The National Association of Chain Drug Stores is a trade association that represents the interests of multiple-pharmacy owners. The organization was founded in 1933 to help improve the operations of multiunit organizations and to represent them in interactions with other segments of pharmacy.[12] The group lobbies on issues related to pharmacy and the commercial interests of chain pharmacies and also continues to serve as a vehicle for interaction with other pharmacy organizations on topics of interest to chain-pharmacy companies. The organization publishes several newsletters and holds an annual meeting each year.

National Pharmaceutical Council (NPC)

The National Pharmaceutical Council was founded in 1953. It consists of more than twenty research-based pharmaceutical manufacturers. The organization publishes an annual comprehensive report on pharmaceutical benefits provided under state assistance programs, primarily Medicaid. It also sponsors a variety of research and education projects.

Pharmaceutical Research and Manufacturers of America (PhRMA)

The Pharmaceutical Research and Manufacturers of America (PhRMA) is an organization of U.S. pharmaceutical companies actively engaged in manufacture and marketing of finished dosage-form pharmaceuticals under their own brand names and engaged in development of new therapies. The organization was originally founded in 1958 as the Pharmaceutical Manufacturers Association or PMA. The organization promotes the roles of the research-based pharmaceutical industry in the prevention and treatment of illness. PhRMA collects and disseminates data on the industry, such as industry investment in research and products being developed.

Pharmaceutical Care Management Association (PCMA)

The Pharmaceutical Care Management Association represents pharmaceutical benefit management companies. It was formed under the name of the National Association of Mail Service Pharmacies (NAMSP) in 1975 and changed its name to the American Managed Care Pharmacy Association in 1989.[13] The organization added pharmaceutical benefit managers to its membership in 1994 and changed its name again in 1996 to the Pharmaceutical Care Management Association to disassociate itself from negative connotations attached to "managed care" and state-level efforts to implement legislation regulating pharmacy benefit managers.[14] As of 2003, only pharmaceutical benefit managers and pharmacy benefit management divisions of health plans were eligible for membership. The organization actively lobbies on the behalf of its member companies and publishes information pieces on mail-order pharmaceuticals. Companies involved in mail delivery of pharmaceuticals may be either active full members or active supporting members. Associate membership is available to pharmaceutical manufacturers that supply prescription or nonprescription drugs to the industry. Affiliate membership is open to other firms or to individuals engaged in business with industry firms.

Education, Regulatory, and Foundation Organizations

United States Pharmacopeial Convention (USP)

The United States Pharmacopeial Convention is the organization that publishes the *United States Pharmacopoeia-National Formulary* (USP-NF) that is recognized by the federal government as the official compendium of drug standards. The organization was formed in 1820 for the purpose of developing a national pharmacopoeia. When the Food and Drugs Act of 1906 was passed, the USP was recognized as an official pharmacopoeia by the federal government. Although the USP publication is recognized as an official document by the U.S. government, the organization is not a government agency, and most of the work of the association is done by volunteer experts representing other organizations in pharmacy, medicine, and related areas.

The 1900 articles of incorporation for the organization describe the purposes of the organization as encouraging and promoting

> the science and art of medicine and pharmacy by selecting by research and experiment and other proper methods and by naming such materials as may be properly used as medicines and drugs with formulas for their preparation: by establishing one uniform standard and guide for the use of those engaged in the practice of medicine and pharmacy in the United States where by the identity, strength, and purity of all such medicines and drugs may be accurately determined, and for other like and similar purposes; and by printing and distribution at suitable intervals such formulas and the results of such and similar selections, names and determinations.[15]

In addition to the USP-NF, a variety of other information resources are published. During the early 1970s, the organization begin a major thrust in publishing patient counseling information, which is now produced as a separate publication, the *USP Dispensing Information*.[16]

American Association of Colleges of Pharmacy (AACP)

Schools and colleges of pharmacy are represented in the American Association of Colleges of Pharmacy, founded in 1900. In addition to institution memberships, individual memberships are available to administrators, faculty, and staff of the pharmacy academic institutions. The association has two main councils, the Council of Faculties and the Council of Deans. The organization maintains a journal which publishes articles on pharmacy education topics and also gathers and publishes data for use by member organizations in comparative analysis of individual programs, identification of trends in pharmacy education and practice, and for consideration in policy decisions related to pharmacy education. The AACP works with other organizations in providing input on development of standards in pharmacy education.

National Association of Boards of Pharmacy (NABP)

The National Association of Boards of Pharmacy is the organization for State Boards of Pharmacy; in other words, the state agencies responsible for licensing pharmacists and regulating pharmacy practice in their respective states. Some agencies external to the United States, such as U.S. territories and Canadian provinces, are also members. A main function of the organization is that is produces a model or standard pharmacy licensing exam called the National American Pharmacist Licensure Examination (NAPLEX), which is used by most of the agencies in testing pharmacists for licensure. The organization also produces an exam on federal drug law and has developed model pharmacy laws that the state agencies can use as guidance and input when legislative changes are under consideration. The organization serves as a clearinghouse for pharmacist transfer of licensure for one state to another and for pharmacy licensure information.

In addition, NABP administers the Foreign Pharmacy Graduate Examination Committee (FPGEC) Certification. This examination is accepted by almost all states as a means to document the equivalency of a foreign pharmacist's education. In states that accept the certification, the FPGEC is considered to partially fulfill eligibility requirements for state licensure. Individual states set their own additional criteria for licensure of foreign pharmacy graduates.

Accreditation Council for Pharmacy Education (ACPE)

The Accreditation Council for Pharmacy Education establishes standards and accredits schools and colleges of pharmacy. It is recognized as an accreditation organization by the United States Department of Education and the Council on Postsecondary Accreditation (COPA). Founded in 1932, it is not a government agency and schools and individuals do not have membership in the organization. However, the ACPE has considerable influence since most state licensing agencies often require, with some exceptions, graduation from an accredited school of college of pharmacy in order to sit for their licensing exams. Much of the ACPE's budget is provided by a philanthropic foundation, the American Foundation for Pharmaceutical Education. The organization also maintains a widely used process for review and approval of continuing education providers, programs, and materials. Its board of directors is made up of individuals appointed by the American Association of Colleges of Pharmacy, the American Council on Education, the American Pharmacists Association, and the National Association of Boards of Pharmacy. The board of directors is responsible for establishing the policies and setting standards for accreditation of professional degree programs and for approval of continuing pharmaceutical education providers. The organization also maintains a public interest panel, which includes at least two representatives of the public who are not pharmacists or involved in pharmaceutical education.

American Foundation for Pharmaceutical Education (AFPE)

The American Foundation for Pharmaceutical Education was formed in 1942 to assist in training teachers for colleges of pharmacy and to help develop scientists for the pharmaceutical industry. Working to attract individuals to the study of pharmacy and to graduate education, the organization provides fellowships for graduate students and more recently has provided financial support for research by new faculty members who were AFPE graduate fellows. In addition to fellowships, the ACPE has provided financial support for the *American Journal of Pharmaceutical Education,* which is published by the American Association of Colleges of Pharmacy, and financial support to the American Council on Pharmaceutical Education, an organization that accredits schools and colleges of pharmacy. Other activities include financial support for teachers' seminars, student recruitment programs, and gathering of data on pharmacy practice and pharmacy education. The organization is supported by gifts from individuals, the pharmaceutical industry, and others.

CURRENT ISSUES FOR PHARMACY ORGANIZATIONS

Multiplicity of Organizations

Today, there are national, state, and local organizations that cover regions, counties, and even single cities. Not only are there multiple organizations based on geographic areas, but organizations have proliferated to represent specific interests of individuals based on varied practice interests or varied practice sites within pharmacy.[17] Each individual is faced with many pharmacy-related organizations that he or she might join and support. As previously explored, organizations exist with a range of geographic broadness. How many organizations should or must individuals support through membership fees, time, and other resources that organizations need? Does the existence of so many organizations benefit the profession or society, or is the existence of so many organizations detrimental to pharmacy and/or to society? These questions have been examined for decades, and there are competing viewpoints.

The argument often is made that the existence of multiple organizations reduces the clout or ability of the profession to affect implementation of policy decisions that would advance the profession and/or improve health care. Varied (and sometimes conflicting) positions on policy issues is said to confuse policymakers and consumers and to cause them to question which organization really represents the views of the profession.

Despite concerns that have been expressed pertaining to the perceived need for pharmacy to speak with one voice, some mechanisms do exist for pharmacy organizations to work together. One example is the Joint Commission of Pharmacy Practitioners (JCPP), which was formed in 1977 as a mechanism for national pharmacy organization to discuss issues. The JCPP's members are other pharmacy organizations, including the Academy of Managed Care Pharmacy, American Association of Colleges of Pharmacy, American College of Apothecaries, American College of Clinical Pharmacy, American Pharmacists Association, American Society of Consultant Pharmacists, American Society of Health-System Pharmacists, National Community Pharmacists Association, National Association of Boards of Pharmacy, and National Council of State Pharmacy Association Executives. The JCPP has organized and sponsored conferences devoted to strategic planning for the future of pharmacy.

During a period in the early 1990s, several pharmacy organizations formed coalitions to work on health care reform. Unfortunately, there was not just one coalition but several speaking for the profession. Interestingly, many members expressed displeasure with the lack of unity and encouraged the organizations to work more closely on health care reform. It seems unlikely that many of the national pharmacy organizations will merge in the near future. However, it would seem wise for the organizations to continue to work toward professional unity.

INDIVIDUAL DECISIONS REGARDING ORGANIZATIONS

How should individuals approach the issue of personal participation in pharmacy organizations? The large number of organizations makes decisions more complex than if only one or two existed. However, the large number of national organizations focusing on specific practice areas also means that each pharmacist should be able to identify at least one national organization that pursues goals consistent with his or her personal interests.

Since pharmacy organizations function on a variety of levels, ranging from the national to the local, it seems that individuals desiring to participate in defining and advancing the role of the profession will want to consider membership within at least one national, one state, and one local organization.

Most pharmacy organizations offer student membership at reduced rates and many have student chapters, so pharmacy students should consider becoming involved in pharmacy organizations while still in school. Involvement in the organizations offers the opportunity to not only network with other students but also with practicing pharmacists. Service on committees or as an officer in the organizations also provides excellent opportunities for development of leadership skills.

Since the profession provides an opportunity for service and for personal reward, many believe each pharmacist has a duty to support the profession by supporting pharmacy organizations. Each individual must make a personal decision on whether to accept this belief. However, if most members of a profession choose not to support its organizations, the existence of the profession and its potential contributions to society will be jeopardized.

NOTES

1. Vollmer, H.M. And Mills, D.L. *Professionalization* (Englewood Cliffs, NJ: Prentice-Hall, 1966).
2. Ibid.
3. Sonnedecker, G. *Kremer and Urdang's history of pharmacy,* Fourth edition (Philadelphia: J. B. Lippincott Company, 1976).
4. Schondelmeyer, S.W. Professional association membership decisions among pharmacists, Doctoral dissertation, The Ohio State University, 1984.

5. Sonnedecker, *Kremer and Urdang's history of pharmacy.*
6. Ibid.
7. Ibid.
8. Ibid.
9. Konnor, D.D. Scientists to the fore. *American Druggist* (1987) May: 90.
10. Konnor, D.D. The state of state associations. *American Druggist* (1995) November: 2828-2830, 2833-2834.
11. Shefcheck, S.L. and Thomas, J. III. The outlook for pharmacist initiation and modification of drug therapy. *Journal of the American Pharmaceutical Association* (1996) NS36(10): 597-604; Punekar, Y., Lin, S., and Thomas, J. III. Pharmacist collaborative practice progress: State laws and perceived impact of collaborative practice. *Journal of the American Pharmaceutical Association* (2003) 43(2): 503-510.
12. Sonnedecker, *Kremer and Urdang's history of pharmacy.*
13. Konnor, D.D. The mail service pharmacy industry: Growing by meeting the needs of managed health care. *Journal of Research in Pharmaceutical Economics* (1990) 2(1): 3014.
14. Konnor, D.D. Managed care pharmacy association focusing on state antimanaged care. *Weekly Pharmacy Reports* (1996) 45(46/November 11): 3.
15. United States Pharmacopeial Convention, Inc., *About USP: People Programs, Policies, and Procedures.* Retrieved March 24, 2005, from United States Pharmacopeial Convention, Inc. Web site. <http://www.USP.org/aboutUSP/p4/ p4_aol.html>.
16. United States Pharmacopeial Convention, Inc. *170 years of USP: The end of the beginning,* Proceedings of the United States Pharmacopeial Convention, Inc. (Rockville, MD: United States Pharmacopeial Convention, Inc., 1991).
17. Rappaport, P. The unity issue. *The Canadian Journal of Hospital Pharmacy* (1992) 45(4): 133-134.

Chapter 7

Emerging Roles

Richard J. Bertin

INTRODUCTION

Today's health care system offers unprecedented opportunities for pharmacists. In the not-too-distant past, pharmacy was seen as a largely undifferentiated profession in which the vast majority of practitioners dispensed prescriptions, written by physicians, from a traditional community or hospital pharmacy setting. A relatively small number of pharmacists deviated from this path to pursue careers in nuclear pharmacy, research, industry, or academia.

The present picture is vastly changed, with pharmacists occupying clinical and managerial/administrative roles at many points in the health system. Certainly, drug distribution is still an important activity that pharmacists perform or supervise. Other chapters in this book have described some of the expanded roles into which more pharmacists are moving. This chapter will explore that phenomenon in more detail, and highlight three topics that are of particular current interest.

The proliferation of nontraditional roles for pharmacists can likely be traced back to the expansion of pharmacist education from the basic chemistry-related courses of the early days of the profession. Courses in business management, accounting, and related subjects were necessary parts of the curriculum when most pharmacists were engaged in community pharmacy or hospital pharmacy practice. In these settings, knowledgeable budgeting, purchasing and inventory management, and staff supervision were often markers of professional acumen, and pharmacists with these skills were frequently selected for higher management positions in the health industry. Of all the health professionals, pharmacists combined (and many still combine) a unique blend of clinical and managerial skills which make them adaptable to a variety of positions.

The addition of greatly enhanced clinical training and experience to the scientific and managerial knowledge base of pharmacists really opened the doors to broader roles in the provision of health care for patients. Courses in anatomy and physiology, combined with formally taught skills in patient history taking, counseling, and physical assessment paved the way. Introduction of the PharmD curriculum in a few schools and therapeutics courses which required that pharmacy students interact with other health-profession students proved that pharmacists could hold their own in a more clinically structured environment. The introduction of new institutional drug distribution systems, which required more direct participation of pharmacists in receiving and interpreting drug orders, also brought many of these practitioners out of their cloistered basement enclaves. The net effect was a sea change in pharmacy practice, beginning in institutions but slowly spreading through the profession. The eventual acceptance of the PharmD degree, traumatic as that step was for many in pharmacy education and practice, marked a change in pharmacy that can never be reversed.

Community pharmacy practice has been particularly affected by the changes in pharmacist roles. Historically, pharmacists have always served as an important portal of entry into the health care system for patients in the community setting, providing counseling on over-the-counter medications and frequently referring patients with serious complaints to physicians. Ironically, however, community pharmacists of not too long ago were ethically forbidden to discuss specific drug therapy with a patient or even to identify the name of a prescribed drug on a prescription container. The pharmacist's only recourse was to refer the patient back to the physician with any questions about the drug or its effects. Obviously, this significantly curtailed the pharmacist's real utility as the "drug expert" in patient care.

By the turn of this century, however, the situation had changed dramatically. Colleagues in the health professions are now accustomed to seeing pharmacists playing a significant role in health care, wherever they practice. With few exceptions, pharmacists in these roles are well accepted by colleagues and patients. Although some older pharmacists still in practice are uncomfortable with these new clinical roles, the profession is clearly changing. Enthusiastic, well-trained pharmacists have more opportunities open to them than ever before. The remainder of this chapter will address some of these opportunities.

ADVANCED PRACTICE CREDENTIALING

As pharmacists have become more clinically involved in patient care, pharmacy has taken note of the practice models that characterize other health professions.[1] An important example of this is the move toward the acquisition of credentials that indicate a pharmacist has the knowledge and skill to perform advanced-level services. Pharmacy, like medicine and the other health professions, is regulated at the state level by state boards of pharmacy. Candidates are licensed to practice after having (1) graduated from a college or school of pharmacy approved by the board; (2) spent a minimum number of hours of experience in structured, supervised practice; and (3) passed a licensing examination.

State licensure is an indication that the individual has attained the basic degree of competence necessary to ensure the public health and welfare will be protected. Individuals who have received a license may use the abbreviation RPh (for "registered pharmacist") or other designation authorized by the board of pharmacy after their names.

Pharmacy practitioners who wish to broaden and deepen their knowledge and skills may participate in a variety of postgraduate education and training opportunities. They include the following.

Academic Postgraduate Education and Training

Pharmacists who wish to pursue a certain field of study in depth may enroll in postgraduate master's or doctor of philosophy (PhD) programs. Common fields of study for master's candidates include business administration, clinical pharmacy, and public health. Common fields for doctoral studies include pharmacology, pharmaceutics, pharmaceutical and medicinal chemistry, pharmacotherapeutics, pharmacy practice, and social and administrative sciences.

Bachelor-level pharmacists who have been in the workforce may also return to a college or school of pharmacy to earn the PharmD degree. These programs, which are tailored to the individual's background and experience, may follow "nontraditional" pathways. However they must produce the same educational outcomes as traditional PharmD degree programs.

Residencies

A residency is an organized, directed postgraduate program in a defined area of pharmacy practice. Pharmacy practice residencies focus on the resident's development of professional competence in the delivery of patient care and practice management activities. Specialized pharmacy practice residencies focus on the knowledge, skills, and abilities needed to provide care in a specialized area of pharmacy practice (e.g., critical care, drug information, pharmacotherapy, or oncology). Residencies are usually twelve months in duration, although certain specialized residencies require an additional twelve (or continuous twenty-four) months for completion. The American Society of Health-System Pharmacists (ASHP) is the recognized accrediting body for pharmacy practice and specialty residency programs in pharmacy. The ASHP Commission on Credentialing (COC), a committee of the ASHP Board of Directors, is responsible for the development of standards for residency programs, administering the accreditation process, and granting accreditation. The COC consists of fourteen appointed pharmacists, who have served as residency program directors and who represent a variety of practice settings, as well as two "public" members. ASHP partners with appropriate organizations, including the Academy of Managed Care Pharmacy (AMCP), the American College of Clinical Pharmacy (ACCP), the American Pharmacists Association (APhA), and the American Society of Consultant Pharmacists (ASCP), in developing standards and/or accrediting residency programs of a specialized or practice-setting-specific nature.

The majority of pharmacists who pursue residency training currently do so by completing a pharmacy practice residency. These residencies are usually based in a particular practice setting or practice type, such as a hospital, ambulatory care clinic, community pharmacy, managed care organization, or home or long-term care practice. Specialized residency training often involves additional education and training experiences beyond the pharmacy practice year, usually in specialized areas of practice such as pharmacokinetics; the care of specific types of patients (e.g., pediatrics); or a focus on specific diseases (e.g., oncology).

The Centers for Medicare & Medicaid Services (CMS), an agency of the federal government, recognizes residency accreditation bodies within the health professions, including ASHP in its role as the accrediting body for pharmacy residency training. Consequently, ASHP-accredited residency programs are eligible for inclusion by a Medicare "provider" (i.e., usually a hospital) in the calculation of (and reimbursement for) the entity's costs for providing services to Medicare beneficiaries. The rules and regulations guiding this reimbursement policy are reviewed regularly by CMS and are subject to change.

Fellowships

A fellowship is an individualized postgraduate program that prepares the participant to become an independent researcher in an area of pharmacy practice. Fellowship programs, like residencies, usually last one to two years. The programs are developed by colleges of pharmacy, academic health centers, colleges and universities, and pharmaceutical manufacturers.

It should be noted that several pharmacy organizations, including the ACCP, the ASHP, and the APA, award the honorary title of "Fellow" to selected members as a means of publicly recognizing their contributions to the profession. A Fellow of ASHP, for example, may write "FASHP" for "Fellow of the American Society of Health-System Pharmacists," after his or her name. The two uses of the word *fellow*—one denoting an individual participating in a postgraduate training program and the other denoting receipt of an honorary title—should be clearly distinguished.

There is no official accreditation body for fellowship programs; however, an official position statement by ACCP on Guidelines for Clinical Fellowship Training Programs can be found online at <http://www.accp. com/position/pos15.pdf>.

Certificate Training Programs

A certificate training program is a structured and systematic postgraduate continuing education experience for pharmacists that is smaller in magnitude and shorter in duration than a degree program. In addition to didactic instruction, the design of certificate programs includes practice experiences, simulations, and/or other opportunities for the demonstration of desired professional competencies. The length of any particular certificate program is determined by its stated goals, desired professional competencies, and outcome measures. This generally requires a minimum of 15 contact hours (1.5 CEUs). Certificate programs are designed to instill, expand, or enhance practice competencies through the systematic acquisition of specified knowledge, skills, attitudes, and behaviors. The focus of certificate programs is relatively focused; for example, the APhA offers programs in such areas as asthma, diabetes, immunization delivery, and management of dyslipidemias.

Certificate training programs are offered by national and state pharmacy organizations and by schools and colleges of pharmacy and other educational groups. The programs are often held in conjunction with a major educational meeting of an organization. The Accreditation Council for Pharmacy Education (ACPE) approves providers of such programs. The Standards and Quality Assurance Procedures for ACPE-Accredited Providers of Continuing Pharmaceutical Education Offering Certificate Programs in Pharmacy are found online at <http://www.acpe-accredit.org/pdf/Certificate. pdf>.

Traineeships

Traineeships, in contrast to certificate training programs, are defined as intensive, individualized, structured postgraduate programs intended to provide the participant with the knowledge and skills needed to provide a high level of care to patients with various chronic diseases and conditions. Traineeships are generally of longer duration (about five days) and involve smaller groups of trainees than certificate training programs do. Some are offered on a competitive basis, with a corporate sponsor or other organization underwriting participants' costs. Pharmacy organizations currently offering traineeships include the American College of Apothecaries (ACA), the ASCP, and ASHP's Research and Education Foundation.

Certification

Certification is a credential granted to pharmacists and other health professionals who have demonstrated a level of competence in a specific and relatively narrow area of practice that exceeds the minimum requirements for licensure. Certification is granted on the basis of successful completion of rigorously developed eligibility criteria that include a written examination and, in some cases, an experiential component. The voluntary, advanced practice certification processes available to pharmacists include those overseen by the Board of Pharmaceutical Specialties, the Commission for Certification in Geriatric Pharmacy, and the National Institute for Standards in Pharmacist Credentialing. Other multidisciplinary certifications are also available to pharmacists. It should be noted that completion of a certificate training program is *not* similar to certification.

The development of a certification program includes the following steps:

1. Defining the area in which certification is offered (role delineation)
2. Creating and administering a psychometrically valid examination
3. Identifying other criteria for awarding the credential (e.g., experience)
4. Identifying recertification criteria

A professional testing consultant or firm typically assists in the development of the role delineation and the examination to ensure that the examination meets professional standards of psychometric soundness and legal defensibility.

Certifying Agencies for Pharmacists Only

Three groups, the Board of Pharmaceutical Specialties, the Commission for Certification in Geriatric Pharmacy, and the National Institute for Standards in Pharmacist Credentialing, offer certification to pharmacists.

Board of Pharmaceutical Specialties (BPS)
<http://www.bpsweb.org/default.shtml>

Established in 1976 by the American Pharmacists Association (then the American Pharmaceutical Association), BPS certifies pharmacists in five specialties: nuclear pharmacy, nutrition support pharmacy, oncology pharmacy, pharmacotherapy, and psychiatric pharmacy. Pharmacists who wish to retain BPS certification must be recertified every seven years.

The recognition of each specialty is the result of a collaborative process between the board and one or more pharmacy organizations, which develop a petition to support and justify recognition of the specialty. This petition must meet written criteria established by the BPS.

A nine-member board that includes six pharmacists, two health professionals who are not pharmacists, and one public/consumer member directs the BPS. A specialty council of six specialist members and three pharmacists not in the specialty direct the certification process for each specialty.

BPS examinations are administered with the assistance of an educational testing firm, resulting in a process that is psychometrically sound and legally defensible. Each of the five specialties has its own eligibility criteria, examination specifications, and recertification process. All five examinations are given on a single day once a year in approximately twenty-five sites in the United States and elsewhere.

In 1997, BPS introduced a method designed to recognize focused areas within pharmacy specialties. A designation of "Added Qualifications" denotes that an individual has demonstrated an enhanced level of training and experience in one segment of a BPS-recognized specialty. Added qualifications are conferred on the basis of a portfolio review to qualified individuals who already hold BPS certification. The first added qualification to receive BPS approval was infectious diseases, which is within the pharmacotherapy specialty.

Commission for Certification in Geriatric Pharmacy (CCGP)
<http://www.ccgp.org>

In 1997, the American Society of Consultant Pharmacists (ASCP) Board of Directors voted to create the CCGP to oversee a certification program in geriatric pharmacy practice. CCGP is a nonprofit corporation that is autonomous from ASCP. It has its own governing board of commissioners. The CCGP Board of Commissioners includes five pharmacist members, one physician member, one payer/employer member, one public/consumer member, and one liaison member from the ASCP Board of Directors.

To become certified, candidates are expected to be knowledgeable about principles of geriatric pharmacotherapy and the provision of pharmaceutical care to the elderly. Pharmacists who meet CCGP's requirements are entitled to use the designation Certified Geriatric Pharmacist, or CGP. Pharmacists who wish to retain their CGP credential must recertify every five years by successfully completing a written examination.

CCGP contracts with a professional testing firm to assist in conducting the role delineation or task analysis and in developing and administering the examination. The resulting process is psychometrically sound and legally defensible; it also meets nationally recognized standards. The CGP certification exams are administered twice a year at multiple locations in the United States, Canada, and Australia. CCGP publishes a candidate handbook that includes the content outline for the examination, eligibility criteria for taking the examination, and the policies and procedures of the certification program.

National Institute for Standards in Pharmacist Credentialing (NISPC)
<http://www.nispcnet.org/>

The NISPC was founded in 1998 by the American Pharmacists Association (then the American Pharmaceutical Association), the National Association of Boards of Pharmacy (NABP), the National Association of Chain Drug Stores, and the National Community Pharmacists Association. The purpose of NISPC is to "create a consolidated, nationally recognized, credential for pharmacists seeking certification in a variety of disease states."[2]

NISPC offers certification in the management of diabetes, asthma, dyslipidemia, and anticoagulation therapy. At the time of its founding, the organization's immediate objective was to design a process that would document the competence of pharmacists providing care for patients with these disease states. The NISPC credential was first recognized in the state of Mississippi, where it was used to enable pharmacists to qualify for Medicaid reimbursement as part of a pilot project in that state. NABP developed the competency assessment examinations and oversees their administration. The NISPC tests are administered nationally as computerized examinations and are available throughout the year.

Multidisciplinary Certification Programs

Some certification programs are available to professionals from many health disciplines, including pharmacists. Areas in which such certification is available include diabetes education, anticoagulation therapy, pain management, and asthma education. Some of these programs are still in the early stages of development.

As of early 2004, fewer than 10 percent of the estimated 200,000 practicing pharmacists in the United States held advanced-practice credentials such as those described previously. This indicates that there remains great potential for growth in participation in the future.

COLLABORATIVE DRUG THERAPY MANAGEMENT

In recent years, many pharmacists have embraced the concept of pharmaceutical care. This concept has been broadly defined as identifying potential and actual drug-related problems, resolving actual drug-related problems, and preventing drug-related problems.[3] This is an appropriate role for well-trained and motivated pharmacists. Pharmacists are considered to be essential resources on medication usage, dosages, interactions, contraindications, and side effects and to be very knowledgeable on cost-effective medications for patients. They are able to identify and avert potential and actual adverse drug reactions. Unfortunately, in many settings, this knowledge is not maximally utilized.

It has been well documented that an unacceptable level of drug-related morbidity and mortality in the United States is a result of medication errors. This has been due in part to the complexity of available medications and the fact that it is not possible for doctors and nurses to be up-to-date with all the information associated with medication safety. About 39 percent of medication errors happen during the prescribing phase, 50 percent happen between the transcription-ordering and medication-administering phase, and the other 11 percent happen during the final dispensing phase. The common link between all these phases is the lack of appropriate pharmaceutical care, resulting in an economic impact on the health care system. Therefore, the logical step in optimizing medication outcomes for patients is for pharmacists to go beyond identifying the problems and come up with ways to prevent these problems. Studies have shown that a reduction of as much as 66 percent is seen when pharmacists are involved in patients' medication processes. One way of accomplishing this is through collaborative drug therapy management (CDTM).

CDTM is "the provision of pharmaceutical care in a collaborative and supportive practice environment that allows the qualified pharmacist legal, regulatory and ethical responsibility to solve drug-related problems when discovered"[4] and can be seen in a wide array of settings. The main components of CDTM are a collaborative practice setting; access to patients' medical records; a competency level of knowledge, skills, and ability of pharmacotherapy; documentation of activities; and reimbursement for these activities. With an established CDTM program, there would be an increase in efficient workflow, improved patient outcomes, and a reduction in medication errors.

In CDTM, pharmacists are not trying to replace physicians. Physicians go through years of training and schooling to be able to diagnose patients. Pharmacists do not. A CDTM proposes that physicians be patients' care managers, whereby they diagnose and make initial treatment decisions, and pharmacists be the medication experts in continuing to select, initiate, monitor, change, or discontinue patients' medications in order to reach therapeutic goals and positive patient outcomes through cost-effective means. With a CDTM, pharmacists would have dependent prescriptive authority, meaning that pharmacists would share with collaborating physicians the risk and responsibilities associated with the patient's overall health outcome. Pharmacists would be able to authorize prescription renewals, adjust dosages, administer immunizations/drugs, initiate, recommend, or discontinue medications, order lab work, and schedule follow-up visits without waiting or hunting down a physician for approval. Also, with dependent prescriptive authority, pharmacists would be assisting physicians, not replacing them, by adding pharmacists' knowledge of drugs to make for a more efficient work environment.

Among health professionals, pharmacists are highly accessible to patients since many pharmacies are in minority communities, in urban centers, and in institutions. The majority of patients seek out pharmacists for advice on not only prescription medications but also over-the-counter medications. With the increase in prescription medications switching to nonprescription status and the cost of physician visits, patients are taking their health-care needs into their own hands. Pharmacists need to be part of this self-care movement to provide information on medications that are cost-effective to patients. They also need to provide information on medications and cost to physicians, who are initially prescribing and diagnosing these patients. Therefore, with the use of a CDTM pharmacists would be optimizing patients' therapeutic regimens in a cost-effective way through appropriate selection of medications and reduction in the incidence of medication errors.

CDTMs are not novel ideas. Pharmacy and therapeutics committees have been part of an implied CDTM through drug formularies or through the identification of therapeutically equivalent drugs. Many health-systems have "site-based protocols," which can be broadly defined under a CDTM between pharmacists and physicians. Usually, these implied CDTMs need to be formally recognized in order to facilitate payments for pharmacists' services, to clearly identify these pharmacists' roles as pharmaceutical care providers, and to increase physicians' awareness of pharmacists as drug experts. As formal recognition of CDTMs develops, pharmacists are seeking to be recognized by the federal Centers for Medicare & Medicaid Services as providers eligible for payment for their services. Currently, states permitting CDTMs between pharmacists and physicians include: Arkansas, California, Florida, Hawaii, Idaho, Indiana, Iowa, Kansas, Kentucky, Michigan, Mississippi, Nebraska, Nevada, New Mexico, North Dakota, Ohio, Oregon, South Dakota, Texas, Vermont, and Washington. This list is expected to increase.

Pharmacists are assuming advanced roles as pharmaceutical care providers through the use of CDTMs. CDTMs allow pharmacists to have dependent prescriptive authority. After the physicians' initial diagnoses and treatment decisions, pharmacists provide drug therapy management such as renewing prescriptions; adjusting dosages; administering immunizations/drugs; initiating, recommending, or discontinuing medications; ordering lab work; and scheduling follow-up visits. In this way, the contribution of the pharmacist's clinical expertise can be maximized to the benefit of patients and health care systems.

PHARMACIST IMMUNIZATION PROGRAMS

An integral part of contemporary pharmaceutical care is the pharmacist's role in promoting health and preventing disease. With this focus in mind many pharmacists are expanding their roles as health care providers through the provision of immunizations to patients.

This new emerging role of pharmacists as immunization providers could not come at a more crucial time. A recognized increased vaccination need exists due to threats of bioterrorism; emerging infectious diseases (e.g., severe acute respiratory syndrome, or SARS); and an alarming rate of 90,000 Americans dying per year of vaccine-preventable deaths that occur despite available vaccines. These events have prompted a renewed emphasis on immunizations and the role of pharmacists and health care providers. The pharmacist can now play one of three immunization roles: educator, facilitator/collaborator, or vaccinator. These roles can be applied to a variety of settings, including hospital, rehabilitation center, emergency department, ambulatory clinic, outpatient pharmacy, nursing facility, and home health care center.

As educators, pharmacists are at the forefront of identifying high-risk patients in need of vaccines and are a constant source of drug information for the public on immunologic drugs and where to get them. They can determine a patients' immunization statuses through gathering immunization histories, advocating the use of vaccine profiles, distributing vaccination records to patients, avoiding immunologic drug interactions, and screening patients for immunization needs. An evaluation can be performed to identify patients most in need of immunizations based on age, diagnoses, or medication use. For instance, if a patient is on theophylline, digoxin, warfarin, or insulin for a chronic cardiovascular disease, lung disease, or diabetes, these medications are indications for immunizations. The pharmacist can then counsel patients, their families, and the public in making the right decision about what immunizations they require. In an organized health care setting, pharmacists are often part of a pharmacy and therapeutics committee and can advocate and recommend vaccines, toxoids, immune globulins for inclusion on the formulary. To increase public awareness of immunizations, pharmacists can organize local observations of National Infant Immunization Week, the last full week of each April, and National Adult Immunization Awareness Week, the second week of each October; hang posters; wear buttons; hand out immunization brochures; and write articles for pharmacy newsletters on preventable infections through vaccinations. Pharmacists should encourage the public to carry their own up-to-date vaccine records, thereby involving them in their own health promotion and disease-prevention process.

As a facilitator/collaborator, the pharmacist provides support services by partnering with those who can immunize. The national Centers for Disease Control and Prevention (CDC) have written guidelines for health care workers to protect themselves against such diseases as hepatitis B, influenza, measles, mumps, rubella, and varicella viruses. It should be noted that all adults should be immunized against tetanus and diphtheria. Special work conditions require immunizations against pneumococcal or other vaccine-preventable diseases. Also in these guidelines are outlines for work restrictions and other administrative implications for infectious diseases. Pharmacists should recommend following these guidelines to protect the health care workers and their patients. These recommendations can be done through infection-control or occupational health committees to advocate vaccines and immunodiagnostic tests to contribute to the well-being of the health care workers. In addition, sending mobile carts to nursing stations, wards, and clinics can increase vaccination rates and employee health.

When reviewing charts, pharmacists can make recommendations to physicians concerning needed immunizations before the patient leaves the facility. Pharmacists can contract with nursing facilities to perform comprehensive immunization assessments on all their residents and provide data on their findings. Pharmacists can also work with their city, county, and state health departments and collaborate with pharmacy organizations, physicians, and like-minded advocators of health promotion to get the word out on the importance of being immunized.

Forty-three states currently allow pharmacists to vaccinate. However, each state's laws and regulations regarding pharmacy practice determine whether or not a pharmacist can administer vaccines. Once the authority is given for pharmacists to immunize, a prescription is typically needed. But in some states, a CDTM agreement can be formed in which the pharmacist has a standing order from the prescriber and a prescription is not needed every time a vaccine is given. A pharmacist must achieve and maintain annual competency through formal training in epidemiology, vaccine characteristics, injection techniques, contraindications, and emergency responses to adverse events, as well as knowledge of recent immunization recommendations, schedules, and techniques. Immunizations are clearly cost-effective when compared with the cost of treating vaccine-preventable illness.

Pharmacists are in a key position to play a role in preventing diseases by promoting and administering immunizations among the public. As more pharmacists and state regulatory agencies recognize the value of this public health role, the practice should grow. This emerging role will do much to solidify the public's perception of the pharmacist as an important contributor to their health.

CONCLUSION

In 2001, the Pharmacy Manpower Project found that the opportunity for improving the quality of drug use, and thus the quality of patient outcomes and quality of life in this country is staggering. This blue-ribbon commission of experts from across the profession further concluded that pharmacy needs to move even more rapidly to redeploy its members from medication order fulfillment to patient care. It is certain that the future of pharmacy as a profession lies in its development and implementation of advanced levels of knowledge and skills in the provision of patient care. The emerging roles described in this chapter and elsewhere in this book are becoming more accepted by pharmacists, patients, and the health care community throughout the country. The advanced-level credentials that document the pharmacist's ability to provide these services are similarly growing in strength throughout the profession. With the prospect of expanded payment opportunities for pharmacists' services, all pharmacists need to ensure that they are prepared to meet the challenges of today and tomorrow.

NOTES

1. Council on Credentialing in Pharmacy. Reference Paper on Credentialing in Pharmacy. Available online at <www.pharmacycredentialing.org>. September 2003.
2. National Institute for Standards in Pharmacist Credentialing (NISPC). <http://www.nispcnet.org/about_NISPC.html#history>.
3. Carmichael, Jannet M. Do pharmacists need prescribing privileges to implement pharmaceutical care? *American Journal of Health-System Pharmacy* 1995; 52 (15): 1699-1701.
4. Barry, Chris P. and Fuller, Timothy S. A Path to Pharmaceutical Care (Part 2): Evolution of Collaborative Drug Therapy Management. *Hospital Pharmacy* 1998; 33(5): 490, 494, 497.

Chapter 8

Political Realities of Pharmacy

Robert I. Field

Drugs have long mixed with controversy and politics. As far back as the Roman Empire, Pliny the Elder warned of adulteration of the natural food and drug supply.[1] Today, pharmacy continues to confront a range of complex political realities whose breadth is constantly expanding. The perennial concern over drug safety raises but one set of issues, while economics, intellectual property, and international trade are among a host of new ones.

This chapter will review the most significant political issues facing pharmacy today. They affect the range of players in the field, from pharmacists to manufacturers to insurers to patients. Many reflect familiar historical themes, but others, particularly economic concerns, are relatively new. The chapter also considers a new set of political issues that are likely to emerge surrounding the growth of genomic medicine. Each issue, old and new, reflects a clash of competing interests and of conflicting values. They challenge us as a society to find the best balance.

Much of the history of food and drug regulation in America repeats a familiar theme. Well-publicized scandals engendered political controversies that prompted new laws and new forms of regulation. The 1904 publication of *The Jungle* by Upton Sinclair[2] raised public awareness of unsanitary conditions in the meatpacking industry and led to the passage two years later of the first comprehensive food and drug law.[3] In 1937, the deaths of over 100 patients, mostly children, from an antibiotic preparation known as elixir of sulfanilamide led to passage the following year of the federal Food, Drug, and Cosmetic Act, which forms the basis for pharmaceutical regulation today.[4] Reports from Europe in 1962 of severe birth defects linked to the drug thalidomide gave impetus to the passage of amendments toughening that regulation scheme later the same year.[5]

Present political controversies, however, are different in important ways. Americans are not so concerned with the safety and efficacy of the drugs they take as with the ability to afford them. Past political controversies led to laws that ensured the quality of drugs; consumers now want guaranteed access. In a sense, the pharmaceutical industry has become a victim of its own success. It has produced many highly effective products that are central to treating a range of conditions, making their cost a cause for concern. Nothing intensifies a political debate more than discussions of the flow of money.

The issues discussed in this chapter are among the most prominent today, but they are only some of the many that create political realities for pharmacy in the United States. Just as they reflect an evolution from past concerns, they will eventually be transformed into new ones. What will not change in the foreseeable future is the central role of pharmacy in American health care. Pharmacists, used to playing a local role in meeting community health care needs, increasingly find themselves in the middle of a highly visible national stage.

GROWTH OF PHARMACEUTICAL USE AND SPENDING: PRELUDE TO INTENSIFYING POLITICAL CONFLICT

The growing role of pharmaceutical products in American health care provides the context for current political debates. The use of medications and consequent spending on them has increased dramatically in recent years. Between 1992 and 2000, overall utilization of prescription drugs in America increased by 52 percent.[6] In 1990, they accounted for 6 percent of health care spending, in 2002 over 9 percent, and by 2012 they are projected to account for 15 percent.[7] Prescription sales rose almost 19 percent and the number of prescriptions dispensed grew by 7.5 percent just between 1999 and 2000. Between 1993-2003, prescription purchases increased by 70 percent in quantity dispensed.[8]

These trends have sent ripples throughout the economy. In the business world, General Motors spent more than $1 billion in 2001 on prescription drugs for active and retired employees.[9] In the world of government, between 2000 and 2002 Medicaid expenditures for prescriptions rose by over 18 percent compared with 5.3 percent for hospital care.[10] For individuals, between 1998 and 2000 premiums for Medicare supplement insurance policies that included prescription drug coverage rose by an average of 37 percent.[11]

The effects are a particular burden for those who do not have prescription insurance coverage. Although the extent of coverage has grown considerably, it is still unavailable to many.[12] In 1990, about 25 percent of all prescription spending was reimbursed through private insurance and 60 percent was paid for out of the patient's pocket. In 2000, insurance covered almost 50 percent, put patients still paid for 30 percent directly.[13] As of

2001, about three-quarters of beneficiaries had some coverage through private insurance policies that supplement Medicare, but the extent of the coverage provided by these policies varies considerably.[14] The remaining one-quarter of Medicare beneficiaries, about 10 million people, were without any prescription coverage at all.

POLITICAL FALLOUT

Financial trends such as these cannot fail to have political consequences. The cost of prescriptions has become a "pocketbook" issue that affects almost everyone. Those who do not feel it themselves often experience it indirectly through its effect on family members. Everyone sees the effects of increasing drug costs in higher overall premiums for health insurance. Politicians have no choice but to listen.

In responding to complaints about the high cost of their products, pharmaceutical companies point to the tremendous expense involved in producing them and to the huge benefits that they provide. The process of bringing a drug from concept to market can take over ten years and, according to some estimates, cost over $800 million.[15] It is estimated that for every 250 drugs that enter initial preclinical testing, only one completes the path to final FDA approval.[16] Without an adequate return on this investment in the form of revenues, companies could not afford the financial risk. However, when there is an adequate return for investing in new drug research, the rewards for society can be great. Pharmaceutical products are credited with a leading role in recent dramatic increases in longevity.[17] They may also help to hold down other health care costs, such as hospitalization. It is not, the industry argues, as if society does not receive great value for its pharmaceutical expenditures.

The combination of tremendous social value and potentially unaffordable costs creates a prescription for political turmoil. Political attention has focused on a range of pharmaceutical industry practices, and in a business this complex, attention to one issue inevitably leads to examination of many others. Therefore, we are seeing much of American pharmacy, from research to manufacturing to marketing to dispensing, come under greater public scrutiny.

Future Conflicts

In coming years, the industry is likely to face even more turmoil from forces beyond economics. Technology is changing the face of every aspect of pharmacy. On the immediate horizon are changes in prescribing and dispensing. With the encouragement of industry, insurers, and hospitals, physicians are increasingly prescribing through computerized systems and hand-held digital devices. Once entered, prescriptions are increasingly being filled in large automated centers through the use of computerized robotics. Some patients are avoiding their physicians altogether and ordering drugs over the Internet. Each of these innovations changes the cost of distributing drugs.

In the long run, an even more fundamental scientific revolution may transform the very meaning of pharmaceutical products. That is the advance in our understanding of genetics. Over the coming decades, the field of genomics will change the basis of drug development and possibly of all health care. As a result, both the effectiveness of medicines and the cost of their development are likely to rise significantly. A range of highly emotional political issues can be expected in response. Our society has begun to grapple with just a few of them, including human cloning, stem cell research, and genetic privacy, but the full brunt of the controversies that the genetics revolution will engender is yet to be felt.

REGULATION, PATENTS, AND POLITICS

Present political realities begin with the existing government structures governing the pharmaceutical industry. The Food and Drug Administration (FDA) oversees the development, testing, marketing, and manufacture of drugs. The Patent and Trademark Office (PTO) issues patents that protect new drug products from competition for a period of time. Until recently, these two agencies and the regulatory laws that they implement operated largely independently, as they were originally designed. Recently their responsibilities have begun to overlap, creating new political pressures for the industry and for the regulators involved.

FDA Regulation

The FDA is the public's guardian of drug safety and efficacy. It is the "police" force that stands between unsafe, useless, or improperly manufactured products and consumers. Unlike almost all other areas of consumer regulation in which rules are enforced for products on the market, drug regulation applies before a product even reaches the market, in fact before it even sees its first tests. This rigorous form of regulation is intended to protect consumers before a disaster has a chance to occur. Some believe, however, that the FDA overdoes its job and holds back many drugs that are safe and needed. The battle between these competing concerns creates a fundamental and perennial political reality for the agency.

In response to fears that valuable new drugs were being kept from consumers through regulatory delays, the Prescription Drug User Fee Act of 1992 directed the FDA to accelerate its review of new drug applications and imposed fees on the companies requesting those approvals to finance the process.[18] Review times have declined since the law was implemented, but some critics contend that reduced vigilance against hazardous products has resulted.[19] Is another thalidomide waiting to sneak through an overstressed review process, or does our overconcern that there will be one keep lifesaving medicines from reaching the market? The agency faces pressure to speed up its approval of new drugs, while also facing the prospect of condemnation if it lets a dangerous drug slip through.

This is a balancing act that the FDA will probably always face. In addition to safety, the balancing also has cost implications. A longer and more intensive review process adds to the expense of developing new drugs. In all sectors of health care, society juggles a perpetual trade-off between quality, cost, and access.[20] We will never find the perfect equilibrium, and the FDA will always find itself caught in the middle.

Intellectual Property

Underlying the economic foundation of the pharmaceutical industry is the law of patents, which protects the financial interests of product innovators. Inventors are entitled to prevent competitors from making or selling their inventions for a period of twenty years from the date they file a patent application with the PTO. This protection applies to new drugs in much the same way as it does to other inventions, although much of the twenty-year protection period can be exhausted during premarket testing, before financial rewards can be realized.

With the protection from competition that a patent affords, a manufacturer becomes a monopolist for a period of time during which it has tremendous leeway in setting the price. Manufacturers argue that this is essential to ensure sufficient profits to compensate for the extreme cost and risk of developing new drugs and bringing them to the market. Industry critics contend that some companies abuse the patent laws by charging exorbitant prices when they can. Prescription drugs are a necessity, they contend, and pricing policies should take their lifesaving nature into account.

In a market-based economy, the answer to monopoly pricing is competition. For pharmaceuticals, this is accomplished through the sale of generic drugs, copies of drugs that are manufactured by competing companies once the original patent has expired. However, bringing these products to market raises a host of difficult questions. When should a generic manufacturer be allowed to begin testing a copy of a patented drug? Must it go through the entire testing and FDA review process? How much of the original product may be copied?

In 1984, the patent rules that apply to new drugs were changed by the Drug Price Competition and Patent Term Restoration Act (commonly known as the Hatch-Waxman Act).[21] This law was intended to strike a balance between two goals. One was to streamline the generic approval process to bring competing forms of existing products to market faster. The other was to maintain sufficient economic rewards to encourage research-based companies to continue to produce new ones. Of particular significance in the evolution of food and drug regulation, it created a mechanism that explicitly tied the FDA regulatory process and the PTO patent process together.

The law implements a complex regulatory scheme. To assist the introduction of generic drugs, products that copy patented drugs can be tested before the original patent has expired, and applications for approval of them can reference safety data that was filed for the original drug. In return, original manufacturers are granted longer patent terms. Other provisions permit further delays in the marketing of generic products under some circumstances when the validity of patents are in dispute and grant exclusive marketing periods for the first generic product to reach the market.

Most observers feel that the Hatch-Waxman Act has fulfilled its original goals of bringing generic drugs to market sooner while protecting the financial returns for brand-name products. However, industry critics argue that patent laws are still too restrictive and that they are open to abuse by manufacturers. They point to filings that protect inactive ingredients, metabolites, and other peripheral aspects of drugs beyond the time when the original patent has expired. They also point to the high cost and consequent unavailability of some lifesaving medications that have patent protection, such as AIDS drugs in many third world countries. The industry responds that any weakening of patent protections would destroy the incentives needed for continued investment in the expensive process of new drug development.

The appropriate length and extent of patent protection is an ongoing debate that goes to the heart of pharmaceutical economics. It continues to play out in many forms. Congress has considered proposals to amend the Hatch-Waxman Act to encourage greater generic competition and has done so with bills that passed such as Senate Bill S.812 which provided for greater access to affordable pharmaceuticals. This bill passed in 2002. Some third world countries have refused to honor pharmaceutical patents on AIDS medications. Many lawsuits have been fought over the validity of individual patents. Because of the large economic implications, achieving the best balance between patent protection and generic competition is likely to remain elusive and politically sensitive for some time.

INSURANCE FOR PRESCRIPTIONS

The growth in private prescription insurance coverage during the 1990s coincided with a period of rapidly rising costs. Which was the cause and which the effect is a matter of debate. As an array of new drugs made prescription medications more central to the treatment of a range of diseases, the need for assistance in affording them grew. At the same time, the availability of financial resources to cover the cost of drugs encouraged more physicians to prescribe expensive ones and more patients to use them. Undoubtedly, these forces have strengthened each other. The result is that prescription coverage has become a financial necessity for most Americans, yet many have no access to it. For those insurance plans that cover prescriptions, controlling costs is a primary concern. Efforts to this end have been inconsistent in their success. For the most part, they have relied on outside administrators rather than the insurers themselves.

The Role of Pharmacy Benefit Managers

Most private prescription insurance plans are administered by companies known as pharmacy benefit managers (PBMs) under contract with insurers. These organizations purchase drugs in bulk from manufacturers on behalf of millions of insured patients. This group purchasing gives them substantial leverage to gain price concessions, which generally take the form of rebates paid to the PBM by the manufacturer. While an individual patient may not have the power to bargain over price, PBMs, which specialize in facilitating group sales, do.

PBMs also try to control unnecessary drug expenditures to further hold down costs. Most insurance companies structure prescription benefit plans around formularies, lists of preferred drugs that patients are encouraged to use. A formulary generally includes one or two medications for each condition, excluding other similar products as duplicative. Often, the drugs chosen for inclusion on a formulary are those for which the insurer or PBM has negotiated the best price. Insurers also encourage patients to use generic substitutes for brand-name drugs whenever possible. The result is that medications fall into one of three financial categories under most insurance arrangements. The cheapest are generics, followed by brand-name drugs on the formulary, followed by other brand-name drugs.

To translate these pricing levels into incentives for patients, most insurers structure their coverage into three tiers of reimbursement, under which patients face the lowest copayment for the cheapest drugs, generics, and the highest copayment for nonformulary brand-name drugs. Under some plans, this copayment may be so large that it is prohibitive for many patients. In some cases, requests for reimbursement for the most expensive drugs are also subject to utilization review by the insurer or the PBM, and reimbursement may be denied altogether.

The Politics of PBMs

PBMs, as the gatekeepers to prescription coverage, have strong opponents. Patients and physicians often resent their role in restricting coverage through formulary development and utilization review. Some insurers feel that they do not effectively help to control costs because they keep much of the savings from manufacturer rebates for themselves. Others argue that PBMs merely add an unneeded layer of bureaucracy to an already complex system.

Of all the opponents of PBMs, none are more passionate than pharmacists. The drugs that PBMs purchase in bulk are often distributed to patients through mail-order, bypassing retail pharmacies entirely. When they do facilitate sales through pharmacies, PBMs often restrict the transaction through utilization review. Those sales that are completed are usually subject to large negotiated discounts. As a result, pharmacists are seeing their profits and their autonomy taken by large bureaucratic companies that never see patients directly.

Against this array of opponents, PBMs also have their supporters. Some politicians see them as the central players in a Medicare prescription benefit. Rather than having the government take on the new and unfamiliar role of administering drug reimbursement, they argue, why not let companies that are expert in this business handle the task? This would make PBMs the central agent for almost everyone's prescription purchasing, under both private and governmental insurance.

The future of PBMs is uncertain. They face resistance from several elements of American pharmacy, but they may also have great political opportunities. Whatever their fate, it seems certain that some form of large, centralized purchasing of drugs will play an important role in the future. Group purchasing is the only form of market discipline that can create effective price pressure, and rising costs will increasingly demand the efficiencies of mail-order and other forms of mass distribution. The days when filling a prescription was a matter between a patient, a physician, and a pharmacist are waning. The growth of insurance coverage complicates the picture in many ways and adds much more than just financial reimbursement.

STATE COST-CONTROL ISSUES: MEDICAID AND THE UNINSURED

State governments are active players in pharmaceutical cost debates in two ways. First, they provide insurance coverage for prescriptions for their poorest citizens under Medicaid through the Centers for Medicare and Medicaid Services (CMS). Costs for this program have been rising rapidly.[22] They reflect the largest single expense in some state budgets, even though they are shared with the federal government.

Some states have also sought to address the prescription needs of uninsured citizens who are not covered by Medicaid. These are citizens who are caught in the middle: they are too wealthy to qualify for Medicaid but too poor to afford insurance or to pay for medications out-of-pocket. Lacking access to private insurance, they not only have no third party to help pay the bill, they also have no group-purchasing leverage through PBMs.

A few states have been particularly aggressive in seeking to control Medicaid drug costs and the burden on uninsured residents. They have established formularies of preferred drugs that include products for which manufacturers have provided significant discounts. Physicians must receive prior approval before prescribing anything else. Some states are also seeking to require drug companies to sell at the discounted Medicaid prices to uninsured residents. Others are seeking to form multistate purchasing cooperatives to bargain for additional discounts under Medicaid and for uninsured residents. Many of these programs have been challenged in court, so their ultimate chances for success are uncertain. However, it is clear that state governments have taken on a new role as major players in the political realities of pharmacy pricing.

OTHER COST-CONTROL ISSUES

A number of other pharmaceutical industry practices have received considerable political attention in the battle over cutting costs. Three are particularly visible at the federal level. These include international pricing, advertising, and consumer sales.

International Pricing and Reimportation

Some industry critics point to the lower prices charged for pharmaceuticals in many foreign countries as evidence that Americans are being overcharged. Drug companies respond that virtually all developed countries other than America directly regulate prices, so the lower prices are maintained artificially. The issue, they argue, is not so much that American prices are too high than that foreign prices are too low.

Whatever the cause, many Americans have found that they can obtain some medications at much lower prices outside of the country. The closest and easiest source for these bargains is Canada, a country that controls drug prices. Some residents of northern states drive across the border for pharmaceutical shopping trips, and others order drugs from Internet-based Canadian pharmacies. The price disparities have not escaped political attention.

Congress responded by enacting the Medicine Equity and Drug Safety Act of 2000, which permits the FDA to let drug wholesalers purchase American drugs at cheaper prices abroad and then "reimport" them back to the United States for sale at lower prices.[23] Proponents argue that this will give Americans the same access to affordable medications that is enjoyed by our geographically closest foreign neighbors. Pharmaceutical manufacturers counter that selling drugs to Americans at artificially maintained lower prices will deny them the revenues needed to continue the expensive process of drug discovery and development. They also warn that adulterated or mishandled drugs could find their way back into the country.

The statutory mechanism for reimportation is complex and cumbersome. For example, to guard against the possibility that mishandled drugs will be sold, the law imposes complex record-keeping requirements to document the chain of custody of products involved. The FDA has not yet implemented it, and it is not clear that it ever will. Nevertheless, international pricing discrepancies will continue to attract political attention. The United States market has become the main source of profits for most pharmaceutical companies.[24] This puts a heavy financial burden on American drug buyers and will create an ongoing source of political friction.

Direct-to-Consumer Advertising

In 1997, the FDA amended a long-standing policy that limited the ability of drug companies to advertise their products directly to patients through television.[25] Direct-to-consumer advertising, commonly referred to as DTC, has since grown into a multibillion-dollar business, with almost $2.5 billion spent in 2000.[26] Although for the most part only a few best-selling drugs are promoted in this way, television commercials have been associated with sizeable sales growth for those products.[27]

Some consumer advocates and some insurance companies complain that DTC advertising inflates utilization of drugs, adding costs for the system overall. Pharmaceutical firms counter that the ultimate decision on utilization rests with each patient's physician, whose professional judgment guards against unnecessary sales. They add that DTC advertising raises awareness of medical conditions and available treatments, resulting in timelier and often more effective care.

The battle over DTC advertising promises to intensify. Some insurers have proposed limiting reimbursement for drugs that are advertised. If patients want medications that they see on television, they will have to pay the cost themselves. However, some drug manufacturers see the ads as leveling the playing field in a different way. They educate consumers about medications that may not be on their insurer's formulary, thereby encouraging them to challenge formulary restrictions or to switch insurers. The power of television advertising as a marketing tool has been clear since the dawn of the medium. It has now come to form a battleground in passionate fights over pharmaceutical costs.

Over-the-Counter Sales to Consumers

When efforts to limit demand by beneficiaries for expensive drugs have failed, some insurers have taken a different tack. Instead of trying to restrict access, they have paradoxically tried to expand it. Health insurance covers the cost of prescription drugs, not those sold over-the-counter (OTC). FDA regulations permit prescription medications to be sold in this way when years of widespread use have shown them to be safe. Most commonly, it is a drug's manufacturer that requests a change in status, after a product's patent has expired. If the status of a widely used prescription drug changes to OTC, then patients have freer access, although with no insurance coverage.

In 2001, for the first time, a health insurance company, Wellpointe HealthWorks of California, petitioned the FDA to change the status of a prescription drug to OTC, in this case three widely prescribed, nonsedating antihistamines.[28] Although initially opposed, the manufacturer of one of these products, Schering-Plough, announced in 2002 that it would acquiesce, and the FDA approved the switch later that year. Switching a drug to OTC status is not unusual, but the active involvement of an insurance company is. It is an example of how cost pressures and insurance coverage are altering the industry's dynamics.

DTC advertising and OTC drug status reflect different aspects of consumer access as a driver of drug costs. In one case, greater access resulting from aggressive marketing may be increasing overall costs, and in the other, greater access at lower prices may be reducing them. The crucial difference in the effects of these practices is insurance. When reimbursement is available, patients will use more high-priced drugs. The irony is that while policymakers are looking for ways to increase coverage as a way to help patients cope with high prices, insurers are seeking to restrict coverage as a means to control costs. The problem of trade-off between access and cost on a societal level will not be easily resolved.

THE DEBATE OVER MEDICARE COVERAGE

Of all the current debates over pharmaceuticals, the most politically charged is overcoverage for prescriptions under Medicare. It is the elderly who need and use prescription drugs the most. There is a growing political consensus that some sort of coverage is needed. It does not seem right that millions of those most in need of drugs to maintain their lives and health are unable to afford them. The difficult part has been deciding how.

Medicare Part D provides some coverage for outpatient prescription drugs for seniors beginning with the roll out of the Drug Discount Card program in 2004-2005, and the full benefit in 2006 for some coverage for seniors in January 2006 has begun the long overdue process of more completely providing drug benefit coverage for the elderly Medicare population.

A basic division exists between proposals that would have added prescription reimbursement as a direct benefit administered by the government in the same manner as existing coverage for hospital and physician services and those that would rely on administration by the private sector. Under the direct government approach, a percentage of the cost of prescriptions has been reimbursed after a patient's annual spending had exceeded a deductible. Claims would be submitted to the government as they are for physician services. The private-sector approach will rely largely on PBMs. They will administer reimbursement under contracts with the government in much the same way that they presently do for private insurers.

Either approach to covering prescriptions under Medicare would be extremely expensive. Estimates of the cost of most proposals are at least $1.3 trillion over ten years.[29] In view of the spiraling level of prescription spending that already exists, controlling costs will be crucial if a program is to succeed. Proponents of a direct government program see deductibles and copayments taking the lead role in holding down utilization. They believe that prices can also be controlled through the government's group-purchasing clout, since by covering prescriptions for the elderly, it will become the largest single purchaser of pharmaceutical products in the country. But the program as it exists now does not allow CMS to negotiate directly with manufacturers.

Proponents of the PBM approach believe that the same techniques to control costs presently used for private insurance could be brought to bear under a Medicare program. PBMs will institute formularies in Medicare Part D within broad CMS-coordinated guidelines, review utilization, and use group-purchasing leverage to extract price concessions from manufacturers. Competition between PBMs will provide Medicare beneficiaries with a choice of differing benefit and administrative structures. PBMs will take financial risk for cost overruns in providing drug benefits as an added incentive to control them. Those that do not meet cost targets would absorb losses, while those that exceed them would reap profits.

With a tremendous amount of money at stake and differing philosophical approaches, each group with an interest in a prospective Medicare prescription benefit has had strong hopes and fears. Organizations representing beneficiaries support the addition of coverage but fear that overly restrictive utilization controls or income restrictions will limit its effectiveness. Pharmacists are concerned about the possibility of greater power accumulating in the hands of PBMs. The pharmaceutical industry is concerned about the eventual possibility of price controls. Although a Medicare drug benefit would increase demand for its products, pressure to limit prices for such a large new market might be inevitable. How else could the government realistically afford it? The Medicare program already controls the prices that it pays to hospitals and physicians, putting them at the mercy of political rather than market forces. For this reason, the industry tends to favor the private-sector approach to extending coverage.

One significant component of the Medicare Part D benefit mandates a program for medication therapy management services (MTMS). Whether this MTMS will provide increasing reimbursement for pharmacists' cognitive services (enhancing patient compliance, disease management of chronic diseases, enhanced drug therapy management) remains to be seen. If these services are managed centrally by PBMs, some pharmacists may be left out of the provision of MTMS. This political and policy decision will be made over the near and long-term future.

In politics, as in many other areas, the level of passion tends to correlate with the amount of money involved. For a Medicare prescription benefit, there is a lot of both. The creation of Medicare in 1965 significantly altered the practice of medicine and the growth and structure of hospitals. For better or worse, American health care was never the same. A Medicare prescription benefit will undoubtedly do the same for the pharmaceutical industry.

PHARMACEUTICAL INDUSTRY
RESEARCH AND MARKETING

As its importance to American health care has grown, various practices of the pharmaceutical industry have come under increasing public scrutiny. Two areas have seen particular attention. One is the conduct of research, through which new products are created and tested, and the other is the promotion of products once they reach the market.

Research

The lifeblood of the pharmaceutical industry is research. It is the engine that creates new products that keep companies going. The validity of the clinical trials that stand behind new drugs is also essential to effective regulation. However, since drug-development research is extremely costly, time-consuming, and financially risky, researchers face pressures not only to maintain the integrity of their investigations but also to help facilitate the development of new drugs. In some cases, investigators own stock or have other financial ties with the companies whose drugs they are studying. This creates a potential conflict between maintaining objectivity and achieving financial gain.

The pharmaceutical industry recently adopted voluntary guidelines to reduce the chance that conflicts of interest will distort clinical findings.[30] Some scholarly journals have adopted policies requiring that authors of articles disclose all financial ties to research sponsors, whether or not related to the study in question.[31] However, some critics contend that these steps are not enough and that external government regulation is also needed. They feel that the risk of compromised results is too great.

Scientific researchers are not used to being regulated. The nature of science is free inquiry without external constraints. However, effective drug regulation requires complete objectivity. Increasingly, clinical researchers must venture out of the ivory tower into the political and legal realms to defend arrangements with sponsors. The business of research has become a visible and contentious area.

Marketing

Unlike other industries that manufacture consumer goods, pharmaceutical companies do not sell most of their products directly to consumers. They sell them to intermediaries who make the actual purchasing decisions.

These intermediaries are physicians, and occasionally other clinicians, whose approval is required before a prescription can be filled. Even DTC advertising directs patients to consult their physician about the decision to use a product. The job of pharmaceutical marketers, therefore, is primarily to influence physicians. They do this in a number of ways, some of which are controversial. Although advertising in professional journals and other media is extensive, information about new drugs is spread primarily by sales representatives known as detailers, who meet individually with potential prescribers to provide product data. Recent predictions of the impending demise of detailing because of Internet marketing, managed care purchasing, and other industry changes have turned out to be wrong. In fact, the number of detailers retained by the American pharmaceutical industry has increased markedly in recent years, with the average American sales force growing by over 40 percent between 1999 and 2001.[32]

The key to pharmaceutical product detailing is gaining access to physicians for personal meetings. Often, this is facilitated with gifts. The items can be relatively trivial, such as a take-out lunch, or can constitute significant practice enhancements, such as a textbook or a continuing education session. However, some have been seen as excessive, such as trips to resorts and tickets to sporting events. Where is the line between information dissemination and improper inducements?

Incentives to physicians to prescribe medications raise both ethical and legal concerns. Federal law prohibits payments of any kind in return for recommending health care products that are reimbursed by Medicare or Medicaid. Recently, the federal Department of Justice has investigated, and in some instances prosecuted, manufacturers of drugs and devices for paying what are alleged to be kickbacks in return for prescribing a product. These actions have significantly raised the political visibility of drug-industry marketing practices. As public concerns about pharmaceutical prices have led politicians to look widely for culprits, marketing inducements have been an attractive target.

THE ROLE OF PHARMACISTS

The role of pharmacists used to be described fairly easily. They filled prescriptions. Sometimes they would dispense advice to patients along with medications and other times they would consult with a patient's physician. However, for the most part, they took a piece of paper with written advice and handed back a bottle containing a drug. Retail pharmacists worked in a corner drugstore and hospital-based pharmacists in an institutional pharmacy department.

The profession is changing. Corner drugstores are being replaced with national chains, and retail sales are moving toward mail-order delivery and Internet-based ordering. Some hospital pharmacists now do rounds in intensive care units. Others are helping to design systems to reduce medication errors.

The most fundamental change of all is the enhanced role of pharmacists in providing advice and counseling to patients, which many pharmacists and patients see as an increasingly important part of the profession.[33] Often, the pharmacist who fills the prescription is the only readily available source of information on side effects, drug interactions, and other crucial issues. Many states now require patients to certify that they have been provided with the chance to ask questions when obtaining a prescription. In hospital settings, pharmacists are often the only ones to check dosages and other aspects of drug orders for appropriateness and errors.

Pharmacists are also seeing their administrative role growing. With most privately insured patients covered by a pharmacy benefit plan, the majority of prescription sales are financed through PBMs. Pharmacists must verify coverage for each insured customer and sometimes serve as the liaison between patient and insurer when coverage is denied because of formulary restrictions or utilization review. Some pharmacists fear that they are becoming business agents as much as clinicians.

In a transformed profession, the old system of reimbursement may no longer be the most appropriate. With financial margins for selling drugs reduced by the group-purchasing power of PBMs and many sales diverted to mail order, pharmacy financial returns from filling prescriptions become shakier. At the same time, pharmacists are increasingly providing something more valuable than technical skill at dispensing; they are providing expert advice. Some pharmacists believe that they should be explicitly compensated for it.

The political battles over reimbursing pharmacists for "cognitive services" such as patient counseling within Medicare Part D are continuing. Who will pay them? Will patients pay out of pocket, will insurers provide reimbursement, or will compensation be included in the cost of drugs? Recognition of patient counseling as a reimbursable service could change the pharmacy profession completely. It could also place pharmacists in competition with other professionals, such as physicians and nurse practitioners, who serve similar roles. Further, it raises the related issue of whether, and to what extent, pharmacists should be permitted to prescribe medications on their own. The pharmacy profession has a tremendous amount at stake in defining its new role.

THE NEXT POLITICAL REALITY: GENETICS

If the political conflicts that we face today seem daunting, those we can expect to face in the years ahead will be formidable. Genomic medicine will transform the industry. We can only speculate about the political consequences of using genetics to design and manufacture drugs, but several concerns are increasingly evident.

Understanding the human genome will have far-reaching consequences throughout society. In pharmacy, gene therapy may permit physicians to alter our genetic makeup to cure defects that cause specific diseases. Genetics will also transform conventional pharmaceutical products. Clinicians will be able to predict with much greater accuracy which drugs will be most effective on which patients and which side effects will most likely occur. Drugs can then be tailored almost to the individual, to optimize therapeutic effectiveness and reduce adverse drug reactions.[34]

The problem, as with much else in medicine, is cost. With each drug customized to a small group of patients, the potential market for each product shrinks to the point where it may not be economically viable for a manufacturer to make it. Every drug almost becomes an orphan drug. Who will be able to afford the development and production costs for a product with such limited potential sales? Clearly, it will not be individual patients. Insurers may find it unfeasible as well. New financing mechanisms will be needed.

The other great challenge posed by genomic medicine will be the protection of intellectual property rights. Who owns the rights to use our genes? Is it the researchers who discover the genes and their uses, the manufacturers that design and develop products that put them to use, or the people who carry them around in all of their cells? Some argue that patent rights are as essential to encourage research and development using genetics as they are for conventional pharmaceutical products. Others are concerned about the consequences of permitting ownership of the natural makeup of individuals. A small number of legal cases to date have forced courts to begin to grapple with these questions, but the most explosive issues are yet to be faced.[35] New concepts of intellectual property may evolve.

The genetics revolution in medicine is not a political reality yet. The full clinical promise still lies on the horizon; however, scientists are bringing us closer each day. Every player in American pharmacy will feel the effects.

LOOKING AHEAD

Within this landscape of familiar themes and emerging controversies, the political realities for pharmacy promise to remain contentious. Drug safety continues as a central focus, but economic concerns have added a significant new element and the looming prospect of genomic medicine has the potential to fundamentally change the entire industry. As we look ahead, a few trends stand out as most likely to shape political debates going forward.

The FDA was created in 1938 to aggressively protect drug consumers by intercepting dangerous products before they reach the market. Few people could evaluate the risks of the drugs that they take on their own. However, how far should the government go in telling us what we can and cannot do? At what point might scientific progress be impeded and valuable medicines denied to patients? The history of drug regulation in America is one of scandals leading to tighter controls, with a gradual loosening of restrictions in between, as the pendulum of regulatory fervor swings back and forth. Congress and the FDA will always struggle to find the best balance.

Debates over the proper role of government intervention also play out with regard to pharmaceutical costs. Although most foreign countries believe that explicit price controls are the answer, America relies on a less-regulated, more market-oriented approach. However, the application of market forces to pharmaceutical products is far from direct, with PBMs, insurance companies, government benefit programs, pharmacies, and FDA safety regulators all involved. The government cannot help but play some role in the market. The hard part that we will always face is defining exactly what it should be.

If government is to play a direct role in making drugs affordable for patients, what cost should it be willing to bear? Government spending on a Medicare prescription benefit is certain to increase utilization, as it did for hospital and physician services. Should we all share the cost through taxes or should the heaviest utilizers pay more? All social programs raise questions concerning the fairness of financing.

The cost issue has also forced us to examine the structure of intellectual property protection. Most agree that patent protection is essential to encourage research and innovation, but also that at some point products should enter the public domain to permit market competition. As debates over the Hatch-Waxman Act have revealed, achieving the balance is not easy. Similar issues are arising in other areas of technology as the Internet has changed the ability to reproduce copyrighted material. Defining ownership rights in ideas will always pose difficult challenges, especially in a field as technologically complex and rapidly changing as pharmacy.

Finally, there will always be conflicts between different players in the industry. Consumers want the best products for the best price. Insurers want to control costs and utilization. Pharmacists want to continue to play a key role in bringing pharmaceutical products to patients. Pharmaceutical manufacturers want to continue bringing products to market and realizing financial rewards for doing so.

Politics is the drama of competing interests as they vie with one another. With a range of players and interests, pharmacy and politics have long gone hand in hand. As pharmaceuticals become increasingly essential to our health and well-being, the drama for pharmacy is certain to stay highly visible and sensitive in the years to come.

NOTES

1. Hutt, P.B. and Merrill, R.A. *Food and Drug Law* (Westbury, NY: The Foundation Press, Inc., 1991), p.1.
2. Sinclair, U. *The Jungle,* Norton Critical Edition (New York: W.W. Norton and Company, 2002).
3. PL 59-384, 34 Stat. 768 (1906).
4. 21 U.S.C. §§301 et seq. (1938).
5. 76 Stat. 780 (1962).
6. Health Care Finance Administration. HCFA Study of the Pharmaceutical Benefit Management Industry. June 2001. Available online at <http://www.cms.hhs.gov/researchers/reports/2001/cms.pdf>.
7. U.S. Centers for Medicare and Medicaid Services. National Health Care Expenditures Projections: 2002-2012. <http://www.cms.hhs.gov/statistics/nhe/projections-2002/highlights.asp?>.
8. Kaiser Family Foundation, Fact Sheet 3057-03. Accessed via: <www.kff.org/rxdrugs/loader.cfm?url=/commonspot/security/getfile.cfm&PageID=48305?>.
9. Barry, P. Drugs and Money: Coverage Crisis Deepens. American Association of Retired Persons Bulletin Online. January 2002. Available online at <http://www.aarp.org/bulletin/>.
10. Kaiser Family Foundation. Medicaid spending: what factors contributed to the growth between 2000 and 2002. <http://www.kff.org/medicaid/upload/22135_1.pdf>.
11. National Institute for Health Care Management. *Prescription Drug Expenditures in 2000.*
12. Kaiser Family Foundation. Medicare: the prescription drug benefit. Fact Sheet 7044-02, March, 2005. Available online at <http://www.kff.org/medicare/loader.cfm?url=/commonspot/security/getfile.cfm&PageID=33325>.
13. Centers for Medicare and Medicaid Services. Health Care Industry Update: Pharmaceuticals. January 10, 2003. Available online at <http://www.cms.hhs.gov/reports/hcimu/hcimu_01102003.pdf>.
14. Kaiser Family Foundation. The Medicare Program: Medicare and Prescription Drugs, May 2001. Available online at <http://www.kff.org/medicare/rxdrug debate.cfm>.
15. Pharmaceutical Research and Manufacturers of America. Pharmaceutical Industry Profile 2002. Available online at <http://www.phrma.org/publications/publications/profile02/index.cfm>.
16. Ibid, p. 20.

17. Lichtenberg, F.R. Sources of the U.S. Longevity Increase, 1960-1997. National Bureau of Economic Research Working Paper No.w8755, January 2002. Available online at <www.nber.org/papers/w8755>.

18. 21 U.S.C. §§101 et seq. (1992).

19. United States General Accounting Office. *Food and Drug Administration: Effect of User Fees on Drug Approval Times, Withdrawals, and Other Agency Activities.* Report No. GAO-02-958, September 2002. Available online at <www.gao.gov>.

20. Kissick, W. *Medicine's Dilemmas* (New Haven, CT: Yale University Press, 1994).

21. Pub. L. No. 98-417, 1984 Stat. 1538 (codified as amended in scattered sections of 21 and 35 U.S.C.) (1984).

22. Kaiser Commission on Medicaid and the Uninsured. Policy Brief: Medicaid: Purchasing Prescription Drugs. January 2002. Available online at <http://www.kff.org/medicaid/4025=index.cfm>.

23. PL 106-387, §1(a), 114 Stat. 1549 (2000).

24. Harris, G. Drug Firms' "Bad" Year Wasn't So Bad. *The Wall Street Journal,* February 21, 2003, p. B4.

25. Food and Drug Administration, Center for Drug Evaluation and Research. Draft Guidance for Industry and Consumer-Directed Broadcast Advertisements. July 1997. Announced in *Federal Register* (August 12, 1997) 62(155): 43171-43173.

26. Competitive Media Reporting, Strategy Report, and IMS Health, National Prescription Audit Plus, cited in Centers for Medicare & Medicaid Services, Health Care Industry Update: Pharmaceuticals, p. 31.

27. Rosenthal, M.D. Promotion of Prescription Drugs to Consumers. *New England Journal of Medicine* (February 14, 2003) 346(7): 498-505.

28. Over-the-counter status for Claritin considered to treat hives. Available online at <http://archives.cnn.com/2002/HEALTH/conditions/04/22/fda.claritin/>.

29. Congressional Budget Office. Issues in Designing a Prescription Drug Benefit for Medicare, October 2002. Available online at <http://www.cbo.gov/showdoc.cfm?index=3960&sequence=1&from=0>.

30. Pharmaceutical Research and Manufacturers of America. *Principles on Conduct of Clinical Trials and Communication of Clinical Trial Results.* Updated 2004. Available online at <http://www.clinicalstudyresults.org/primers/2004-06-30%201035.pdf>.

31. Kassirer, J.P. and Angell, M. Financial Conflicts of Interest in Biomedical Research. *New England Journal of Medicine* (August 19, 2003) 329(6): 570-571.

32. Pharmaceutical Online. Detailing ROI is falling, but sales forces keep growing. July 18, 2001. <http://www.pharmaceuticalonline.com/content/news/article.asp?docid={0f83ec0d-7aed-11d5-a772-00d0b7694f32}>.

33. See Amsler, M.R., Murray, M.D., Tierney, W.M., et al. Pharmaceutical Care in Chain Pharmacies: Beliefs and Attitudes of Pharmacists and Patients. *Journal of the American Pharmaceutical Association* (2001) 41(6): 850-855.

34. Weinshilboum, R. Inheritance and Drug Response. *New England Journal of Medicine* (2003) 348(6): 529-537.

35. One of the few cases to address issues related to intellectual property rights in genetic information is *Moore v. Regents of the University of California* (51 Cal.3d 120, 271 Cal.Rptr.146, 793 P.2d479 [Cal. 1990]), which dealt with ownership rights to a therapeutic product derived from tissue from a patient's body that was obtained after a medical procedure.

Chapter 9

Hospital and Health Care Institutions

Charles E. Daniels

INTRODUCTION

The concept of a hospital or house of healing is an ancient idea. The modern concept of a hospital is much newer, with changes that have accompanied over two hundred years of advances in science. Since the middle of the twentieth century the hospital has seen radical changes. It has changed from the location where poor people went to die to the high-tech setting that we know today. The changes in technology and chances for cure over that time are matched by the complexity of organization and ownership that is seen in the modern health care setting. The typical hospital of the early 1900s was a large inner-city institution run by a religious charity or the city or county. Another hospital snapshot of that time showed the "sanitarium" concept, where chronic disease patients went for long-term treatment of mental illness or infectious disease. In either case the focus was on supportive care, as there were only a few tested surgical procedures or medications to treat diseases.

The Hill-Burton Act[1] (1946) changed the face of the hospital industry by providing federal government funds to build new hospitals. The initial intent was to address underserved areas, and the acceptance of funding through this program required that the hospital also agree to provide service to those unable to pay, as well as irrespective of race, color, national origin, creed, or related characteristics. The focus of the act was to bolster the nonfederal hospital sector. Under the funding support of the act the number of nonfederal, short-term general and specialty hospitals grew to a peak of 5,814 in 1984.[2] The increased number and broader geographic distribution of hospitals throughout the 1940s, 1950s, and 1960s made the use of hospitals more functional for most physicians and patients (Figure 9.1). Over nearly thirty years new hospitals and extended care facilities were built, in part from Hill-Burton funds. In addition, these funds paid for modernization of many older facilities. The lack of modern hospital beds that sparked

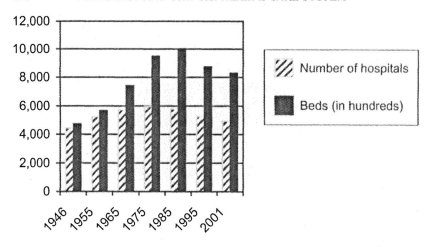

FIGURE 9.1. Number of Hospitals and Staffed Beds by Year

the original enactment was replaced with a different situation in many hospitals: more inpatient beds than were necessary.

Hospitals became more of a community resource following the Hill-Burton–related growth; there were also radical changes in diagnostic and treatment technologies that presented the prospect of cure or functional control for many illnesses. Infectious diseases from simple bacterial infections were no longer likely to end in death. The availability of safe and effective agents for many chronic diseases made it likely that patients with diabetes, hypertension, and many other conditions would live long and productive lives if treated properly. Specific and less-toxic antipsychotic agents allowed patients who had been committed to state mental hospitals for life to become functional members of society. In this context, the U.S. institutional health care environment of today is a significantly different place than just a generation ago.

Hill-Burton progress in hospital growth addressed one aspect of the problem of access to health care. It also spotlighted another problem, the shortage and maldistribution of trained health care providers, physicians, nurses, pharmacists, and several others. Federal funding to expand training programs for these health care workers in the 1970s resulted in rapid growth of physicians but has not yet addressed the uneven geographical distribution of providers. Another aspect of this distribution problem is the concentration of specialty-trained physicians in some major metropolitan regions and a lack of such providers in rural centers.

In the 1980s a different issue took center stage for the hospital and health care institution: the soaring costs of health care. The availability of hospital rooms, trained providers, and new diagnostic and therapeutic options led to the growing realization that sustained growth of health care costs were consuming an unacceptable portion of the national economy at the expense of other important sectors. Because most medical expenses are funded by the federal and state governments or employers through health care benefits, pressure grew from all three of these sources to curb the growth in total hospital cost. This pressure led to rounds of significant cost-cutting efforts within organizations that took the form of downsizing some programs and elimination of some unprofitable services. This also set the stage for consolidation and merger of health care organizations. Application of classic and creative business concepts resulted in the next major change in the environment of the health care institution.

SCOPE OF THE U.S. HEALTH CARE INSTITUTION

The hospital stands as the most physically distinguishable element of the U.S. health care system, but health care in the United States is provided in a variety of locations, not just hospitals. The traditional inpatient hospital setting is one part of a complex web of providers and locations that are interlinked to provide preventive and ill-care services. This includes long-term skilled nursing facilities, large and small office-based medical practices, ambulatory surgical centers, chiropractors, outpatient diagnostic laboratory and imaging facilities, the clinic or community pharmacy, and many others (see Figure 9.2). The complexity of this web of providers has influenced patients' access to service, cost of care, and quality of care in both positive and negative directions. Data from the Medical Expenditure Panel Survey showed that 36 percent of the direct spending in health care went for inpatient care. Table 9.1 shows the distribution of the $596 billion spent on health care in 1999.[3] Inpatient expenditure is the single greatest expense.

In order to address access to service, cost of care, and quality of care, hospitals or related organizations have tried to integrate several components of the system in different ways over the past twenty years. The hypothesis is that the segmentation of the health care industry makes it difficult to manage toward improved performance on those three dimensions. Integration of providers has meant that hospitals are often not simply the traditional stand-alone organizations that were the hallmark of bygone years. More frequently, the hospital is owned by a larger organization that owns clinics, laboratories, community or mobile imaging facilities, home infusion services, and perhaps one or more outpatient pharmacies. The same three driv-

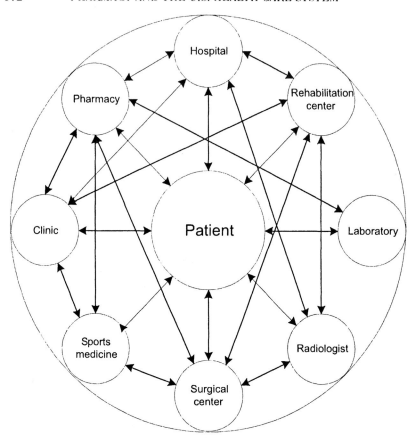

FIGURE 9.2. Relationship Between Various Elements in the Health Care System (Patient interacts with several elements of the system, each of which interacts dependently with other relevant providers.)

ers, with emphasis on costs, have changed the nature of hospital ownership. The reorganizations of the 1980s and 1990s have resulted in the consolidation of the hospital industry and near extinction of the independent, free-standing, single-facility hospital. Few hospitals are able to survive without the value and resources available under the mantle of multihospital systems. The economies of scale, which come from partnerships with other hospitals, make it advantageous to collaborate through joint ownership or other formal affiliations to share information technologies, administrative support services such as human resources, purchasing, billing, and some-

TABLE 9.1. Direct Expenditures for Health Care in 1999 (MEPS)

Expense category	Percent of expenses
Ambulatory	31.2
Dental	8.8
Home health	5.3
Prescribed medicines	15.8
Inpatient care	36.1
Other	2.8

Note: Total ≠ $596 billion

times even clinical services such as radiology and pharmacy. The hospital industry has historically been owned by "not-for-profit" corporations, which are incorporated with the mission to provide a public benefit. The evolutionary changes in the industry and application of business to health care have created opportunities for "for-profit" corporations to thrive in large and small niches.

TYPES OF HOSPITALS

Since hospitals and their related health care organizations take on such a wide variety of roles in the medical care of Americans, it is useful to think about them based upon several different dimensions: size, mission, ownership, or several other characteristics. The American Hospital Association (AHA) is a nongovernmental agency that represents and registers hospitals. It maintains comprehensive information on the characteristics, operations, and ownership of hospitals and health care organizations in the United States. This information is published in *Hospital Statistics* and the *AHA Guide.*[4]

The AHA may register an organization if it is accredited by the Joint Commission on Accreditation of Healthcare Organizations (JCAHO) or is certified under federal regulations as a provider of acute care by the Centers for Medicare & Medicaid Services (CMS) under Title 18. Alternatively, an organization may be registered if it is licensed as a hospital by the state government and meets specific requirements listed in the *AHA Guide* (see Appendix A). Osteopathic hospitals, which meet the other criteria, are also registered within the AHA database.

The AHA statistics provide valuable information for health care providers, planners, and researchers. Organizations are classified using different characteristics. These characteristics include type of ownership, size, location, and types of services provided. The most frequently used classification is by service. Hospitals are classified by service type, such as general hospitals, specialty hospitals, psychiatric hospitals, rehabilitation hospitals, chronic disease hospitals, and teaching hospitals. Based upon December 2003 data, there were 5,794 AHA-registered hospitals in the United States, with 975,962 staffed beds.[5] The majority of these hospitals (84 percent) are considered to be community hospitals within the AHA definition. Community hospitals are the dominant provider of hospital care, accounting for 95 percent of all hospital admissions. The community hospital is defined by AHA as a nonfederal, short-term general, or other specialty hospital. Specialty hospitals include obstetrics and gynecology; eye, ear, nose, and throat; rehabilitation; orthopedic; and other individually described specialty services. Academic medical centers are included on the list of community hospitals if they meet the other criteria (e.g., nonfederal short term). Hospitals that are not accessible to the general public, such as college infirmaries or prison hospitals, are not included.

HOSPITAL ORGANIZATION AND SERVICES

Every hospital has an organization and governance structure to support its mission. Governance of the hospital is intended to assure that the organization accomplishes what it intends to do. The JCAHO accreditation manual's section on leadership includes a standard on governance.[6] This standard requires that the hospital clearly define how it is governed and the lines of authority for key planning, management, and operations activities. It also requires the hospital to identify who is responsible for the governance of the organization and how the medical staff will participate. Importantly, JCAHO expects the governing structure to annually evaluate its performance related to the vision, mission, and goals of the hospital.

In health care organizations there are many variations on the organizational structure, but most begin at the prototype structure shown in Figure 9.3. This represents a high-level picture of the organization. The first critical element is the existence of a board of directors or a board of governors who are responsible for the overall performance of the organization. The members of the board are often a mix of members from the health care community, local business leaders, community representatives, and other key stakeholders in the success of the enterprise. The board of directors is expected to be aware of and sensitive to the external environment and community expectations along with the mission and owner long-term objectives. The second critical element is a group of physicians, dentists, or other inde-

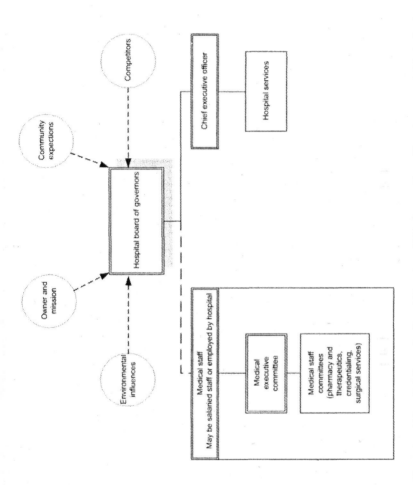

FIGURE 9.3. Macrolevel Hospital Organizational Structure (Chief executive officer is accountable to the board for operational and financial issues.)

pendent health care providers who serve as the medical staff and admit patients to the hospital and other services. They are responsible for several elements of oversight and direction of the organization and typically are represented on the board of directors. The third critical element of the hospital organization is a chief executive officer, or CEO. The CEO is typically hired by the board to direct the entire operation, including patient care services, financial operations, and all other functions of the corporation. The CEO is responsible for the translation of expectations of the board of directors and medical staff into a functional and financially sound organization.

From within the operational-level view of the hospital organization, the office of the CEO is at the top. The CEO maintains the authority and responsibility to run the day-to-day and month-to-month operations of the hospital. This is typically done through distribution of responsibilities to one or more senior managers, often called vice presidents or associate directors. In some large hospital organizations a chief operating officer (COO) may be in place to manage daily operations and allow the CEO to spend more time on strategic or long-term issues. Figure 9.4 shows the typical hospital organizational structure from an operations-level perspective. It is typical to have senior managers in positions of the chief financial officer and chief information officer, plus senior managers with similar titles for patient care services (including nursing and other clinically focused departments); hospital operations (including nutrition, housekeeping, maintenance, etc.); and a division to manage public relations, volunteer services, and so on. The actual distribution of service departments will vary from hospital to hospital, but this example provides a picture of how it might be organized in a medium-sized organization. The chief medical officer (CMO), also frequently called the chief of staff, may have a staff/consultant relationship with the CEO or may be a line manager with responsibility for some of the functional programs, such as safety or quality assurance. In most cases, the CMO is the liaison to the medical staff and deals with a wide range of medical staff and patient care issues such as physician competency and credentialing. As hospitals have begun to address the quality of clinical practices and have engaged the medical staff, the CMO role has become more important than in prior years.

The pharmacy director often reports to a senior hospital manager at the vice president or associate director level. Pharmacists, technicians, and other support staff usually report to one of the pharmacy managers or to the director of pharmacy. Figure 9.5 is a sample of the organizational structure at the hospital pharmacy level.

The scope of services provided by each hospital is selected to allow them to accomplish their mission. They are developed to meet the unique combi-

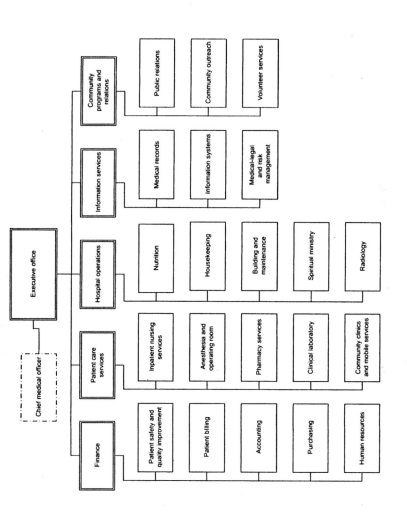

FIGURE 9.4. Example Hospital Organization of Services (Larger hospitals may have more levels of management and greater diversification.)

177

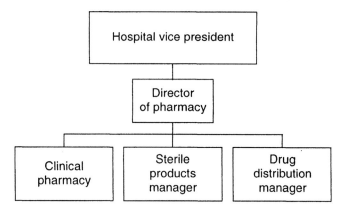

FIGURE 9.5. Example Hospital Pharmacy Service Organization

nation of needs of the patient population served by the organization. Specific services to be provided by the hospital are partially determined by the requirements of the various accrediting agencies, but how they are provided is influenced by the mission, operational needs, and medical staff composition. For instance, a county hospital with a focus on the underserved, low-income population may provide a different menu of services than a for-profit hospital in a wealthy suburban setting.

HEALTH CARE STAFFING

Safe and effective operation of a hospital or any health care facility depends on many people to work as a team. Some of the key players of the hospital team are physicians and other independent licensed health care providers, nurses, and pharmacists. A brief description of the special role of each follows.

Medical Staff

The organization's medical staff may include physicians (including osteopathic physicians), dentists, podiatrists, and several other categories of licensed independent practitioners. The physician members of the medical staff may include generalists, surgeons, radiologists, pathologists, and several other categories of licensed physicians. The medical staff may be a limited or closed staff, such as physicians at a military hospital, or an open staff, which allows community physicians to apply for privileges to admit patients and provide care. In most community hospitals the physicians who practice medicine are not employed by the hospital but by a physician practice group or are in independent practice. Although this is the long-standing model, it has made some aspects of patient care subject to discontinuity. It also makes it more complicated to create and implement standards of care throughout the hospital. Recent trends in hospital personnel planning have included hiring more dedicated hospital physicians on a salaried basis to assure quality care in such areas as the intensive care units (intensivists) or for general hospital care (hospitalists). The intent is to enhance the consistency and quality of care.

Nurse practitioners, physician assistants, and some other groups (e.g., acupuncturists) are considered to be independent licensed practitioners. The rules governing the rights of these groups are usually determined on a state-by-state basis, with more latitude in some places than others. Although their scope of practice is typically more limited by law than the physician, they have made significant impact in the health care organization and often have rights to write medical orders within the limits of the law in that state. Nurse practitioners and physician assistants are routinely employed in hospital emergency rooms and ambulatory clinics.

Nurses

Nurses are the backbone of clinical care in most hospitals. They provide and coordinate care on the minute-by-minute basis for hospitalized patients. In the ambulatory setting, they have a similarly important function. Typically, there are more nurses employed by hospitals than any other category of employee, usually by a wide margin. Nursing shortages or nursing strikes can quickly reduce the function of an organization. New hospital wings have been completed but not opened due to the lack of trained nurses.

Nurses in hospitals and health care organizations have a wide variety of training and educational backgrounds, from vocational school to nursing diploma to college degree. State laws also govern what functions can be done by licensed personnel versus unlicensed. In an effort to assure quality care, some states have passed, or attempted to pass, laws which govern the minimum nurse-to-patient ratio. In many hospitals, key administrative positions are held by nurses as a result of their detailed understanding of the workings of the organization.

Pharmacist

The hospital pharmacist is a critical player in the health care team. Over the past several years, hospitals have increased the presence of the pharmacist in the patient care areas. This follows literature purporting that pharmacists can reduce prescribing errors and costs when they are actively involved in patient care beyond traditional dispensing activities. Pharmacists are expected to review all medication orders, solve problems, and supervise medication distribution activities. The American Society of Health-System Pharmacists maintains minimum standards for pharmacy services, which in conjunction with accreditation and government regulations provide the pharmacist with a framework for services to be provided.

HOSPITAL OWNERSHIP

It seems unusual to the novice to consider who owns the hospital. In the most general sense, hospitals seem to be a community resource to relieve pain and suffering and prolong life. Although it is true that it is a community resource, each hospital has a formal ownership structure, which determines many things, most critically its vision, mission, and medical focus. Hospitals founded by religious or faith-based organizations were the most traditional early purveyors of hospital care, and therefore have become the legal owners of many hospitals in operation today. Local, county, or state governments are also major hospital owners. More recently "for-profit" corporations have become leading investors and owners in the hospital industry. These corporations typically have stockholders who have invested in anticipation of a dividend or return on the investment. Table 9.2 provides more detail on the ownership characteristics of the spectrum of hospitals on the U.S. health care landscape. Not-for-profit community hospitals continue to dominate the hospital industry based upon their number. Table 9.3 looks more specifically at community hospital ownership by category. The federal government, primarily through the U.S. armed forces and the Veterans Administration, also owns 240 hospitals that serve the focused needs of their patient populations.

Not-for-Profit Hospitals

Not-for-profit hospitals are incorporated as charitable organizations and have protected ownership and tax advantages. They include hospitals founded or built with funds from philanthropic or religious organizations. These hospitals are by far the most common types in the U.S. hospital industry. Many of these hospitals are now part of organized systems that provide care to their target population. A system is defined by AHA as either a multihospital or diversified single-hospital system. When two or more hospitals are owned, leased, sponsored, or contract-managed by a central organiza-

TABLE 9.2. Ownership of Hospitals in the United States

Type of hospital	Owners	Examples
Not-for-profit (voluntary)	Religious affiliation	
	Independent	
	Other organizations	Corporate (e.g., oil companies, lumber companies)
		Shriners, etc.
		Managed care organizations
Investor-owned (for-profit)	Proprietorship	
	Partnership	
	Corporation	
Government	Local	City
		County
	State	University hospital
		Psychiatric
		Prison
		Chronic disease
	Federal	Department of Defense (Army, Navy, etc.)
		Veterans Administration
		Department of Health and Human Services
		Department of Justice (federal prisons)

Source: Adapted from Wilson, F.S. and Neuhauser, D. *Health Services in the United States* (Cambridge, MA: Blalinger Publishing Co., 1985).

TABLE 9.3. Ownership of Community Hospitals

Community hospital ownership	Number	Percentage
Not-for-profit (nongovernment)	3,025	61
Local, county, or state government	1,136	23
Investor owned (for-profit)	766	16
Total	4,927	100

tion, they are considered to be a multihospital system. Single freestanding hospitals that include several owned or leased nonhospital programs, such as clinics, urgent care centers, and soon, are also considered to be hospital systems.

Investor-Owned Hospitals

Although not-for-profit hospitals have been the most dominant ownership group, investor owned, for-profit hospitals have existed for a long time. Individual physicians or small groups of physicians have opened their own hospitals to assure that they would have conveniently located, high-quality facilities in which to treat their private patients. Larger corporate hospital organizations have come to dominate the for-profit segment of the hospital industry. For-profit hospital corporations often own several dozen hospitals and manage them from regional headquarters. The principles of economy of scale and shared resources provide a strong base to provide a similar-quality product at the lowest cost possible. Several attempts have been made to compare the quality of care and costs between not-for-profit and for-profit hospitals, but the published evidence is conflicting.[7] At least one study concluded that in areas where for-profit hospitals influence the competitive market they have driven down the expenditures of all hospitals in that region.[8] It is clear that investor-owned hospitals play an important role in the provision of hospital care and have leveraged their position so that they influence aspects of hospital care in all other segments of the industry.

Federal Hospitals

Federal hospitals are a numerically small element in the provision of care to the U.S. public (240 hospitals). However, the role and influence of that small group is important. Because they are present in most major U.S. cities in the form of Veterans Administration (VA) and military hospitals, they influence the hospital environment in several important ways. Army, Navy, and Air Force hospitals provide care to a large group of active and retired military personnel and dependents. VA hospitals and clinics provide care to a large number of former military. In 2004 there were 1,127 VA hospitals and related facilities in urban and rural settings all across the United States and in U.S. possessions.[9] These include several important teaching and research centers. To qualify for care in a VA hospital the patient must have service-related medical problems or be a wartime veteran without the ability to pay for care in a civilian facility.

Many federal hospitals are actively involved as training sites for post-graduate medical education (i.e., medical residencies). Many renowned medical and health professions schools rely on VA hospitals for primary training sites. It is noteworthy that the VA has led the way for other U.S. hospitals through its effort to improve patient safety through reduction in medal errors in hospitalized and ambulatory patients. They have led the nation as early adopters of automated prescribing and bar-coded patient identification before medication administration. They have also demonstrated options for developing a "culture of safety" as well as the value of disclosure to patients when medical errors have occurred. In addition to military and VA hospitals, the federal government also operates hospitals for special populations, including the American Indians, Alaska Natives, and federal prisoners.

Rural Hospitals

There were 2,261 rural community hospitals in 2003. This represents 44 · percent of all community hospitals. Rural hospitals have a different character than urban hospitals. They are smaller, with a median size of 58 beds compared to 186, and the populations they serve are older, making them more dependent on Medicare reimbursement.[10] Between 1990 and 1999, 186 rural hospitals closed. In 1999, 34 percent were operating with a negative financial margin. A larger proportion of care was moved to the ambulatory setting. These financial realities have led many rural hospitals to make difficult choices about what services to offer and what to close. For the small hospital, it may be necessary to close an emergency room or cardiology unit in order to minimize losses for those small-volume services. Another challenge in the rural setting is recruiting and retaining key physicians and trained health care providers such as registered nurses, radiology technicians, and pharmacists. To combat the challenges of providing service in the rural environment, many hospitals have joined with multihospital systems in an ownership or management arrangement. This has allowed many of them to gain some of the advantages and economies of larger urban hospitals. It has also allowed them to offer resources that would be difficult to install and maintain as independents. Shared access to such things as sophisticated mobile imaging and treatment facilities, as well as the ability to contract with subspecialized consultants who will come to the rural location on a regular schedule, are feasible for small hospitals in larger alliances. High-tech programs such as telemedicine also promise a future for quality medicine in the rural setting.

Specialty Hospitals

Specialty hospitals provide focused care for a particular portion of the population or a special disease state. Over 700 nonfederal specialty hospitals were in the United States in 2001. Many of these specialty hospitals are affiliated with and may share some facilities with general hospitals or other specialty hospitals. Pediatric hospitals are intended to provide specialized care for children and frequently neonates. Traditional hospital settings often are not well suited to provide care to children. Facilities and equipment needs differ for children and newborns. Consider the difference in furniture in a kindergarten classroom and a college classroom. This scale of variation exists in the hospital facilities, from beds and chairs to room decorations and recreation. It is also clear that the supportive resources for a pediatric environment are different, including social workers and teachers. Finally, the clinical expertise required for children is different. Pediatric anesthesiologists, nurses, neonatal ICU staff, pediatric pharmacist expertise, and medication use issues are different. Given this, it seems very appropriate to create specialty hospitals for this population.

For similar reasons, several other specialty hospitals have evolved, the most numerous of which are cancer centers, eye or ENT centers, rehabilitation hospitals, and behavioral-health specialty facilities (including alcohol and chemical dependency programs). Each of these specialty hospitals addresses the same spectrum of issues as other hospital types. Pharmacy services in these specialty hospitals are increasingly focused and involved in meeting the needs of the patients.

REGULATION

Because health care provides services that are not easily evaluated and assessed by the general public, it is difficult for the layperson to know the difference between a good and bad provider. For that reason, limits and rules are needed on the practice of health care. Hospitals and health care providers in general are quite heavily regulated in order to address this dilemma. Figure 9.6 is a representation of the regulatory environment in which the hospital operates. Some of these regulatory connections are more significant than others. The Centers for Medicare & Medicaid Services (CMS) provides reimbursement for federal health care patient care. In most hospitals, federal reimbursement is a significant component of revenue—in some health care organizations it accounts for over 50 percent—making CMS's regulations critical for most hospitals. Furthermore, because federal reimbursement regulations influence many other payers, their decisions on

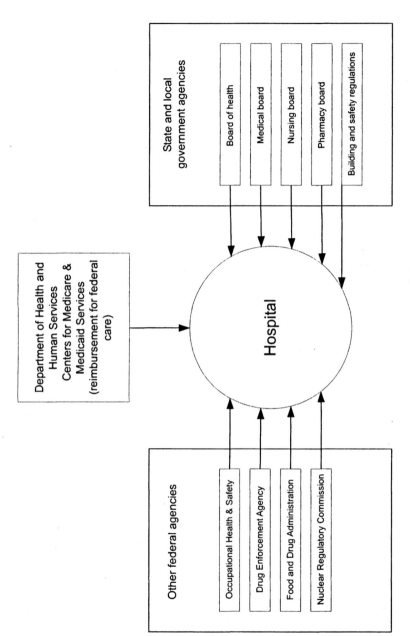

FIGURE 9.6. Regulatory Interfaces for U.S. Hospitals

185

what must be provided and how much they will pay strongly affects the financial well-being of the hospital. Regulations from federal, state, and local agencies impact facility design and construction; patient, staff, and property security; food handling requirements; waste management rules; drug-use activities; and many other aspects of daily operations in the health care organization.

Other regulations that influence health care organization operations also come from federal, state, county, and city agencies. These include health and safety rules, such as dealing with hazardous substances, and may also include clinical service requirements, such as required staffing ratios. State or regional facility planning regulations may also dictate what type of services must be offered or limit development of new programs that are resource intensive, in order to decrease duplication of existing programs.

ACCREDITATION

Most hospitals are accredited by the Joint Commission on Accreditation of Healthcare Organizations, commonly known as JCAHO (see Appendix B). Although this accreditation is voluntary, it is considered to be the standard method to demonstrate compliance with generally accepted principles for good care in the inpatient environment. JCAHO also accredits long-term and ambulatory care elements of the health care organization. In this field they compete with other organizations, such as the National Committee on Quality Assurance (NCQA), that are more commonly used to accredit services in the ambulatory and managed care environment.

JCAHO accredits health care organizations based upon the degree of compliance with a series of standards. As previously mentioned, leadership of the organization is one group of standards. There are also groups of standards that focus on ethics and patient rights, provision of care to patients, nursing care, medical staff expectations, medication management, and performance measurement. Obtaining accreditation from JCAHO or another agency does not guarantee that no harm can happen as a result of care, it simply provides a yardstick by which the organization is measured and compared with other similar facilities. There is still much work to be done in the concepts and measures of quality in health care.

It is the expectation of accreditation groups that pharmacy services will include preparation of dosage forms that are in unit-of-use and ready to administer. It is also expected that pharmacies will prepare IV admixture products in a controlled and sterile environment. Recent new JCAHO standards require that medication orders be reviewed by a pharmacist prior to administration of the medication. These expectations have partially guided the scope and content of hospital pharmacy services. Although there is still substantial diversity in how modern pharmaceutical services are provided, the role of the pharmacist in the health care organization has continued to take on substantially more prominence over the past thirty years.

FUTURE DIRECTIONS
AND CHALLENGES FACING HOSPITALS

The hospital and health care organization of the early twenty-first century faces many challenges to financial and patient care objectives. The AHA has identified six critical issues that will affect the future of hospitals and the statistics that support them.[11] The first of those challenges is payment shortfalls for Medicare and Medicaid. In the complex world of hospital reimbursement, it is not easy to determine the "real" costs associated with an episode of care. It is clear that many hospitals rely heavily on revenue generated from this patient group. A series of changes in Medicare and Medicaid reimbursement formulas has resulted in potential financial disasters for many hospitals. This will continue to be an important issue for all hospitals.

The next challenge is a shortage of trained workers. The shortage of nurses is well known, but similar shortages of imaging technicians, pharmacists, and laboratory technicians are also cited by AHA hospitals as impacting the provision of quality care.

Rising demand and limited capacity is the result of several things, including downsizing or closing hospitals in many multihospital systems. Reduced capacity comes in the face of an upswing in inpatient admissions and outpatient services in community hospitals (e.g., ambulatory surgery). Furthermore, hospital emergency departments are becoming busier in the face of staff shortages. Seventy-nine percent of urban hospitals were reported to be at or over capacity in 2002.[12]

Other challenges for the health care organization are increases in regulatory burdens, such as environmental and physical plant regulations, and documentation requirements (paperwork) for many activities that are not directly related to patient care. Hospitals are also challenged with rapidly growing costs. Increasing labor costs, increasing supply and medication costs, and increasing costs for equipment and technology make it difficult to meet all of the expectations of patients and payers. Hospital facilities are also growing older, which means that many facilities will need to be remodeled or replaced.

In spite of these challenges, the hospital system in the United States has shown a great resilience over the past fifty years as major changes in the environment have arisen. For that reason, it is safe to assume that the challenges faced over the next decade will be addressed with the same creativity and determination.

APPENDIX A: REQUIREMENTS FOR INCLUSION IN AHA GUIDE IF NOT JCAHO OR CMS CERTIFIED

Function: the primary function of the institution is to provide patient services, diagnostic and therapeutic, for particular or general medical conditions.

1. The institution shall maintain at least six inpatient beds, which shall be continuously available for the care of patients who are nonrelated and who stay on the average in excess of twenty-four hours per admission.
2. The institution shall be constructed, equipped, and maintained to ensure the health and safety of patients and to provide uncrowded, sanitary facilities for the treatment of patients.
3. There shall be an identifiable governing authority legally and morally responsible for the conduct of the hospital.
4. There shall be a chief executive to whom the governing authority delegates the continuous responsibility for the operation of the hospital in accordance with established policy.
5. There shall be an organized medical staff of fully licensed physicians that may include other licensed individuals permitted by law and by the hospital to provide patient care services independently in the hospital. The medical staff shall be accountable to the governing authority for maintaining proper standards of medical care, and it shall be governed by bylaws adopted by said staff and approved by the governing authority.
6. Each patient shall be admitted on the authority of a member of the medical staff who has been granted the privilege to admit patients to inpatient service in accordance with state law and criteria for standards of medical care established by the individual medical staff. Each patient's general medical condition is the responsibility of a qualified physician member of the medical staff. Where nonphysician members of the medical staff are granted privileges to admit patients, provision is made for prompt medical evaluation of these patients by a qualified physician. Any graduate of a foreign medical school who is permitted to assume responsibilities for patient care shall possess a valid license to practice medicine, or shall

be certified by the Educational Commission for Foreign Medical Graduates, or shall have qualified for and successfully completed an academic year of supervised clinical training under the direction of a medical school approved by the Liaison Committee on Medical Education.

7. Registered nurse supervision and other nursing services are continuous.
8. A current and complete medical record shall be maintained by the institution for each patient and shall be available for reference.
9. Pharmacy service shall be maintained in the institution and shall be supervised by a registered pharmacist.
10. The institution shall provide patients with food service that meets their nutritional and therapeutic requirements; special diets shall also be available.

APPENDIX B: JOINT COMMISSION ON ACCREDITATION OF HEALTHCARE ORGANIZATIONS

The mission of JCAHO is to continuously improve the safety and quality of care provided to the public through the provision of health care accreditation and related services that support performance improvement in health care organizations

JCAHO evaluates and accredits more than 15,000 health care organizations and programs in the United States. Since 1951, JCAHO has developed standards and evaluated the compliance of health care organizations against these benchmarks.

JCAHO's evaluation and accreditation services are provided for the following types of organizations:

• General, psychiatric, children's, and rehabilitation hospitals
• Health care networks, including managed care plans, preferred provider organizations, integrated delivery networks, and managed behavioral health care organizations
• Home care organizations, including those that provide home health services, personal care and support services, home infusion and other pharmacy services, durable medical equipment services, and hospice services
• Nursing homes and other long-term care facilities, including subacute care programs, dementia special care programs, and long-term care pharmacies

- Assisted-living facilities that provide or coordinate personal services, twenty-four-hour supervision and assistance (scheduled and unscheduled), activities, and health-related services
- Behavioral health care organizations, including those that provide mental health and addiction services and services to persons with developmental disabilities of various ages, in various organized service settings
- Ambulatory care providers, for example, outpatient surgery facilities, rehabilitation centers, infusion centers, group practices, and office-based surgery
- Clinical laboratories, including independent or freestanding laboratories, blood transfusion and donor centers, and public health laboratories

JCAHO is an independent, not-for-profit organization. It is governed by a board of commissioners that includes nurses, physicians, consumers, medical directors, administrators, providers, employers, a labor representative, health plan leaders, quality experts, ethicists, a health insurance administrator, and educators. Its corporate members are the American College of Physicians, the American College of Surgeons, the American Dental Association, the American Hospital Association, and the American Medical Association.[13]

NOTES

1. PL 79-725, Hospital Survey and Construction Act (1946).
2. American Hospital Association. *Hospital Statistics* (Chicago, IL: Health Forum, 2003).
3. Olin, G.L. and Machlin, S.R. *Chartbook #11: Health Care Expenses in the Community Population, 1999.* (Rockville, MD: Agency for Healthcare Research and Quality, 2003). Available online at <http://www.meps.ahrq.gov/Papers/CB11_03-0038/CB11.htm>.
4. American Hospital Association. *AHA Guide* (Chicago, IL: American Hospital Association, 2003); American Hospital Association. *Hospital Statistics.*
5. American Hospital Association. *AHA Resource Center Fast Facts on U.S. Hospitals* (Chicago, IL: American Hospital Association, 2003).
6. JCAHO. *Comprehensive Accreditation Manual for Hospitals* (Oakbrook Terrace, IL: Joint Commission on Accreditation of Healthcare Organizations, 2004). P LD-7.
7. Sloan, F.A., Trogdon, J.G., Curtis, L.H., and Schulman, K.A. Does the ownership of the admitting hospital make a difference? Outcomes and process of care of Medicare beneficiaries admitted with acute myocardial infarction. *Med Care* (2003) 41(10): 1193-1205; Devereaus, P.J., Schunemann, H.J., Ravindran, N., et al. Com-

parison of mortality between private for-profit and private not-for-profit hemodialysis centers: A systematic review and meta-analysis. *JAMA* (2002) 288: 2449-2457.

8. Kessler, D.P. and McClellan, M.B. The effects of hospital ownership on medical productivity. *Rand J Econ* (2002) 33: 488-506.

9. Department of Veterans Affairs. *Department of Veterans Affairs Facility Directory* (Washington, DC: Department of Veterans Affairs, 2004). Available online at <http://www1.va.gov/directory/guide/home.asp?isFlash=1>.

10. The Lewin Group/American Hospital Association. *TrendWatch: Challenges Facing Rural Hospitals* (report) (Chicago, IL: American Hospital Association, 2002).

11. Steinberg, C. *Overview of the United States Health Care System.* (Chicago, IL: American Hospital Association, 2005 <http://www.aha.org/aha/Nhcp/content/overview.ppt>.

12. The Lewin Group Analysis of AHAED and Hospital Capacity Survey, 2002.

13. JCAHO. About us. 2004. Available online at <http://www.jcaho.org/about+us/index.htm>.

Chapter 10

Pharmacist Involvement
in Long-Term Care for Seniors

Tanya C. Knight-Klimas
Richard G. Stefanacci

The number of elderly persons in the industrialized world and in the
United States is growing at such an unprecedented rate that several phrases
used to describe this population explosion have been coined, including the
"aging of America" and the "graying of America." This increase in the
number of elderly has and will continue to drive important changes in the
health care delivery and payment systems in the United States. This chapter
describes the growth of the elderly population, the utilization of health care
by elders, and the role of the clinical pharmacist in caring for seniors in
various health care settings.

DEMOGRAPHICS OF THE ELDERLY POPULATION

Since the very first census of the United States population was conducted
in 1790, data on senior demographics has been available. However, it was
not until 1870 that data on the senior population was first published.[1] Since
this first report we have been able to track an increased life expectancy,
which has changed the very nature of the elderly population, and the most
significant effects will soon be upon us.

Since 1900, the number of elderly persons (arbitrarily defined as those
sixty-five years and older) has increased by tenfold, and since 1960 the
number of elders in the United States has grown at a faster rate than any
other segment of the population.[2-4] In 1960, the elderly comprised approximately 9.1 percent of the U.S. population, today the elderly comprise approximately 12.4 percent of the population, and by the year 2030 it is estimated that 20 percent of the nation will be elderly.[5] See Figure 10.1.

Because women have a longer life expectancy than men, women out-
number men in the sixty-five-and-over population. Presently about 21 mil-

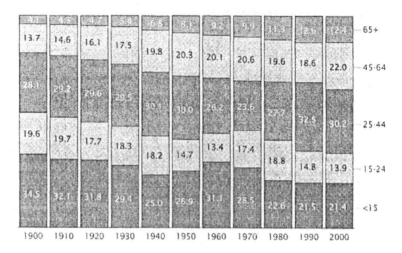

FIGURE 10.1. Percent Distribution of the Total Population by Age, 1900 to 2000 (*Source:* U.S. Census Bureau, decennial census of population, 1900 to 2000. Available online at <http://www.census.gov/prod/2002/pubs/censr-4.pdf>, p. 56.)

lion women and 14 million men are aged sixty-five and over, yielding a male-female ratio of 67. This means there are 67 males for every 100 females. This ratio steadily declines with age. In the sixty-five to seventy-four age range the male-female ratio is about 82, in the seventy-five to eighty-four age range the ratio is about 65, and in the over eighty-five age group the ratio is about 41.[6] Two additional findings are worthy to note. First is that diversity is less evident among the older population than among the younger population. The percentage of non-Hispanic white people increases with age. For example, 80 percent for those sixty-five to seventy-four years of age, 86 percent for those seventy-five to eighty-four, and 87 percent for those eighty-five and over are non-Hispanic whites. Second, the living arrangements and marital status of the older population differs considerably between men and women as they age. Men are more likely than women to be married and living with their spouses (74 versus 50 percent, respectively). Not surprisingly, as a result of these facts, the vast majority of our oldest seniors are widowed, non-Hispanic, white females living alone.[7]

The main reason for the increase in the elder segment of the population is a decrease in mortality rates. Figure 10.2 depicts the downward trend in the nation's mortality rate since 1900. Factors contributing to the decline include: improvements in sanitation and nutrition; medical advances such as the introduction of better diagnostic techniques and surgical procedures; the discovery of novel medications such as antibiotics and insulin and, more

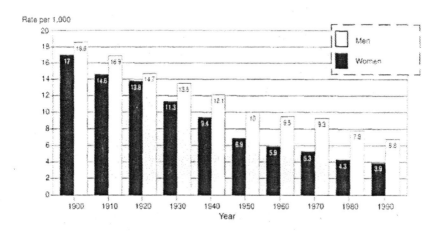

FIGURE 10.2. U.S. Death Rates by Gender from 1900 to 1990 (*Sources: National Center for Health Statistics: Vital Statistics of the United States, 1982, Volume II, Mortality, Part A, DHHS Pub. No. [PHS 86-1112]. Public Health Service, Washington, DC, U.S. Printing Office, 1985; U.S. Bureau of the Census, Historical Statistics of the United States, Colonial Times to 1970, Bicentennial Edition, Part 1, Washington, DC, 1975.*)

recently, the development and use of chronic medications that have been shown in clinical studies to measurably decrease mortality, such as beta-blockers, angiotensin-converting enzyme inhibitors, and 3-hydroxy 3-methyl glutaryl coenzyme reductase inhibitors; better management of acute and chronic disease states; preventive medicine; and other socioeconomic and environmental factors.[8-18] A growth spurt in the elderly cohort is expected between 2010 and 2030, when the first of the baby boomers will reach age sixty-five. The baby-boom generation is defined as the generation born between 1946 and 1962. In fact, 2000 Census data suggest that the most rapid increase in any age group was that of the 45 to 54 age bracket, due mainly to the start of the baby-boom generation.[19] By 2030, the total number of persons aged 65 and older will reach 70 million.[20] Meanwhile, as the elderly population grows by 75 percent during this period, the under-sixty-five population will increase by only 7 percent. The fastest-growing segment of the elderly population is and will continue to be the over-eighty-five population. Census data from 2000 suggest about 1.5 percent of the total national population is eighty-five years or older. By the year 2050, nearly one-fourth of all seniors will be over age eighty-five, and at least one in thirteen Americans will be eighty or older. The growth rates of those turning senior and those turning "old-old" (defined as those eighty-five years and older) have staggering implications on the delivery of health care because not only is the percent of senior persons growing, but the fastest-growing segment of seniors is the "old-old," or those who tend to suffer from more disease and disability and will therefore require more health care services.

DEMAND FOR HEALTH CARE SERVICES

This rapid expansion of seniors will have a profound impact on our health care system. For example, the incidence and cost of chronic conditions associated with long-term care such as hip fractures and Alzheimer's disease will increase dramatically. It is estimated that by the year 2040, 840,000 hip fractures will be treated at a cost of $6 billion, compared to a quarter of that cost in 1987. The number of patients with Alzheimer's disease is predicted to increase from 4 million to 10 million by 2040, with a cost of treatment near $150 billion annually.[21,22]

By 2030 it is expected that 14 million seniors will require some type of long-term care. Of those 14 million just over 5 million will reside in nursing homes while the remaining 9 million will receive alternative forms of long-term care.

The Pareto principle has been applied to describing the demand for health care services. This principle was first described in the seventeenth century by an Italian economist who noted that 80 percent of the land was owned by 20 percent of the population. It has been noted that similar applications apply to senior health services. In one report it was noted that about 10 percent of the older population incurs about 70 percent of all health care costs, which suggests that the minority consume the majority of resources.[23] The importance of this finding is that by being better able to identify high resource utilizers, one can potentially improve health-related outcomes and decrease cost.

One method of identifying those at high risk is a screening method developed at the University of Minnesota called the Probability of Repeated Admission (PRA), which is used to predict hospitalization. The PRA assigns a numerical value of 0 and 1 from the answers to questions. A score of 0.5 means that the individual has a 50 percent chance of being hospitalized multiple times in the following years. In addition to predicting hospital admission, the PRA tool has been shown to be effective in identifying chronic illness, risk of functional decline, nursing home use, doctor visits, and total cost of care.[24] When the items on the PRA tool were evaluated, the one question with the highest correlation to risk of utilization was, not surprisingly, "self-description of one's own health status." Those that described their health as poor held the highest likelihood of hospitalization within one year.

Pharmaceutical expenditures have also increased. This growth is arguably largely attributable to changes in utilization as opposed to changes in prices.[25] Increased utilization stems from an increase in demand secondary to a growing number of seniors with comorbidity and an increased availability of new and effective medications. This increase in drug use and drug cost will present several challenges in caring for the elderly.

SPECIAL CONSIDERATIONS IN THE PROVISION OF HEALTH CARE TO THE ELDERLY

Elder adults are the most heterogeneous segment of the population with respect to physical, social, and health status.[26] The rate at which an individual ages is variable; how well an individual ages is also variable and is dependent upon both genetic and environmental factors.[27] For instance, one seventy-year-old gentleman may be viewed as being a frail elder if he is suffering from chronic disease and disability, whereas another seventy-year-old gentleman may be viewed as having aged "successfully" if he has limited disease and disability.[28,29] Frailty refers to a loss of physiologic reserve that makes a person susceptible to disability from minor stresses,[30] whereas successful aging has been described as a process by which deleterious effects are minimized and function is preserved.[31] Therefore, chronological age is not as descriptive as physiological age when assessing the health status of an individual.

The elderly have the highest rate of acute illness, as well as chronic illness and disability.[32,33] The prevalence of chronic disease states increases with age; 80 percent of the elderly population having at least one chronic condition at any point in time.[34,35] Chronic conditions that lead to disability include heart disease, stroke, chronic obstructive pulmonary disease, diabetes, arthritis, osteoporosis, and visual and hearing impairments.[36]

The use of medications can often accomplish prevention, cure, or palliation of disease, but they can also cause adverse effects. Because the elderly are often afflicted with multiple chronic disease states, they use a disproportionate amount of medication, increasing their risk of adverse drug events.

Medication Usage in the Elderly

Older adults use approximately 33 percent of the nation's prescription and nonprescription medications, even though they comprise only about 13 percent of the U.S. population.[37] A newer statistic suggests the average senior uses 40 percent of all over-the-counter (OTC) medications sold in the United States.[38]

Data on drug use in the elderly varies with the age of the cohort studied and with the clinical setting studied. A survey of both institutionalized and ambulatory elderly conducted nearly two decades ago revealed that drug use was significantly higher in the former, with 9 percent taking ten or more drugs daily.[39] The average number of agents used increases with age, with an average of 4.4 drugs per day for those eighty years old and above. Recent data indicate that 91 to 94 percent of ambulatory adults age sixty-five and older use medications, 44 to 57 percent use five or more, and 12 percent use ten or more medications.[40] The type of medication most commonly used by the elderly also depends upon the setting. Studies examining community-dwelling elders found they use analgesics, diuretics, cardiovascular medications, and sedatives often, whereas nursing home residents use psychoactive medications most often, followed by diuretics, antihypertensives, analgesics, cardiovascular medications, and antibiotics.[41-43]

One investigation sought to examine the pharmacoepidemiology of prescription medication use in community-dwelling elderly living in rural Pennsylvania. The authors found that among more than 900 participants, over 71 percent reported taking at least one prescription medication. The "old-old" participants reported taking more cardiovascular agents, anticoagulants, vasodilating agents, potassium supplements and diuretics than the younger elderly cohort.[44]

Self-treatment with OTC medications is common, especially for chronic disease states whose prevalence increases with age, such as arthritis and constipation. The most frequently used OTC medications are analgesics, such as nonsteroidal anti-inflammatory drugs (NSAIDS), insulin, and gastrointestinal products such as laxatives. In addition to high utilization of prescription and OTC medications, use of dietary supplements is also increasing. Common dietary supplements include multivitamins, vitamin E, vitamin C, calcium, gingko, ginseng, garlic, saw palmetto, and St. John's wort.[45-48] Reasons listed for increasing popularity and utilization of dietary supplements include high prices of medications and patient dissatisfaction with conventional medications and treatment. [49.50]

One study that investigated the use of dietary supplements in older veterans found that 50 percent of respondents reported using one or more such products (vitamins, minerals, and herbals) within the past three months.[51] Given the large number of medications consumed by the elderly, their potential risk for adverse drug events may be significant.

Barriers to Health Care

Although the use of medication can benefit elders, the aged are presented with many barriers to health care, such that they are not able to take advantage of some of these available therapies. These barriers include lack of transportation; being too ill and immobile to seek treatment; misperception that certain symptoms and problems are normal with aging; perceived unresponsiveness by the medical system (inadequate parking, abbreviated encounters with clinicians, inconvenient office locations); depression; denial; isolation; and atypical presentation of illness leading to underrecognition and underreporting of disease.

Another significant barrier to health care is the lack of adequate health insurance. In 2000 it was estimated that the national *outpatient* retail prescription medication cost was approximately $131.9 billion, as reported by the National Institute for Health Care Management Research and Educational Foundation.[52] Compare this to data from 1991 in which a total of $36 billion was spent on both inpatient and outpatient prescription medications.[53] What is more is that a significant percent of prescription costs is paid out-of-pocket or through cost-sharing (deductibles, copayments, out-of-pocket expenses after expenditure caps are exceeded) so that a large burden is placed on the individual. One survey conducted in 1996 suggests that 51 percent of prescription costs were paid by the patient through out-of-pocket payment and cost sharing.[54] Elderly individuals with limited income and poor or no insurance are at the greatest risk of paying large out-of-pocket expenses. Moreover, these costs are likely to continue to increase as people are living longer and with more chronic conditions that require long-term prescription therapy.

Drug-Related Problems in the Aged

In addition to the aforementioned general barriers to health care, the elderly are also at risk of specific drug-related problems (DRPs). These can include withdrawal events, medication error, overdose, therapeutic failure, nonadherence, inappropriate medication use, drug interactions, and adverse drug events.[55,56] An adverse drug event (ADE) is an adverse event, expressed as a sign, symptom, or laboratory abnormality in which a drug is suspected and plausible.[57] The geriatric population is at a particularly high risk of developing ADEs for several reasons. In fact, in 1995 Dr. Gurwitz made a statement that is still true today. He stated, "any symptom in an elderly patient should be considered a drug side effect until proved otherwise."[58] The most consistently reported risk factor for ADEs in the literature is polypharmacy, and the risk of ADE increases exponentially as the number of medications increases.[59-63] Other associated or suspected risk factors for ADEs include comorbidity history of ADE; changes in pharmacokinetics (the way in which the body handles medication) and pharmacodynamics (the way in which a medication affects the body); nonadherence; and fragmented health care.[64-66] It is controversial whether age, in and of itself, is a risk factor for ADEs; though it probably is not.[67,68] The prevalence rates of ADEs in the community has been shown to range from 2.5 percent to as high as 50.6 percent, in long-term care 9.5 to 67.4 percent, and in the hospital setting 1.5 to 44 percent.[69-74] The cost of ADEs has also been studied. It is estimated that for every dollar spent on medication in a nursing facility, an additional $1.33 is spent treating DRPs, and in the ambulatory setting the cost of DRPs was approximated to be $76.6 billion.[75,76] Clearly, DRPs are common in the elderly and are costly to the health care system.[77] Fortunately, many ADEs are thought to be preventable. A study of hospitalized elderly showed that, compared to their younger counterparts, the elderly had a higher rate of preventable ADEs (5.3 percent versus 2.8 percent in their younger counterparts, p = 0.001). The authors suggest this was due to more complex medical issues in the elderly rather than to less aggressive or appropriate care.[78]

Medication Appropriateness

Because the elderly utilize a disproportionate percentage of medications and are at risk of developing a host of DRPs, several methods of assessing the appropriateness of a medication have been proposed. The Medication Appropriateness Index (MAI) is a valid and reliable tool used to implicitly determine medication appropriateness by taking into consideration specific patient characteristics.[79] Medication appropriateness can also be evaluated explicitly using the Beers criteria. The Beers criteria are a list of medications evaluated by Dr. Beers and colleagues who specialize in geriatric medicine and determined best to be avoided in the elderly.[80,81] Medication appropriateness in the elderly is a concept popular with the provision of pharmaceutical care.[82-89]

Recognizing the benefits and risks associated with medication therapy, the goal of pharmacotherapy is to promote successful aging by maintaining functional independence, preventing disability and iatrogenic disease, and increasing patients' health-related quality of life. As mentioned earlier, polypharmacy and changes in physiology, pharmacokinetics, and pharmacodynamics can potentially lead to the development of DRPs. The geriatric pharmacist is well positioned to optimize utilization and to decrease expenditures associated with pharmacotherapy. The role of the geriatric pharmacist in various geriatric health care settings will be discussed in the following sections.

LONG-TERM CARE

Long-term care is not synonymous with nursing home care. Long-term care encompasses a wide variety of care environments that can offer improved outcomes and utilize less resources than traditional nursing home care.[90] With an increased demand both from consumers and payers for higher quality at reduced costs we have and will continue to see a stimulated growth of long-term care facilities that are alternatives to nursing homes. In addition, although long-term care can be provided to patients of all ages, 70 percent of patients utilizing it are elderly.[91]

Long-term care is simply and most appropriately defined as care that is provided for an extended period of time. These services can be provided in a range of settings outside of the nursing home environment and are listed in Table 10.1.

The Spectrum of Long-Term Care

- Hospital-based nursing facility
- Subacute care
- Nursing facility
- Psychiatric hospital
- Intermediate care facility for the mentally retarded
- Community-based care
- Adult congregate living
- Adult day services
- Home health care
- Community mental health center
- Hospice
- Senior center
- Retirement housing
- Home care
- Independent community living[92,93]

TABLE 10.1. Long-Term Care Organizations

Type of facility	Number of facilities/agencies	Parties responsible for medication costs
Assisted living facilities (ALF)	11,500	Individuals
Licensed boarding homes	32,000	Individuals/Medicaid
Adult day care centers	10,000	Individuals/Medicaid
Home health care	6,880	Individuals/Medicaid
Nursing facilities (NF)	17,000	Individuals/Medicaid
Skilled nursing facilities (SNF)	14,815	The skilled nursing facility
Hospice	2,332	Individuals/Medicaid/ Medicare for hospice-related diagnosis only
Continuing care retirement communities (CCRC)	1,000	Individuals/Medicaid
Program for all-inclusive care for the elderly (PACE)	42	The PACE program

Sources: Simonson, W. Consultant Pharmacy Practice, Second Edition (Nutley, NJ: Hoffman LaRoche, 1995); Hawes, C., Rose, M., and Phillips, C. A National Study of Assisted Living for the Frail Elderly, Executive Summary: Results of a National Survey of Facilities (Beachwood, OH: Meyers Research Institute, 1999); Congressional Budget Office. Annual Report of the Board of Trustees of the Medicare Trust Funds, 2003; Krauus, N. et al. Nursing Home Update—1996: Characteristics of Nursing Facilities and Residents (Rockville, MD: Agency for Health Care Policy and Research, 1997). MEPS Highlights, Number 2, AHCPR Pub. No. 97-0036; Long Term Care Education.com, available online at <http://www.longtermcareeducation.com/A1/e.asp>; National PACE Association, available online at <http://www.npaonline.org>.

The Role of the Geriatric Pharmacist in Long-Term Care

Pharmacists who specialize in geriatrics are well positioned to provide clinical or consulting services to elderly patients in a variety of geriatric practice settings. Pharmacists can complete a postdoctoral residency or fellowship in geriatric pharmacy practice available through twelve institutions throughout the United States and can attain certification as certified geriatric pharmacists (CGP) through the American Society of Consultant Pharmacists (ASCP). Consultant pharmacy practice is a discipline within the profession of pharmacy that has its roots in the provision of pharmacy services to nursing homes—now referred to as nursing facilities (NFs)—and other long-term care (LTC) environments.[94] It is noteworthy that although the concept of consultant pharmacy originated less than four decades ago, today more than 10,000 consultant pharmacists provide a broad range of services.[95]

Pharmacists can consult in many practice settings, including nursing facilities (such as nursing homes, skilled nursing facilities, and intermediate care facilities), subacute care and assisted living facilities, psychiatric hospitals and intermediate care facilities for the mentally retarded, correctional facilities, adult day care, continuing care retirement communities, PACE programs (Program of All Inclusive Care for the Elderly), home care, and hospice.

NURSING FACILITIES

Nursing Facilities (NFs) typically describe a facility in which long-term care is provided to residents within that facility. State Medicaid programs predominantly pay for such long-term services. Data from the National Nursing Home Survey indicate that there are currently over 1.6 million nursing home residents.[96] Studies suggest medication use in NFs is significant and increasing. One such study revealed that individual nursing home residents received an average of 6.7 routine prescription medications per day and 2.7 additional medications on an as needed basis. The percentage of nursing home residents using nine or more prescription medications per day has continued to rise from 18 percent in 1997 to 27 percent in 2000.[97,98] The most common medications prescribed include gastrointestinal agents, analgesics, cardiovascular medications, vitamins and supplements, and psychoactive medications.[99] A recent survey of pharmacists showed that routine medication orders in nursing homes increased by 14 percent from 1997 to 2000. This trend is expected to continue both because of the increased acuity of residents and the increased availability of innovative medications to treat chronic conditions. As noted, the demographic trend is expected to significantly increase the demand for medications while the supply is also expected to see sizable increases. A recent survey conducted by the Pharmaceutical Research and Manufacturers of America indicated that there are 261 drugs in development to treat diseases of aging, as well as 122 medications for heart disease and stroke, plus an additional 402 medicines for cancer.[100]

The majority of NF services are paid by state Medicaid funds. In some cases residents that do not yet qualify financially for Medicaid use their own private funds until they "spend down" to meet the Medicaid requirement. Payment for pharmaceuticals is made separately from payment for residents' care in the NF. In all states, with the exception of New York, the risk for medications belongs to the state Medicaid program. New York is the first state to shift this risk to the facility in a similar manner as the federal government has shifted risk to skilled nursing facilities (SNFs), through Medicare. In New York, the majority of medications are lumped into the Medicaid daily rate for the NF. As a result, the NF provider is at risk for the medication costs. Medicaid typically reimburses institutional pharmacy providers based on the average wholesale price (AWP) minus a percentage plus a dispensing fee. As a result of this payment system, states (with the exception of New York) find that their NFs have no economic incentive to control drug utilization, and in fact pharmacy providers benefit when more medications are prescribed.

The majority of nursing home medications are provided by institutional pharmacy providers. At the present time over 80 percent of the U.S. nursing home beds are covered by institutional pharmacies.[101] The remainder is served by independent community pharmacies or retail chains. Federal and state laws require pharmacy providers of nursing facilities to maintain extended drug control and distribution systems that exceed the standards for pharmacies dispensing only to outpatients. The reason for a dominance in the use of institutional pharmacy providers is that expanded services are offered by these pharmacies to cover the special needs of NFs, including twenty-four-hour drug delivery, maintenance of medication profiles and drug inventory systems, repackaging of drugs from bulk supplies into unit doses, as well as maintenance of emergency kits.

Federal law requires all nursing homes to have a contract with a consultant pharmacist. The role of the consultant pharmacist is to be responsible for ensuring that resident drug use is safe and effective and that facilities are in compliance with federal and state regulatory requirements. A more detailed description of the role of the geriatric pharmacist in long-term care will be discussed in a subsequent section.

Skilled Nursing Facilities (SNF)

By definition, skilled nursing facilities provide twenty-four-hour skilled care for acute patients. Patients generally rely on assistance for most or all of their activities of daily living (ADLs). ADLs are commonly defined as activities such as bathing, dressing, and toileting. Skilled nursing facilities consist of both hospital-based and freestanding enterprises that provide skilled nursing care and rehabilitative services. Certification by Medicare is required to receive payment for the provision of these services. Approximately 75 percent of these facilities are freestanding or operate independently of an acute-care hospital, and nearly 50 percent of all facilities are owned or operated by nursing facility chains.[102] The majority of SNF services are paid by Medicare.

Payments to SNFs are made predominately through the Medicare program. Medicare pays for short-term, postacute care for up to 100 days per benefit period per calendar year for patients who meet certain criteria and maintain ongoing programs of rehabilitation. These services can begin only after a three-day acute hospitalization stay. In direct contrast to Medicaid, Medicare pays for medications and the SNF services in one aggregated bundle, placing the NF at risk for the medications. Using this approach the SNF may benefit when fewer medications are prescribed, shifting dollars from the SNF bottom line to the pharmacy provider.

A paradigm shift occurred on July 1, 1998, when skilled nursing facilities delivering Medicare-reimbursed postacute services began operating under a Prospective Payment System (PPS) using Resource Utilization Groups (RUGs) to calculate payments. This was a major shift for SNFs that had previously been paid on the basis of "average costs" and had not been responsible for medication costs. Under RUGs each resident falls into one of forty-four specified RUGs with a prospectively calculated reimbursement. One problem that exists with this payment system is that although nursing home operators are unable to directly oversee the prescribing of these medications, they are held accountable for pharmaceutical costs.[103]

Skilled nursing facility providers have responded to PPS in several ways. The Office of the Inspector General (OIG) has completed surveys demonstrating that SNFs

1. increase scrutiny of a patient's health status related to admission;
2. place renewed emphasis on utilization management once a patient has been admitted;
3. develop preferential admissions policies for patients for whom they believe the PPS rate is adequate or better; and
4. improve internal utilization, monitoring, and documentation.[104,105]

One can see that the pharmacy consultant will play an important role in each of these areas.

The Role of the Geriatric Pharmacist in the Nursing Facility

Pharmacists play a very critical role in the optimization of pharmacotherapy in the NF. Federal law requires all nursing homes to have a contract with a consultant pharmacist. The consultant pharmacist is responsible for ensuring that resident drug use is safe and effective and that facilities are in compliance with federal and state regulatory requirements. The Department of Health and Human Services' (DHHS) regulations state that NFs must employ or obtain the services of a licensed pharmacist who

1. provides consultation on all aspects of the provision of pharmacy services in the facility;
2. establishes a system of records of receipt and disposition of all controlled drugs in sufficient detail to enable an accurate reconciliation; and
3. determines that drug records are in order and that an account of all controlled drugs is maintained and periodically reconciled.

Most institutional pharmacy providers offer consultant services as part of their agreement with the NF.

The American Society of Consultant Pharmacists (ASCP) developed standards for the consultant pharmacist which state that

the range of a consultant pharmacist's responsibilities include: participating in the drug therapy decision making process, including recommendation of appropriate drug and non-drug therapies; assisting physicians, other prescribers, and patients in selection of appropriate treatment, and evaluating patient response to drug therapy.[106]

Consultant pharmacists can be self-employed, employed by the institution, or employed by a pharmacy provider. Only the state of New Jersey prohibits the consultant pharmacist from being employed by the dispensing pharmacy. This is done to avoid any potential conflict of interest.

The Drug Regimen Review

First, pharmacists are required to perform a comprehensive drug regimen review (DRR). The DRR is a medical chart review of each resident in the facility and its purpose is to ensure ongoing quality pharmaceutical care. The consultant pharmacist must perform an on-site DRR at least monthly for every resident in the facility and must document any actual or potential medication irregularity in the chart. The pharmacist must assess the appropriateness of the medication regimen. Pharmacists should therefore ensure there is an indication for each medication; that the medication is effective and safe for the condition; that the dose, route, and directions are appropriate and practical; that the regimen is free from clinically relevant drug interactions; that no adverse event exists; that necessary laboratory measures are available to monitor the effectiveness and toxicity of the medication; that the duration of therapy is appropriate; that the goal of therapy is being met; and that the medication has a favorable cost-benefit ratio.[107] The interpretive guidelines mandate the pharmacist specifically address and ensure that the resident's medication regimen is free from any unnecessary medications, and if psychoactive medications are used, there must be frequent, documented attempts to taper and discontinue the medication in addition to the implementation of behavioral modifications. Evidence exists that these regulations have been effective; the OIG found that 85 percent of NF residents' psychotropic medications were medically appropriate under these regulations.

Federal efforts to optimize medication management in long-term care are not limited to psychotropic medications. The DHHS presently requires that NF residents' drug profiles be free from unnecessary drugs. The definition used for unnecessary medications is "any drug used in excessive dose, for excessive duration, without adequate indications for its use or in the presence of adverse consequences."[108]

In an effort to extend regulations to optimize medication management, the DHHS incorporated the Beers criteria into the DRR process. The Beers criteria are a published list of medications best avoided in the elderly. These criteria have been widely accepted as a standard for appropriate geriatric medication use. Yet despite these regulations research suggests room for improvement—some 50 percent of nursing home residents in an Agency for Healthcare, Research and Quality-funded study were found to have at least one potentially inappropriate medication prescription as defined by the Beers criteria.[109]

The consultant pharmacist, in his or her DRR, is responsible for identifying irregularities regarding medication appropriateness that must then be communicated to the attending physician and the director of nursing.

The performance of the DRR has greatly evolved over time. The role of the consultant pharmacist in performing DRRs in the nursing home began in the 1960s with the enactment of Medicare and Medicaid, in which supervision of pharmaceutical services by pharmacists was established.[110] In 1974 the importance of pharmacy in medication oversight in long-term care became even more evident, as pharmacists were designated the professional health care providers responsible for evaluating and monitoring the drug therapy of patients residing in skilled nursing facilities and it was *mandated* that pharmacists review the medication regimens of patients.[111] In 1980 the General Accounting Office developed *indicators* for surveyor assessment on the DRR, and in 1982 the State Operations Manual provided surveyors and pharmacists with specific instructions about how the DRR was to be performed. This was also an important undertaking because the development of the indicators gave pharmacists specific guidelines as to what must be included in a DRR and held the pharmacist responsible for the content of the DRR. In 1984 and 1986, the evaluation of medication administration procedures and accuracy were included, as was the evaluation of drug therapy outcomes. Now not only was a pharmacist evaluating the medical chart, he or she was observing a nurse administer medications to the residents and assessing whether medication administration was accurate. The pharmacist was now also responsible for ensuring through chart review that the medications used were achieving their goal.

As a result of the landmark Institute of Medicine report in 1986 that highlighted quality problems and the need for stronger federal regulations, Congress passed the Nursing Home Reform Act as part of the Omnibus Budget Reconciliation Act (OBRA) of 1987.[112,113] A large portion of OBRA 1987 related to improving the provision of pharmaceutical care in the nursing home, including limits on chemical restraints, limits on other unnecessary or harmful drug use, efforts to discourage polypharmacy, and initiatives to disseminate geriatric best practice information to medical providers. OBRA 1987 mandated that pharmacy recommendations made on DRR must be followed by action. This did not mean that the physician needed to accept the recommendation, but he or she did need to acknowledge it and address it. The Act also provided guidelines regarding the use of unnecessary medications and antipsychotics. The result was the most far-reaching revision to the standards, inspection process, and enforcement system since the passage of Medicare and Medicaid in the mid-1960s. The new standards spoke to the evolving role of the consultant pharmacist, the process of care that is expected, and the requirement that care will promote "the maximum practicable functioning" for each individual resident.

The Nursing Home Reform Act of 1987, as part of OBRA 1987, also mandated requirements for regular resident assessment. The law mandated that eighteen areas of health assessment be conducted via the Resident Assessment Instrument (RAI) that provided a comprehensive, accurate, standardized, reproducible assessment of a resident's medical, functional, and psychological needs.

In 1996, the Minimum Data Set (MDS) was implemented. The MDS is a standardized instrument that health care professionals fill out for each resident on admission and yearly. A shortened version is also completed quarterly and when there is a change in a resident's status. It is designed to provide insight into the patient's cognition, function, and well-being and to thereby standardize the assessment of residents and to improve quality of care. Portions of the MDS are related to the purpose and effects of medications. The MDS is part of the larger RAI. The RAI is a form that is used to help guide the development of individualized care plans for residents.

Today the Centers for Medicare & Medicaid Services (CMS) has moved to monitoring data that nursing homes report via the MDS and administrative data from the Online Survey, Certification, and Reporting System (OSCAR). The CMS can use these aggregated data sets to provide a comprehensive view of the individual receiving care in the nursing home. Pharmacists can use information elicited from the MDS to identify potential or actual drug-related problems or to optimize medication. Pharmacists can also help complete the MDS as two sections of it directly pertain to recent medication use, recent medication changes, and frequency of medication administration.[114,115]

In 2002, the CMS implemented a new quality initiative in an effort to provide the public with more information about the quality of nursing homes.[116] It conducted a pilot study and is now preparing for the national launch of the nursing home quality initiative, with ten identified quality indicators (QIs) regarding worsening of ADLs, pressure ulcers, chronic pain and postacute pain, new infections, physical restraints, improvements in walking in postacute-care patients, and delirium. Although not currently part of the facility survey, the presence of these QIs will expand the role of the consultant pharmacist for several reasons. First, many of these QIs are affected by medication use, as is the case with underutilization of pain medications, the use of medications that may contribute to weight loss, or the use of medications that contribute to delirium. Second, the consultant pharmacist is often part of an interdisciplinary quality assurance committee that oversees quality of care issues in the nursing home by evaluating policies and procedures, clinical practice guidelines, algorithms and protocols, and providing staff education.

Other Functions of the Consultant Pharmacist
in the Nursing Facility

In addition to the DRR, the consultant pharmacist can develop and conduct medication use evaluations; may sit on quality assurance committees or other committees, such as the formulary committee; may work closely with the medical team to prepare the facility for annual surveys from licensing bodies; shall assess medication distribution, delivery, dispensing, and storage; shall assess medication administration to ensure accuracy and freedom from significant medication errors; and can also provide education to patients, families, and staff by providing in-services, medication administration training, and other programs.[117]

Evidence of Positive Outcomes Associated
with Consulting Pharmacy

Literature suggests that consultant pharmacy services are associated with positive clinical and economic outcomes.[118-121] The largest study ever conducted to analyze the benefits of consulting pharmacy is the Fleetwood project. The Fleetwood Project is an ongoing landmark initiative begun in 1995 by the ASCP's Research and Education Foundation, in collaboration with different geriatric care providers during three different phases, to demonstrate the value of consultant pharmacy services and to improve patient outcomes. The first phase, Fleetwood I, was a pharmacoeconomic analysis of the cost of medication-related problems and the impact of consultant pharmacy intervention on their costs. Fleetwood I found that consultant pharmacy intervention improved therapeutic outcomes and saved 3.6 billion annually.[122,123] Fleetwood II tested the feasibility of a prospective DRR, which focused on patients at highest risk of a medication-related problem.[124,125] Fleetwood III will examine the prospective DRR and the effects of consultant pharmacy services on reducing medication inappropriateness, adverse drug events, and undertreatment of chronic diseases.[126] The overall goal of the project is to improve health outcomes, to decrease cost and medication-related problems in nursing facilities, and to shift the focus of the consultant pharmacist from retrospective chart review to an integral member of the interdisciplinary care team.[127]

THE ROLE OF THE GERIATRIC
PHARMACIST IN OTHER SENIOR SETTINGS

Assisted Living Facilities

Assisted living facilities (ALFs) are difficult to define. In fact, after several thousand hours of committee work the Assisted Living Workgroup could not come up with a definition. In their most basic form ALFs are residential settings that offer choices in personal care and health-related services.

Assisted living is a relatively new model of care in the United States, and so currently consultant pharmacy services are not federally mandated in these facilities, although Congress is examining the need for federal oversight.[128] One of the main reasons why residents enter an ALF is difficulty managing their medications. Therefore, medication management is a large issue in assisted living. State laws regarding medication administration in the assisted living facility vary widely. Some allow staff to assist with self-administration of medications, others require staff to administer the medication to patients. Some states allow unlicensed staff to administer certain medications, while other states mandate a licensed nurse administer medications. Moreover, unlike in NFs, little research about medication optimization has been done in the assisted living arena.

The consultant pharmacist is well positioned to help optimize medication prescribing and medication administration in an ALF. Although one of the primary goals of an ALF is to optimize the health of patients and to keep them living independently, maximizing their function is also a wise business goal because it allows facilities to retain these patients by delaying the need for skilled twenty-four-hour care. This is also desirable because it is less costly for society to keep patients out of a NF. Therefore, maintaining patients' functional independence, including their ability to manage medications with supervision and the aid of the pharmacist, may assist the movement toward keeping patients in the ALF and out of a skilled NF for as long as possible.

One study that evaluated the appropriateness of medication regimens of 588 residents in 163 ALFs found that 28.8 percent of residents were receiving a potentially inappropriate medication, based on the Beers criteria.[129] Several other studies have suggested that the use, documentation, and monitoring of psychoactive medications in ALFs was suboptimal.[130-133]

One author's review of the literature on assisted living suggests that several trends exist in the literature: the number of medications taken by patients in assisted living is similar to that in NFs, the proportion of patients on psychoactive medications in assisted living is similar to that in NFs, the use of potentially inappropriate medications is a problem in assisted living, depression may be undertreated, and proper documentation of medication indication is lacking.[134] This suggests that there is a role for consultant pharmacy services in these facilities. Innovative pharmacists, often self-employed, can create a business for themselves in assisted living. Consultants can provide similar services to assisted living as they do in NFs. Chart reviews and patient interviews can be performed and recommendations made. The evolving role of consultant pharmacists in any setting is to focus on caring for the patient by being an active member of the interdisciplinary care team, as opposed to restricting one's services to retrospective chart review. The successful consultant pharmacist will make therapeutic recommendations on behalf of the patient and will provide ongoing monitoring and follow-up to ensure positive outcomes are obtained. Patient, family, and staff education should be provided as part of the pharmacist's plan of care for the patient.

Adult Day Services

Adult day services are community-based group programs designed to meet the needs of functionally and/or cognitively impaired adults through an individual plan of care. These structured, comprehensive programs provide a variety of health, social, and other related support services in a protective setting during any part of a day, but less than twenty-four hours. As a result, these services provide respite to family caregivers as well as therapeutic care for cognitively and physically impaired older adults. Adult day centers generally operate programs during normal business hours five days a week. Some programs do offer services in the evenings and on weekends.[135]

Much of the recent increase in the popularity of adult day services is the direct result of the advent of home and community long-term care Medicare and Medicaid waiver programs, which support alternatives to institutional long-term care and rehabilitation. Currently, the funding for adult day services is about 51 percent Medicaid and other public funds, 47 percent private funds, and the remainder long-term care insurance.

Medication use in the adult day service center is regulated by most states. As one can imagine, oversight of medication in a center serving frail elders that attend on an irregular basis and who receive a large portion of their medications at home can lead to confusion. Since the adult day service provider is not financially responsible for medications, it is up to each participant to bring his or her own medications to the center if they need to be administered during center hours. Because only one bottle and label are given with each prescription and the original vial must be used by the center to distribute medications in compliance with dispensing laws, this often results in unlabeled medications left at home for administration on noncenter days and weekends. A role for the geriatric pharmacist can easily be envisioned in this setting, given the complications of medication management in such a subset of patients.

Intermediate Care Facilities for the Mentally Retarded or Developmentally Disabled

The consultant pharmacist can perform similar functions in an intermediate care facility for the mentally retarded as he or she does in a nursing facility. For example, the pharmacist can participate in mandatory surveys, can educate the staff, family, and patient about drug therapy, participate in quality assurance committees, develop organizational policies and procedures, oversee medication administration, and conduct DRRs. DRRs must be conducted by a pharmacist at least quarterly in such facilities, and at least monthly in a nursing facility.

Continuing Care Retirement Communities

A continuing care retirement community (CCRC) is a community that offers several levels of assistance, including independent living, assisted living, and nursing home care. CCRCs are also known as life care communities in some regions. Religious organizations, fraternal groups, and other nonprofit agencies sponsor most CCRCs. It is different from other housing and care facilities for seniors because it usually provides a written agreement or long-term contract between the resident and the community that offers a continuum of housing, health care, and other services, most commonly on one campus or site.[136]

Commonly, CCRCs require a one-time entrance fee and monthly payments thereafter. Fees vary from one community to another depending on the type of housing and services each offers and the extent to which long-term care is covered. Other communities operate on a rental basis, in which residents make monthly payments but do not pay an entry fee. In still other communities, residents own instead of rent their units in arrangements similar to condominium ownership.[137]

Programs of All Inclusive Care for the Elderly

The Program of All Inclusive Care for the Elderly (PACE) is an innovative practice setting that provides comprehensive health, social, and medical care to frail elders who are nursing home eligible but do not wish to live in a nursing home.[138-141] It is a community program designed to serve as an alternative to nursing home living for many elders. PACE is based on the belief that it is better for the well-being of seniors with chronic care needs and their families to be served in the community when possible. PACE serves individuals who are fifty-five or older, certified by their state to need nursing home care, able to live safely in the community at the time of enrollment, and live in a PACE service area. If a PACE participant does need nursing home care, the PACE program pays for it and continues to coordinate care. Nationally, only about 7 percent of PACE participants do reside in a nursing home.[142]

PACE programs receive a lump payment from Medicare and Medicaid for delivering all needed medical and supportive services. The program is able to provide the entire continuum of care and services to seniors with chronic care needs while maintaining their independence in their homes for as long as possible. These services are provided by an interdisciplinary team and include the following:

- Adult day services
- Medical care
- Home health care and personal care
- Prescription drugs
- Social services
- Respite care
- Hospital and nursing home care when necessary[143]

Early in the 1970s when the Chinatown-North Beach community of San Francisco realized the pressing needs of elders whose families had immigrated to the United States, the PACE model of care was born. A community group of leaders formed a nonprofit corporation, On Lok Senior Health Services, to create a community-based system of care. On Lok is Cantonese for "peaceful, happy abode."[144]

PACE offers benefits to all the principle stakeholders in the following manner:

1. For participants, PACE provides the following:
   - Caregivers who listen to and can respond to their individualized care needs
   - The option to continue living in the community as long as possible
   - Coordination of their health care services
2. For health care providers, PACE provides the following:
   - Capitated funding arrangement, rewarding providers that are flexible and creative in providing the best care possible
   - Ability to coordinate care for participants across settings and medical disciplines, including clinical pharmacy
3. For Medicare and Medicaid programs, PACE provides the following:
   - Cost savings and predictable expenditures
   - Comprehensive services emphasizing preventive care
   - A model of choice focused on keeping seniors at home and out of institutional settings

Outcomes from PACE programs have been positive in the areas of consumer satisfaction, reduction in institutional care, controlled utilization of medical services, and cost savings to public and private payers of care, including Medicare and Medicaid.[145-147]

Medication management in a PACE program is especially difficult to monitor, because unlike a nursing home setting, patients in the PACE program attend the health center during the day but return home in the evening and remain home on weekends, when they are not supervised by health staff. Therefore, the effectiveness and toxicity of medications may not be identified as readily and appropriate prescribing at the outset is crucial. Currently thirty-three PACE and pre-PACE programs exist in the United States and the number of such programs is expected to increase.[148] With the advent of new PACE programs and with the knowledge that medication monitoring in the PACE program presents a unique challenge, it is especially important to ensure appropriate medication prescribing at the outset. One pilot study detailed the prevalence and consequence of potentially inappropriate medication use in a PACE program. Although the great majority of prescriptions reviewed (96.6 percent) were considered appropriate by the Beers criteria, over one-third of patients (36.1 percent) were prescribed a potentially inappropriate medication.[149] Thus, the geriatric pharmacist can play a large role in evaluating the outcomes of potentially inappropriate medication use by monitoring drug therapy and bringing therapeutic issues regarding the use of these medications to the attention of the prescribing physician.

Home Health Care

The American Society of Health-System Pharmacists has issued guidelines on the pharmacist's role in home care.[150] They state that the pharmacist should ensure that each patient referred to home care is an appropriate home care candidate based on admission criteria. In doing this, the pharmacist should assess whether the patient and family agree with the provision of home health care services, that they are willing to be educated about the patient's medication, that the home environment is suitable for the provision of services, that the medical condition and prescribed medication therapy are appropriate for home service, that the goals of therapy are documented, and that all components of the medication regimen are appropriate.

The pharmacist should collaborate with the health team to develop an appropriate care plan for each patient. In doing so, the pharmacist should maintain a complete patient database to use for ongoing monitoring of the patient's drug therapy and as an evaluation tool for measuring patient outcomes. The database would include all pertinent subjective and objective information, including demographics, emergency contact information, diagnoses, location and type of intravenous access, pertinent laboratory measures, pertinent historical and physical findings, nutrition screening test results, allergy history, a complete medication history, pertinent social and functional limitations, and appropriate pharmaceutical assessments and plans.

The pharmacist should collaborate with other health care providers to select products, devices, and ancillary supplies. Common examples would be selection of appropriate medications, assessment of stability and compatibility of prescribed medications and infusion device reservoirs, appropriate infusion devices, fluid admixtures, and appropriate administration sets. The pharmacist should also consider the patients' and families' abilities to learn to operate the infusion devices, and should consider patient convenience and cost in his or her recommendations. The pharmacist is responsible for providing education to the patient, family, and staff. The pharmacist should also work with the team to determine which medications should be included in an emergency supply kit.

The pharmacist should also be responsible for ensuring acquisition, proper compounding, dispensing, storage, delivery and administration of all medications and supplies, and tracking adverse drug events and medication errors. The pharmacist should also be involved in developing organizational policies and procedures and be an active member of performance improvement activities.[151]

Hospice Care

Hospice care presents a challenging and unique opportunity for the consultant pharmacist because the goals of therapy and therefore the monitoring of therapy are different; the goal of therapy is to support terminal patients and families and to provide comfort care, as opposed to preventive or curative care.[152] The hospice pharmacist can serve on an interdisciplinary team that is to provide compassionate, comprehensive, innovative care to patients *and* their families. In the hospice setting probably more than any other, the family is treated along with the patient.

The pharmacist in collaboration with the whole hospice team is challenged with

1. identifying all discomforting symptoms quickly,
2. providing only care that serves to increase comfort,
3. providing all care effectively and rapidly, and
4. providing care that is practical, not complex, and without adverse event.

Syndromes that a pharmacist in the hospice setting will observe include pain, weakness, fatigue, early satiety, anorexia and vomiting, and dry mouth and constipation. Many of these can be medication-induced. For instance, dry mouth and constipation can be secondary to the use of opioid analgesics, and weakness, fatigue, anorexia, and vomiting can be due to many disease states, such as cancer, as well as to many medications. It is now recognized that pain is often undertreated; patients should not live or die in pain. Thus, the hospice team should take great care to ensure that pain is effectively and aggressively managed. Delirium can be due to a myriad of causes such as pain, infection, electrolyte abnormalities, unfamiliar environments, and medication. The consultant pharmacist can work with the team in identifying and treating delirium. Other common conditions in which the consultant pharmacist can play a role in managing is cachexia, which may be due to medications and may be managed with some medications. In general, the consultant pharmacist should assess and monitor drug therapy and develop a care plan in collaboration with the rest of the health team. He or she should work to prevent and manage drug-related problems. The pharmacist may dispense and deliver drugs and related devices such as · spacers, nebulizers, intravenous supplies; he or she may compound medication preparations, provide analgesic dose conversions, perform pharmacokinetic drug dosing calculations, and provide education to the patient, family, and staff. The pharmacist should monitor the outcome of pharmacotherapy by utilizing pain scales and other quality-of-life measures.

FUTURE PAYER INITIATIVES

Two major movements initiated by senior care payers are expected to affect medication management for U.S. seniors. First, payers will increasingly move the risk of medication management from themselves to the providers of care. Just as New York Medicaid did in moving the risk for NF residents from themselves to the NF owners, other payers will do the same. As a result, increasing press will be placed upon providers to utilize all means possible to manage medications appropriately; one of these resources is the use of the pharmacy consultant.

The second movement is the Medicare Part D outpatient pharmacy benefit in 2006. Currently Medicare pays for a very limited number of outpatient medications, so implementation of an outpatient Medicare pharmacy benefit package is sure to have a major impact on seniors and their health care providers. One can expect advantages and disadvantages with the passage of such a prescription benefit. The obvious advantage for seniors is a shifting of costs from their pockets to Medicare. Even with private insurance, many elders still bear the brunt of medication costs due to high copayments, large deductibles, and annual limits on coverage. The Medicare prescription benefit would help absorb some of these prescription costs to seniors. The advantage of providing a Medicare pharmacy benefit has been argued for some time. Some point to the fact that after the New Jersey pharmaceutical assistance program was initiated, the number of medications per capita increased; however, the total cost of health care for this population decreased.[153]

The disadvantages of this law include an increased incidence of polypharmacy and adverse drug events, so it is imperative that the proposed benefit package includes services to monitor polypharmacy. Pharmacists are well positioned to play an integral role in preventing polypharmacy and adverse drug events and optimizing medication prescribing and utilization. To that end, Medicare Part D adds a new outpatient pharmacy benefit with inclusion of pharmacist-provided medication therapy management services (MTMS) as an integral component of the benefit. This means that plans must provide medication management services by pharmacy providers, targeting beneficiaries who have multiple disease states and who are on multiple medications.[154]

CONCLUSION

The only constant is change. Those words cannot ring any truer than with regard to the delivery of health care. The number of elderly people in the U.S. and worldwide is growing at an unprecedented rate. With an increased number of elderly patients needing health services, our goals for managing geriatric disease have greatly changed over the years. We are increasingly aware that illness in the elderly should not be thought of as inevitable and we are instituting more appropriate curative, preventive, and palliative care in elders with the goal of maximizing health and function and minimizing disease and disability. Although the majority of elderly people live independently in the community, the number of those needing long-term care is expected to grow. Traditional nursing facilities are still available options, but they are no longer the only option. Many different forms of long-term care exist and geriatric pharmacists have a role in each of these settings.

Pharmacists have been providing consulting services in traditional nursing homes for years, but *change is constant,* as is evidenced by the continually expanding role of the pharmacist in senior healthcare. Now more than ever, geriatric pharmacists have the ability to improve health outcomes and decrease cost in many geriatric settings, where they can serve as integral members of a health team.

NOTES

1. U.S. Department of Commerce, U.S. Census Bureau. *The 65 years and over population: 2000*. Issued October 2001. C2KBR/01-10. Available online at <http://www.census.gov/prod/2001pubs/c2kbr01-10.pdf>.

2. Federal Interagency Forum on Aging-Related Statistics. *Population: Older Americans 2000: Key indicators of well-being*. Available online at <http://agingstats.gov/chartbook2000/olderamericans2000.pdf>.

3. U.S Census Bureau. Available online at <http://www.census.gov>.

4. Shepherd, M. Pharmacists' involvement in nursing home facilities and home health care. In Fincham, J.E. and Wertheimer, A.I. (eds.), *Pharmacy and the U.S. health care system*, Second edition (Cincinnati: Harvey Whitney Books, 2001), pp. 269-296.

5. U.S Census Bureau. Available online at <http://www.census.gov>.

6. U.S. Census Bureau. Available online at <http://www.census.gov>; U.S. Census Bureau. Census 2000, Summary file 1; 1990 Census of Population. General Population Characteristics: United States (1990 CP-1-1).

7. U.S. Department of Commerce, U.S. Census Bureau. The older population in the United States: March 2002. Issued April 2003. P20-546. <http://www.census.gov/prod/2003pubs/p20-546.pdf>.

8. Shepherd, Pharmacists' involvement in nursing home facilities.

9. National Center for Health Statistics. *Vital Statistics of the United States, 1982*, Volume II, Mortality, Part A. DHHS Pub. No. (PHS 86-1112). Public Health Service (Washington, DC, U.S. Printing Office, 1985).

10. AGS Clinical Practices Committee Guidelines abstracted from consensus recommendations for the management of chronic heart failure. *J Am Geriatr Soc* (2000) 48: 1521-1524.

11. AGS Clinical Practices Committee The use of oral anticoagulants in older people. *J Am Geriatr Soc* (2000) 48: 224-227.

12. Mendelson, G., Ness, J., and Aranow, W.S. Drug treatment of hypertension in older persons in an academic hospital-based geriatrics practice. *J Am Geriatr Soc* (1999) 47: 597-599.

13. Gattis, W.A., Larsen, R.L., Hasselblad, V., et al. Is optimal angiotensin-converting enzyme inhibitor dosing neglected in elderly patients with heart failure? *Am Heart J* (1998) 136: 43-48.

14. Luzier, A.B. and DiTusa, L. Underutilization of ACE inhibitors in heart failure. *Pharmacotherapy* (1999) 19(11): 1296-1307.

15. Pahor, M., Shorr, J.I., Somes, G.W., et al. Diuretic-based treatment and cardiovascular events in patients with mild renal dysfunction enrolled in the systolic hypertension in the elderly program. *Arch Intern Med* (1998) 158: 1340-1345.

16. Smith, N.L., Psaty, B.M., Pitt, B., et al. Temporal patterns in the medical treatment of congestive heart failure with angiotensin-converting enzyme inhibitors in older adults, 1989 through 1995. *Arch Intern Med* (1998) 158: 1074-1080.

17. Krumholz, H.A., Radford, M.J., Wang, Y., et al. Early beta-blocker therapy for acute myocardial infarction in elderly patients. *Ann Intern Med* (1999) 131: 648-654.

18. Krumholz, H.M., Radford, M.J., Wang, Y., et al. National use and effectiveness of beta-blockers for the treatment of elderly patients after acute myocardial infarction. *JAMA* (1998) 280(7): 623-629.

19. U.S. Census Bureau. Available online at <http://www.census gov>.

20. U.S. Department of Commerce, Bureau of Census. *Projections of the population of the United States by age, sex, and race: 1988 to 2080* (Washington, DC: U.S. Government Printing Office, 1989).

21. Schneider, E.L. and Guralnick, J.M. The aging of America. *JAMA* (1990) 263: 2335-2340.

22. Max, W. The cost of Alzheimer's disease. *Pharmacoeconomics* (1996) 9: 5-10.

23. Boult, C. Systems for identifying and managing high-risk seniors. *Annals of Long-Term Care* (1998) 6(6): 79-86.

24. Pacala, J.T., Boult, C., Boult, L. Predictive validity of a questionnaire that identifies older persons at risk for hospital admission. *J Am Geriatr Soc* (1995) 45: 374-377.

25. Chernew, M.E., Smith, D.G., Kirking, D.M., and Fendrick, A.M. Decomposing pharmaceutical cost growth in different types of health plans. *Am J Manag Care* (2001) 7: 667-673.

26. Oskvig, R.M. Special problems in the elderly. *Chest* (1999) 115(5): 158-164.

27. Ibid.

28. Simonson, W. Introduction to the aging process. In Delafuente, J.C. and Stewart, R.B. (eds.), *Therapeutics in the elderly,* Third edition (Cincinnati: Harvey Whitney Books, 2001), pp. 1-39.

29. Basics of geriatric care: Biology of aging. In Beers, M.H., Berkow, R. (eds.), *The Merck manual of geriatrics,* Third edition (Whitehouse Station, PA: Merck Research Laboratories, 2000), pp. 3-9.

30. Basics of geriatric care: Prevention of disease and disability. In Beers, M.H. and Berkow, R. (eds.), *The Merck manual of geriatrics,* Third edition (Whitehouse Station, PA: Merck Research Laboratories, 2000), pp. 46-53.

31. Basics of geriatric care: Biology of aging, pp. 3-9.

32. Devone, C.A.J. Comprehensive geriatric assessment: Making the most of the aging years. *Curr Opin Clin Nutr Metab Care* (2002) 5: 19-24.

33. Lassila, H.C., Stoehr, G.P., Ganguli, M., et al. Use of prescription medications in an elderly rural population: The MoVIES project. *Ann Pharmacother* (1996) 30: 589-595.

34. Saini, A., Birrer, R., Harghel, C., et al. Polypharmacy, complementary and alternative medicine in the elderly. *P&T* (2001) 26(12): 616-620, 627.

35. Delafeunte, J.C. Perspectives on geriatric pharmacotherapy. *Pharmacotherapy* (1991) 11(3): 222-224.

36. Basics of geriatric care: Demographics. In Beers, M.H. and Berkow, R. (eds.), *The Merck manual of geriatrics,* Third edition (Whitehouse Station, PA: Merck Research Laboratories, 2000), pp. 9-23.

37. Baum, C., Kennedy, D.L., Forbes, M.B., et al. Drug use in the United States in 1981. *JAMA* (1984) 25: 1293-1297.

38. Coons, J.S., Johnson, M., and Chandler, M.H.H. Sources of self-treatment information and use of home remedies and over-the-counter medications among older adults. *J Geriatr Drug Ther* (1992) 7: 71-82.

39. Chen, L.H., Liu, S., Cook-Newell, M.E., and Barnes, K. Survey of drug use by the elderly and possible impact of drugs on nutritional status. *Drug-Nutr Interact* (1985) 3: 73-86.

40. Kaufman, D.W., Kelly, J.P., Rosenberg, L., et al. Recent patterns of medication use in the ambulatory adult population of the United States: The Slone survey. *JAMA* (2002) 287: 337-344.

41. Lassila et al., Use of prescription medications in an elderly rural population.

42. Avorn, J., Soumerai, S.B., Everitt, D.E., et al. A randomized trial of a program to reduce the use of psychoactive medications in a nursing home. *N Engl J Med* (1992) 327: 168-173.

43. Beers, M.H., Baran, R.W., and Frenia, K. Drugs and the elderly, Part 1: The problems facing managed care. *Am J Manag Care* (2000) 6: 1313-1320.

44. Lassila et al., Use of prescription medications in an elderly rural population.

45. Hanlon, J.T., Fillenbaum, G.G., Ruby, C.M., et al. Epidemiology of over-the-counter drug use in community-dwelling elderly: United States perspective. *Drugs Aging* (2001) 18(2): 123-131.

46. Fanning, K.D., Ruby, C.M., Twersky, J.I., et al. The prevalence of dietary supplement and home remedy use by patients in a geriatric outpatient clinic. *Consult Pharm* (2002) 17(11): 972-978.

47. Anderson, D.L., Shane-McWhorter, L., Crouch, B.I., et al. Prevalence and patterns of alternative medication use in a university hospital outpatient clinic serving rheumatology and geriatric patients. *Pharmacotherapy* (2000) 20(8): 958-966.

48. Dolder, C., Lacro, J., Dolder, N., et al. Alternative medication use: Results of a survey of older veterans. *Consult Pharm* (2002) 17: 653-662.

49. Zeilmann, C.A., Dole, E.J., Skipper, B.J., et al. Use of herbal medicine by elderly Hispanic and non-Hispanic white patients. *Pharmacotherapy* (2003) 23(4): 526-532.

50. Anderson, D.L., et al. Prevalence and patterns of alternative medication use.

51. Dolder et al., Alternative medication use.

52. The National Institute for Health Care Management Research and Educational Foundation. *Prescription drug expenditures in 2000: The upward trend continues.* May 2001. Available online at <http://www.nihcm.org>.

53. Shepherd, Pharmacists' involvement in nursing home facilities.

54. McKercher, P.L., Taylor, S.D., Lee, J.A., et al. Prescription drug use among elderly and nonelderly families. *J Manag Care Pharm* (2003) 9(1): 19-28.

55. Strand, L.M., Morley, P.C., Cipolle, R.J., et al. Drug-related problems: Their structure and function. *DICP* (1990) 24(11): 1093-1097.

56. Hanlon, J.T., Shimp, L.A., and Semla, T.P. Recent advances in geriatrics: Drug-related problems in the elderly. *Ann Pharmacother* (2000) 34: 360-365.

57. Hanlon, J.T., Gray, S.L., Schmader, K.E. Adverse drug reactions. In Delafuente, J.C. and Stewart, R.B. (eds.), *Therapeutics in the elderly*, Third edition (Cincinnati: Harvey Whitney Books, 2001), pp. 289-314.

58. Gurwitz, J., Monane, M., Monane, S., Avorn, J. Polypharmacy. In: Morris, J.N., Lipsitz, L.A., Murphy, K., Bellville-Taylor, P., eds. *Quality Care in the Nursing Home*. St. Louis, MO: Mosby-Year Book; 1997:13-25.

59. Hanlon, Gray, and Schmader, Adverse drug reactions.

60. Nolan, L. and O'Malley, K. Prescribing for the elderly, Part 1: Sensitivity of the elderly to adverse drug reactions. *J Am Geriatr Soc* (1988) 36: 142-149.

61. Fields, T.S., Gurwitz, J.H., Avorn, J., et al. Risk factors for adverse drug events among nursing home residents. *Arch Intern Med* (2001) 161(3): 1629-1634.

62. Montamat, S.C. and Cusack, B. Overcoming problems with polypharmacy and drug misuse in the elderly. *Clin Geriatr Med* (1992) 8(1): 143-158.

63. Grymonpre, R.E., Mitenko, P.A., Sitar, D.S., et al. Drug-associated hospital admissions in older medical patients. *J Am Geriatr Soc* (1988) 36: 1092-1098.

64. Hanlon, Gray, and Schmader, Adverse drug reactions.

65. Fouts, M., Hanlon, J., Pieper, C., et al. Identification of elderly nursing facility residents at high risk for drug-related problems. *Consult Pharm* (1997) 12: 1103-1111.

66. Schneider, J.K., Mion, L.C., and Frengley, D. Adverse drug reactions in an elderly outpatient population. *Am J Hosp Pharm* (1992) 49: 90-96.

67. Thomas, E.J. and Brennan, T.A. Incidence and types of preventable adverse events in elderly patients: Population-based review of medical records. *BMJ* (2000) 320: 741-744.

68. Beers, M.H. Aging as a risk factor for medication-related problems. *Consult Pharm* (1999) 14(12): 1337-1340.

69. Hanlon, Gray, and Schmader, Adverse drug reactions; Nolan and O'Malley, Prescribing for the elderly; Fields et al., Risk factors for adverse drug events among nursing home residents; Montamat and Cusack, Overcoming problems with polypharmacy; Grymonpre et al., Drug-associated hospital admissions in older medical patients; Schneider, Mion, and Frengley, Adverse drug reactions in an elderly outpatient population.

70. Hanlon, J.T., Schmader, K.E., Koronkowski, M.J., et al. Adverse drug events in high-risk older outpatients. *J Am Geriatr Soc* (1997) 45: 945-948.

71. Chrischilles, E.A., Segar, E.T., Wallace, R.B. Self-reported adverse drug reactions and related resource use. *Ann Intern Med* (1992) 117: 634-640.

72. Cooper, J.W. Probable adverse drug reactions in a rural geriatric nursing home population: A four-year study. *J Am Geriatr Soc* (1996) 44: 194-197.

73. Gerety, M.B., Cornell, J.E., Plichta, D.T., et al. Adverse events related to drugs and drug withdrawal in nursing home residents. *J Am Geriatr Soc* (1993) 41: 1326-1332.

74. Bates, D.W., Leape, L.L., Petrycki, S., et al. Incidence and preventability of adverse drug events in hospitalized adults. *J Gen Intern Med* (1993) 8: 289-294.

75. Bootman, J.L., Harrison, D.L., and Cox, E. The health care cost of drug-related morbidity and mortality in nursing facilities. *Arch Intern Med* (1997) 157: 2089-2096.

76. Johnson, J.A., Bootman, J.L. Drug-related morbidity and mortality: A cost-of-illness model. *Arch Intern Med* (1995) 155: 1949-1956.

77. Hanlon, Shimp, and Semla, Recent advances in geriatrics.

78. Thomas, E.J. and Brennan, T.A. Incidence and types of preventable adverse events in elderly patients.

79. Schmader, K., Hanlon, J.T., Weinberger, M., et al. Appropriateness of medication prescribing in ambulatory elderly patients. *J Am Geriatr Soc* (1994) 42: 1241-1247.

80. Beers, M.H., Ouslander, J.G., Fingold, S.F., et al. Inappropriate medication prescribing in skilled-nursing facilities. *Ann Intern Med* (1992) 117: 684-689.

81. Beers, M.H. Explicit criteria for determining potentially inappropriate medication use by the elderly: An update. *Arch Intern Med* (1997) 157(14): 1531-1536.

82. Schmader et al., Appropriateness of medication prescribing in ambulatory elderly patients; Beers et al., Inappropriate medication prescribing in skilled-nursing facilities; Beers, Explicit criteria for determining potentially inappropriate medication use.

83. Hanlon, J.T., Schmader, K.E., Boult, C., et al. Use of inappropriate prescription drugs by older people. *J Am Geriatr Soc* (2002) 50: 26-34.

84. Dhall, J., Larrat, P., and Lapane, K.L. Use of potentially inappropriate drugs in nursing homes. *Pharmacotherapy* (2002) 22(1): 88-96.

85. Hanlon, J.T., Fillenbaum, G.G., Schmader, K.E., et al. Inappropriate drug use among community-dwelling elderly. *Pharmacotherapy* (2000) 20(5): 575-582.

86. Zhan, C., Sangl, J., Bierman, A.S., et al. Potentially inappropriate medication use in the community-dwelling elderly: Findings from the 1996 medical expenditure panel survey. *JAMA* (2001) 286: 2823-2829.

87. Stuck, A.E., Beers, M.H., Steiner, A., et al. Inappropriate medication use in community-residing older persons. *Arch Intern Med* (1994) 154: 2195-2200.

88. Willcox, S.M., Himmelstein, D.U., and Woolhandler, S. Inappropriate drug prescribing for the community-dwelling elderly. *JAMA* (1994) 272: 292-296.

89. Pitkala, K.H., Strandberg, T.E., and Tilvis, R.S. Inappropriate drug prescribing in home-dwelling, elderly patients: A population-based survey. *Arch Intern Med* (2002) 162: 1707-1712.

90. Institute of Medicine. *Improving the quality of long-term care* (Washington, DC: National Academy Press, 2001).

91. U.S. Bipartisan Commission on Comprehensive Health Care. *A call for action, Executive summary* (Washington, DC: U.S. Government Printing Office, 1990).

92. Kane, R.L. and Kane, R.A. A nursing home in your future? *N Engl J Med* (1991) 324: 627-629.

93. Porter, L. What significant changes can long-term care providers anticipate in the next decade? *Contemp Long Term Care* (1994) 17: 39-41.

94. Webster, T.R. A perspective on consultant pharmacy's future: Changing information into dollars. *Consult Pharm* (1989) 4: 8-12.

95. Goldman, B.J. Ancillary health care professionals: Extending the reach of consultant pharmacy. *Consult Pharm* (1991) 6: 212-220.

96. Gabrel, C.S. An overview of nursing home facilities: Data from the 1997 National Nursing Home Survey. *Advance data from vital and health statistics;* No. 311. (Hyattsville, MD: National Center for Health Statistics, 2000). Available online at <http://www.cdc.gov/nchs/data/ad/ad311.pdf>.

97. Tobias, D.E. and Sey, M. General and psychotherapeutic medication use in 328 nursing facilities: A year 2000 national survey. *Consult Pharm* (2001) 16: 54-64.

98. Tobias, D.E. and Pulliam, C.C. General and psychotherapeutic medication use in 878 nursing facilities: A 1997 national survey. *Consult Pharm* (1997) 12: 1401-1408.

99. Avorn, J. and Gurwitz, J.H. Drug use in the nursing home. *Ann Intern Med* (1995) 123: 195-204.

100. Pharmaceutical Research and Manufacturers of America. New Drugs in Development Increases to 785 for Diseases Affecting Older Americans. 2001 survey:

New Medicines in Development for Older Americans. PhRMA, Washington DC, 2001. Available online at <http://www.phrma.org/newmedicines/resources/older_americans_2001.pdf>.

101. Long-Term Care Pharmacy Alliance. Available online at <http://www.ltcpa.org/public/memberinfo/default.asp>.

102. General Accounting Office. *Skilled nursing facilities: Medicare payment changes require provider adjustments but maintain access* (Washington, DC: General Accounting Office, 1999).

103. Stefanacci, R.G. Case study: Optimizing medication use in skilled nursing facilities. *Journal of Quality Healthcare* (2003) 2(2): 1-4.

104. Office of the Inspector General. *Medicare beneficiary access to skilled nursing facilities* (Washington, DC: U.S. Department of Health and Human Services, 2001).

105. Office of the Inspector General. *Early effects of the prospective payment system on access to skilled nursing facilities* (Washington, DC: U.S. Department of Health and Human Services, 1999).

106. Clark, T.R. (ed.). *ASCP policies, standards, and guidelines 2002*, Fifth edition. (Alexandria, VA: American Society of Consultant Pharmacists, 2001), pp. 1-250.

107. Ibid.

108. Social Security Act, Title 19, Sec. 1919. (b)(4)(A)(iii).

109. Denys Tsz-Wai Lau. Potentially inappropriate medication prescriptions among geriatric nursing home residents: Preliminary findings on its scope and associated resident and facility characteristics. Poster presentation: 129th Meeting of the American Public Health Association. Atlanta, GA. October 23, 2001.

110. Shepherd, Pharmacists' involvement in nursing home facilities.

111. Ibid.

112. Institute of Medicine. *Improving quality of care in nursing homes* (Washington, DC: National Academy Press, 1986).

113. Social Security Act, Title 19, Sec. 1919.

114. Clark, T.R. *ASCP policies, standards, and guidelines, 2002.*

115. Meade, V. Tips and insights from a veteran MDS educator. *Consult Pharm* (2002) 17(3): 201-208.

116. Clark, T.R. Quality indicators and the consultant pharmacist. *Consult Pharm* (2002) 17(11): 925-943.

117. Clark, *ASCP policies, standards, and guidelines, 2002.*

118. Bootman, Harrison, and Cox, The health care cost of drug-related morbidity and mortality in nursing facilities; Johnson and Bootman, Drug-related morbidity and mortality.

119. Furniss, L., Burns, A., Craig, S.K.L., et al. Effects of a pharmacist's medication review in nursing homes. *Br J Psychiatr* (2000) 176: 563-567.

120. Gupchup, G.V., Vogenberg, F.R., and Larrat, E.P. Assessing outcome of pharmaceutical care service by consultant pharmacists, Part one: Review and research recommendations. *Consult Pharm* (2001) 16: 844-850.

121. Larrat, E.P., Vogenberg, F.R., and Gupchup, G.V. Assessing outcomes of pharmaceutical care services by consultant pharmacists, Part II: Integrating outcomes research into practice. *Consult Pharm* (2001) 16: 1127-1136.

122. Bootman, Harrison, and Cox, The health care cost of drug-related morbidity and mortality in nursing facilities.
123. Riley, K.Y. The Fleetwood Project phase one. Available online at <www.ascp.com/public/pubs/tcp/1997/jan/fleetwoodproj.html>.
124. Ibid.
125. Harms, S.L. and Garrard, J. The Fleetwood model: An enhanced method of pharmacist consultation. *Consult Pharm* (1998) 13: 1350-1355.
126. Riley, K.Y. The Fleetwood Project phase one. Available online at <www.ascp.com/public/pubs/tcp/1997/jan/fleetwoodproj.html>.
127. Harms, S.L., Garrard, J. The Fleetwood Model: An enhanced method of pharmacist consultation. *Consult Pharm* (1998) 13: 1350-1355.
128. Clark, T.R. Medication use in assisted living: A review of published reports. *Consult Pharm* (2001) 16(11): 1037-1044.
129. Rhoads, M. and Thai, A. Potentially inappropriate medications ordered for elderly residents of assisted living homes and assisted living centers. *Consult Pharm* (2002) 17: 587-593.
130. Spore, D.L., Mor, V., Larrat, P., et al. Inappropriate drug prescriptions for elderly residents of board and care facilities. *Am J Pub Health* (1997) 87L: 404-409.
131. Spore, D.L., Mor, V., Hiris, J., et al. Psychotropic drug use among older residents of board and care facilities. *J Am Geriatr Soc* (1995) 43: 1403-1409.
132. Hyde, J., Segelman, M., Feldman, S., et al. Medication management in Massachusetts assisted living settings. *Consult Pharm* (1998) 13: 1001-1014.
133. Williams, B.R., Nichol, N.B., Lowe, B., et al. Medication use in residential care facilities for the elderly. *Ann Pharmacother* (1999) 33: 149-155.
134. Clark, Medication use in assisted living.
135. Available online at <http://www.nadsa.org>.
136. Available online at <http://www.alfa.org>.
137. Available online at <http://www.cms.gov>.
138. Shannon, K. and Van Reenen, C. PACE: Innovative care for the frail elderly. *Health Progress* (1998) September-Ocboter 79(5): 41-45.
139. Eng, C., Pedulla, J., Eleazer, G.P., et al. Program of all-inclusive care for the elderly: An innovative model of integrated geriatric care and financing. *J Am Geriatr Soc* (1997) 45(2): 223-232.
140. Bodenheimer, T. Long-term care for frail elderly people—The On Lok model. *N Engl J Med* (1999) 341(7): 1324-1328.
141. Available online at <http://www.npaonline.org>.
142. Shannon and Van Reenen, PACE; Eng et al., Program of all-inclusive care for the elderly; Bodenheimer, Long-term care for frail elderly people; Available online at <http://www.npaonline.org>.
143. Shannon and Van Reenen, PACE; Eng et al., Program of all-inclusive care for the elderly; Bodenheimer, Long-term care for frail elderly people; Available online at <http://www.npaonline.org>.
144. Bodenheimer, Long-term care for frail elderly people.
145. Pacala, J.T., Kane, R.L., Atherly, A., et al. Using structured implicit review to assess quality of care in the Program of All Inclusive Care for the Elderly. *J Am Geriatr Soc* (2000) 48: 903-910.

146. Lee, M.A., Brummel-Smith, K., Meyer, J., et al. Physician orders for life-sustaining treatment: Outcomes in a PACE program. *J Am Geriatr Soc* (2000) 48: 1219-1225.

147. Wieland, D., Lamb, V.L., Sutton, S.R., et al. Hospitalization in the Program of All Inclusive Care for the Elderly: Rates, concomitants, and predictors. *J Amer Geriatr Soc* (2000) 48(11): 1373-1380.

148. Pacala, J.T., Boult, C., Boult, L. Predictive validity of a questionnaire that identifies older persons at risk for hospital admission. *J Am Geriatr Soc* (1995) 45: 374-377.

149. Knight, T., Wertheimer, A.I., and Stefanacci, R. Identification of potentially inappropriate medication use in a Program of All Inclusive Care for the Elderly. *Consult Pharm* (2002) 17: 1035-1039.

150. ASHP guidelines on the pharmacist's role in home health. *Am J Health Syst Pharm* (2000) 57(13): 1252-1257.

151. Ibid.

152. Zanni, G.R. and Wick, J.Y. Hospice care: A noble calling for the consultant pharmacist. *Consult Pharm* (2001) 16(9): 821-835.

153. Lavizzo-Mourney, R.J. and Eisenberg, J.M. Prescription drugs, practicing physicians, and the elderly. *Health Affairs* (1990) fall: 20-35.

154. Available online at <http://www.ascp.com/MedicareRx/>.

ONLINE RESOURCES

Administration on Aging: <www.aoa.dhhs.gov>
Agency for Healthcare Research and Quality: <www.ahrq.gov>
Alzheimer's Association: <www.alz.org>
Alzheimer's Research Forum: <www.alzforum.org>
American Geriatrics Society: <www.americangeriatrics.org>
American Medical Directors Association: <www.amda.com>
American Society of Consultant Pharmacists: <www.ascp.com>
Assisted Living Federation of America: <www.ALFA.org>
Centers for Medicare & Medicaid Services: <http://cms.hhs.gov>
ElderWeb: <www.elderweb.com>
Federal Food and Drug Administration: <www.fda.gov>
Federal Interagency Forum on Aging-Related Statistics: <http://www.aoa.dhhs.gov/agingstats/default.htm>
Institute for Safe Medication Practices: <www.ismp.org>
National Chronic Care Consortium: <www.nccconline.org>
National Family Caregivers Association: <www.nfcacares.org>
National Institute on Aging: <www.nia.nih.gov>
National PACE Association: <www.natlpaceassn.org>
National Parkinson Foundation: <www.parkinson.org>
U.S. Census Bureau: <www.census.org>

Chapter 11

The Pharmaceutical Research Manufacturing Industry

Patrick McKercher

INTRODUCTION

The U.S. pharmaceutical research manufacturing industry is a significant participant in the discovery and development of innovative chemical and biological agents used in the treatment of human and animal diseases. The industry is distinguished from other industry sectors because the evolution and continued success of the industry rely more heavily on partnerships with universities than other industries. The successful pharmaceutical market thrives best within societies that embrace innovation, with the corresponding respect for the protection of intellectual property. In addition, the industry enjoys success in economic environments that are relatively free from government price controls, albeit laden with market-driven cost containment. Consequently, the United States is the most conducive environment, accounting for the largest proportion of both pharmaceutical innovations and corresponding profits.

Demand for pharmaceuticals is disease-driven. Therefore, the industry is not susceptible to usual business cycles with fluctuating demands from year to year. Investors consider the industry a sound growth investment that has historically provided predictable returns that are favorably compared to other industries. In addition, the industry employs highly technically competent employees and is a relatively clean industry. Many countries and states actively pursue pharmaceutical manufacturers, and several regions have created a concentration of start-up biotechnology companies.

ECONOMIC IMPACT

The Fortune 500 pharmaceutical manufacturing companies generated $195.8 billion in 2003 sales (see Figure 11.1) and $30.4 billion in profits,

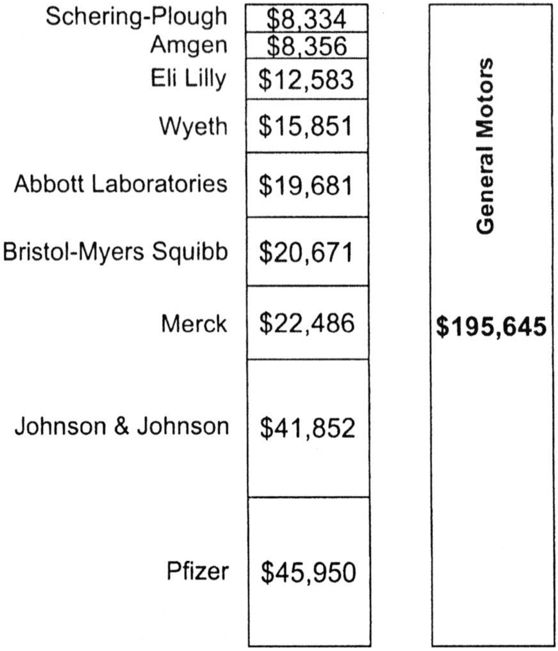

Schering-Plough	$8,334	
Amgen	$8,356	
Eli Lilly	$12,583	General Motors
Wyeth	$15,851	
Abbott Laboratories	$19,681	
Bristol-Myers Squibb	$20,671	
Merck	$22,486	**$195,645**
Johnson & Johnson	$41,852	
Pfizer	$45,950	

FIGURE 11.1. 2003 Sales for Nine Top Pharmaceutical Manufacturers

earning the status of the third most profitable sector in Fortune 500. The pharmaceutical industry ranked third in return on revenue (14.3 percent), second in return on assets (10.3 percent), and fourth in return on shareholder equity (22.1 percent).[1] Pharmaceutical manufacturers totaled nearly 50 percent of worldwide pharmaceutical sales.

In addition, the three major pharmaceutical wholesalers generated $171.2 billion in sales with $2.6 billion in earnings, and the major retail pharmacy chains realized $79.4 billion sales and $1.9 billion in profits (see Table 11.1). Equally significant is the $70.7 billion and $1.1 billion in profits generated by the four pharmaceutical benefit management companies. The total of all public-traded Fortune 500 pharmacy companies including pharmacy benefit managers (PBM)s, retail chains, wholesalers, and manufacturers accounted for 6.9 percent to the total Fortune 500 sales and 8.1 percent of profits. The larger proportion of profits compared to the proportion of sales reflects the relative profitability of the industry to total industry.

TABLE 11.1. Pharmaceutical Sales, Profits, and Employees, 2003

Company	Revenue[a]	Profits[a]	Employees
PBMs	70,738	1,135	32,945
Retail	79,421	1,941	292,060
Wholesale	171,214	2,594	99,845
Manufacturer	195,764	30,423	553,830
Total	517,137	36,093	978,680

Note: Public-traded companies in *Fortune.*
[a]In millions of dollars.

Although large, the pharmaceutical manufacturers are relatively small compared to the leading industry sectors. For example, General Electric is as large as the combined sales of the Fortune 500 pharmaceutical manufacturers and has $11.5 billion in health care sales. Financial metrics for the top companies are presented in Table 11.2.

The combined size of the Fortune 500 pharmaceutical manufacturers, as measured in sales, is comparable to General Motors, the third largest company in 2003. In Figure 11.2 a comparison of sales, profits, and number of employees is presented to illustrate the different character of pharmaceutical versus automobile manufacturers.

COMMON CRITICISMS

Historically, critics of the industry have attacked its profitability, heavy promotional efforts, and pricing policies. These "three Ps" were attacked for most of the previous century and expectations are that critics will continue their enthusiastic efforts to modify the industry's traditional business model. Pharmaceutical manufacturers are faced with unusually high risks in the discovery and development process because the Food and Drug Administration requirements for safety and proven efficacy are more stringent than in other industries. The complexity of the disease process and pharmaceutical interventions imposes a large information dissemination challenge and it is difficult to differentiate between marketing hype and information exchange. Consequently, manufacturers with low success in innovation and relatively weak market penetration have not survived, resulting in consolidation of the industry in fewer and larger companies. Globalization of the economy will change the U.S. pharmaceutical industry such that its financial ratios (i.e., pricing and profitability) will be increasingly similar to

TABLE 11.2. 2003 Sales, Profits, and Employees

Company	Rank	Revenues[a]	Profits/ earnings[a]	Employees
Wal-Mart	1	258,681	9,054	1,400,000
Exxon Mobil	2	213,199	21,510	88,300
General Motors	3	195,645	3,822	325,000
Ford Motor	4	164,496	495	327,531
General Electric	5	134,187	15,002	305,000
McKesson	16	57,129	555	24,500
Pfizer	25	45,950	3,910	122,000
Medco Health Solutions	41	34,265	426	13,000
Walgreen	45	32,505	1,176	130,000

[a]In millions of dollars.

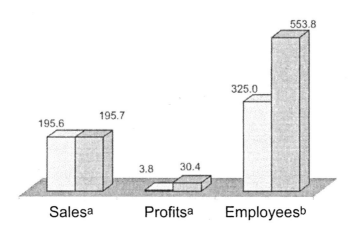

FIGURE 11.2. Top Nine Fortune 500 Pharmaceutical Manufacturers versus General Motors (GM is represented by the lefthand bars; the top nine pharmaceutical manufacturers are represented by the righthand bars; [a]in billions of dollars; [b]in thousands.)

large, capitalized, consumer product companies. The end result will be less concentration of R&D in the United States, smaller work forces, and a shifting research agenda addressing worldwide health challenges, with less priority on the U.S. aging population.

Additional segments of the pharmaceutical manufacturing industry include the generic manufacturers, biotechnology, and niche research manufacturers that tend to develop pharmaceutical agents for licensure to major Pharmaceutical Research and Manufacturers of America (PhRMA) manufacturers. These are important segments that add significantly to the economics of the industry. However, these segments tend to escape criticism or are held in higher regard because they are newer to the economic landscape, smaller, and do not tend to drive pharmaceutical expenditures and budgets. Biotechnology, for example, enjoys a more favorable stature with the public and Congress than the large, capitalized, traditional pharmaceutical manufacturers.

The unique characteristics of the industry, the high level of risk associated with marketing, and the aggressiveness of marketing attract considerable attention, making it an interesting employment environment. Drug recalls are unavoidable since some unknown effects of medications are often revealed with large-scale and long-term use after market launch. These highly visible negative events laden with suspicions of profit seeking and aggressive promotion make this an interesting and exciting industry. Pricing power, an admirable characteristic according to the investment community, is a frustration to the payer community. Pharmacists, insurance, employer payers, and consumers resent price increases and the perceived high cost of a relatively small purchase compared to hospitalization and physician services.

The chemical and pharmaceutical industries are inordinately sensitive to erosion of intellectual property and pricing regulation.[2] Some studies have documented the relationship between pricing regulation and decreased levels of innovation. Wall Street assesses the value of a pharmaceutical manufacturer based on its research pipeline and the expected value of innovations. Consequently, PhRMA, the industry trade association, is very aggressive in combating state and federal initiatives that contain any hint of price controls. The level of lobbying effort has drawn criticism from consumer advocate groups.

Medication expenditures are driven by price increases, increases in the number of patients treated, growing disease candidates appropriately treated with innovative pharmaceuticals, more aggressive medication therapies involving multiple agents and aging demographics of the U.S. workforce, and general population. Payers and administrators of health plans are frustrated by this conspicuous source of health expenditures. Price increases are visible and promotional efforts are obvious. Therefore, although the bulk of expenditure growth is attributable to factors other than price increases, this is the most prevalent source of criticism.

VULNERABILITY

Most R&D investments are made in the United States. Some major manufacturers are not U.S. companies but maintain major R&D and sales functions in the United States because policy and economic environment are most favorable. Prior to the past few decades, pharmaceutical innovation was more evenly distributed among industrialized countries. Growth in R&D tends to exceed general inflation and averages about 7.5 percent[3] compared to inflation, which is generally below 4 percent. This level of enthusiasm for research is driven by a society that has embraced new technology and welcomed new therapies.

The risks to society and its conventions are

1. implied societal agreement to a reduction in technological advancement,
2. policy development shifting the economy away from a free market with few price controls, and
3. failure to respect and enforce intellectual property.

Societal endorsement of reduced innovation is exerted indirectly through payer, employer, and consumer hesitation to pay. Evidence of increased government subsidy in the recent passage of the Medicare Modernization Act[4] including coverage for prescription medications for persons eligible for Medicare coverage sets a pattern of less free market latitude. Therefore, government policies reflecting resistance to payment for some innovations or extension of existing price controls, such as the Federal Upper Limit prices for generic pharmaceuticals, are exerting downward pressure on the level of R&D. Private reimbursement policy exerts similar pressures. However, slowing research progress is invisible because consumers are unaware of treatments that are delayed or not developed.

An example of shifting free-market policies is the current inclusion of provisions for reimportation of pharmaceuticals. In effect, this represents the importation of de facto price controls from countries with these public policies. Estimates are that widespread importation of pharmaceuticals from countries with lower prices will slow innovation because of lost cash flow generally used to finance R&D and reduced enthusiasm for investment in innovations when the return on investment in products in the pipelines is lowered.

Intellectual property rights are being challenged in all business sectors. Considerable interest in anticounterfeiting technology attests to the growing challenge to manufacturers to protect the market exclusivity presumed to be associated with patents, trademarks, and copyrights. Niche research manufacturers rely on the expected value of products eventually licensed to major manufacturers and attract venture capital based on these expected values. The expectation that patents will be protected is key to estimating the future value of innovations.

The pharmaceutical industry could become considerably less robust if consumers are, indirectly, less willing to pay for innovations; products are priced at levels consistent with prices in price-controlled environments; and if compromised intellectual property rights become more prevalent. It is doubtful that a manufacturer will publicly acknowledge slowing research on lifesaving innovations, for fear of public hostility. Slower, less profitable research pipelines will exert downward pressure on stock prices, making the industry less attractive to investors. *Fortune* magazine has predicted a shift in the home of pharmaceutical innovation from the United States to Asian countries in the next fifty years. It is conceivable that our national leadership in pharmaceutical innovation could follow the fate of the automobile industry if economic environmental conditions change dramatically.

THE FUTURE

The pharmaceutical industry is an exciting and promising industry in spite of the criticisms and vulnerabilities mentioned in this chapter. More sophisticated pharmaceutical product screening is increasing the efficiency of research and development. In addition, discoveries in genomics will facilitate the identification of targets for pharmaceutical intervention. Stronger patient advocacy will counter payer and employer resistance to payment. Biotechnological intervention will equal or exceed traditional chemical pharmaceutical dominance in medication therapies.

A stronger partnership with pharmacists and the pharmaceutical manufacturing industry will evolve as diagnosis and treatment becomes more tailored to individual patient needs. More expensive medications, precise diagnosis, and cost-containment pressures bode well for pharmacist intervention, assuring the efficient and effective use of more sophisticated treatments. Promotional efforts are shifting from the physician to include consumers, patient advocacy groups, and other health providers, including pharmacists and nurse practitioners.

The demand for pharmaceuticals and biopharmaceuticals should accelerate as new technologies facilitate discoveries. In addition, the shifting demographics of the world population from infrequent medication users to common users of medications provide significant reason to expect growth in the pharmaceutical market that will exceed growth in the general economy. Personal enhancement and cosmetic pharmaceuticals will continue to enhance the demand outside the traditional price regulatory and cost-containment environment. Higher profitability in these areas will be associated with high promotional efforts. The private-pay and insured pharmaceutical markets will be determined by the therapeutic class of pharmaceuticals such that individual consumers will be both insured consumers and private-pay consumers based on treatment. Today, consumers are insured or not insured based on employment status or eligibility for government programs.

The future for the pharmaceutical manufacturing industry is promising and, because of its complexity, exciting.

NOTES

1. *Fortune,* April 5, 2004, p. F-26.
2. Vernon, J. The relationship between price regulation and pharmaceutical profit margins. *Applied Economics Letters.* 2003b:10:467-470.
3. Scherer, F.M. The link between gross profitability and pharmaceutical R&D spending. *Health Aff.,* (2001), 20: 216-220.
4. Public Law No. 108-173, 21 U.S.C. § 804.

Chapter 12

Drug Distribution

Sheryl L. Szeinbach
Earlene E. Lipowski

INTRODUCTION

The number of pharmaceutical products currently on the market reminds us of the intricacies and complexities of the U.S. drug distribution system. Efficient distribution increasingly relies on advances in automation, bar coding, computerized inventory systems, and information technology. Compared to other countries, distribution channels for U.S. pharmaceuticals represent one of the most complex systems available for medication processing in the world.[1] The underlying support structure for health-related products exists to ensure the delivery of pharmaceutical products to patients and health professionals throughout the United States. Manufacturers, distributors, and retailers are the major firms responsible for product supply and distribution. Manufacturers supply raw materials to develop and produce pharmaceutical products. Distributors ensure that medications, medical devices, health and beauty aids, and other products reach pharmacies and retailers in the pipeline. Retailers distribute these products to the end user or patient. Regardless of the channel used for product delivery, products gain value as they proceed through the distribution network.

As described by Porter, the value chain (see Figure 12.1) represents a collection of activities (product delivery system) performed by the manufacturers, distributors, and retailers to produce, market, deliver, and support its products.[2] The total package can be broken down into core services, which consist primarily of production and delivery functions, while facilitative or ancillary services relate to product marketing and support functions that comprise value-added services.[3,4] Thus, the value chain not only reflects company strategy and its success in maintaining a competitive advantage but also reflects value-added services that contribute to service

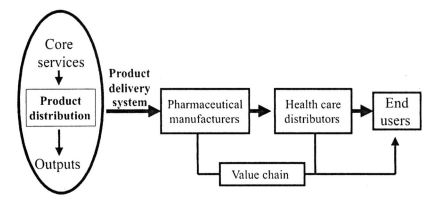

FIGURE 12.1. Customer Core Services and Value Chain for Pharmaceutical Distribution

quality as perceived by customers. The purpose of this chapter is to explore the various functions performed by these organizations regarding the distribution of pharmaceutical products. Specific issues addressed include the mechanisms used by these organizations to achieve operational efficiency, external forces affecting the distribution network, and future directions for the industry.

DISTRIBUTION AND MARKETING STRATEGY

The target of all marketing efforts is the customer. According to McCarthy and Perreault, companies maintain a competitive advantage through four strategic areas known as the marketing mix.[5] The marketing mix includes the product, place, promotion, and price of a product. Product considerations include physical features, packaging, and service. Distribution or place is concerned with all the intermediaries involved in directing the product to the appropriate target market. The product reaches the customer through established channels of distribution, as shown in Figure 12.2. Promotional efforts consist of advertising, publicizing, and selling. Pricing strategies weigh factors such as discounts, allowances, and geographic influences. Each player in the distribution channel determines which marketing mix strategy is most likely to accomplish organizational goals as well as meet the needs of its customers.

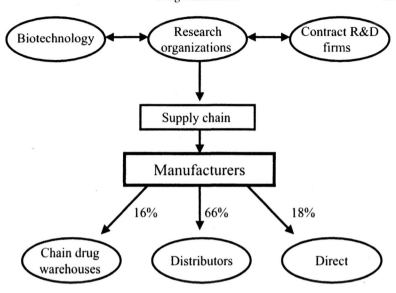

FIGURE 12.2. Distribution Network Used by Manufacturers

PHARMACEUTICAL MANUFACTURERS

The U.S. pharmaceutical industry leads the world in the discovery, development, production, and sales of drugs. The U.S. pharmaceutical industry and the $1.3 trillion health care industry account for about 13 percent of the nation's economic output. It is expected to reach 16 percent by 2010 and could exceed 20 percent by 2040.[6] In 2001, manufacturer prescription drug sales reached $174.4 billion, a 17 percent increase from 2000.[7] According to the Pharmaceutical Research and Manufacturers Association (PhRMA), it takes ten to fifteen years and an average investment of $802 million to discover and develop a new drug.[8] Prescription drugs in 2000 accounted for only about nine cents of every health care dollar, compared to six cents for administrative costs, seven cents for nursing-home care, twenty-two cents for physician services, and thirty-two cents for hospital care.[9] Drug expenditures increased 14.7 percent in 2000, primarily due to an aging population and more therapies for chronic diseases. Only 3.9 percent of the overall increase are accounted for by actual price increases.[10]

Core services for manufacturers evolve from the development of innovative products such as medications, diagnostics, biologicals, technologies, agricultural products, and household products. Support services include well-organized procurement systems to obtain raw materials, tracking programs, marketing campaigns, and educational programs.[11] As major participants in the value chain, manufacturers strive to meet customer expectations by producing high-quality and innovative products, creating positive and beneficial customer relationships, and participating in the network to improve operational efficiency through electronic support systems and electronic data exchange. Changes in health care delivery have a direct influence on pharmaceutical manufacturers and their ability to produce and supply new products (see Figure 12.3).

One aspect of change in health care delivery stems from the interaction of managed care organizations with pharmaceutical manufacturers. For example, some managed care groups, including health maintenance organizations (HMOs), preferred provider organizations (PPOs), and large employer groups negotiate directly with manufacturers. In exchange for manufacturer discounts, providers will use formularies, tiered copayments, generic substitution, cost-effectiveness studies, and drug utilization review

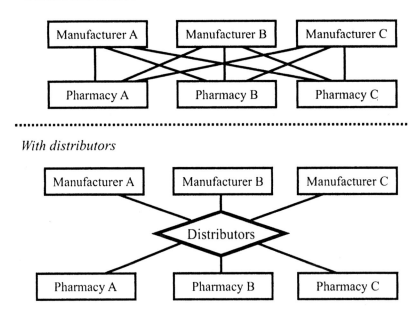

FIGURE 12.3. Value of Health Care Distributors in Reducing the Number of Transactions

to control costs internally and help shift market share to manufacturers. Other distributors and large chain stores gain discounts and rebates from manufacturers through volume purchasing. Group purchasing organizations use competitive bidding to obtain price concessions.

Despite continued changes in the health care market, the industry has more than 1,000 new medications either in human clinical trials or at the FDA awaiting approval.[12] These medications are targeted for AIDS, congestive heart failure, Alzheimer's disease, stroke, many forms of cancer, osteoarthritis, Parkinson's disease, Crohn's disease, urinary incontinence, depression, and many other conditions. Estimates from the Congressional Joint Economic Committee reveal substantial value gains of $2.4 trillion a year resulting from increased life expectancy alone.[13] The industry itself is responsible for company patient-assistance programs that provided prescription medications directly to more than 3.5 million uninsured patients in 2001, up from 1.1 million in 1997. The number of patients receiving assistance through these programs increased more than 50 percent from 1997 to 2000.[14]

HEALTH CARE DISTRIBUTORS IN THE UNITED STATES

The basic function of the drug distribution industry is providing economies of scale to ensure smooth, safe, and cost-efficient distribution of health care products. Distributors select, purchase, and store manufacturers' goods in close proximity to community and hospital pharmacies, as well as many other pharmaceutical service providers. Their core service consists of sorting functions and concentrating functions whereby goods produced by the manufacturer are distributed in economic quantities to retailers who dispense or sell the goods to the end user (see Figure 12.4). By performing this function, wholesalers are able to reduce the total number of transactions required to service the pharmaceutical distribution system. Other general services associated with distributors include storage, transportation, accounting services, financing, and bearing risk for product integrity against theft, damage, spoilage, and expiration.

In the United States, the Healthcare Distribution Management Association (HDMA) represents the firms engaged in health care distribution. Cardinal Health, McKesson, and AmerisourceBergen are the major distributors, but according to HDMA reports more than 72 distributor companies operate approximately 242 distribution centers that cover virtually all distribution needs in the United States.[15] In the past year, total aggregate sales of distributed pharmaceutical products increased by 11.1 percent from $117.7 billion in 2000 to $126.3 billion in 2001.[16] A breakdown of cus-

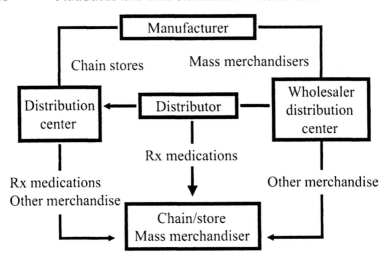

FIGURE 12.4. Distribution in Large Community Pharmacies

tomer markets reveals that 32 percent of the sales went to independent pharmacies and 26 percent went to hospitals. The trend is a reduction in sales through distributors to chain pharmacies and chain warehouses, along with an upward trend in sales through distributors to clinics, nursing homes, and mail-order pharmacy services.[17]

CONTRIBUTIONS OF THE DISTRIBUTOR INDUSTRY

Changing demographics of the U.S. population coupled with new technological advances will ensure a continued and stable role for pharmaceutical distributors. Advances in biological research and gene therapy provide additional opportunities for distributors, as these products require special handling, tracking, and maintenance procedures. As government-licensed operations, full-line distributors adhere to stringent storage and handling procedures designed to ensure the integrity of the medications they distribute. Some of these functions include

1. record keeping,
2. security,
3. temperature and humidity control,
4. returned-goods handling, and
5. emergency planning.

Examples of such materials subject to strict handling requirements include controlled substances, temperature-sensitive medications, hazardous materials, and precursor chemicals. Distributors also foresee growth as suppliers to residential facilities, specialty clinics, and alternative care programs.

Distributors offer valuable management services to their customers, including inventory control systems, staff training, facility design services, and cooperative advertising programs. Support programs of particular value in pharmacies include electronic transmission and online adjudication of third-party claims, private-label merchandise, distribution of orphan drugs; computer systems that provide patient counseling information and screen for drug-drug interactions, drug allergies, and Rx to OTC interactions.[18] Distributors provide point-of-sale (POS) scanning equipment to retail customers and are responsible for maintaining the database. Distributors also interact with third-party programs to reduce errors, improve bidding practices, and provide processing capabilities. The distributors take advantage of the latest advances in automation and economies of scale to improve the operational efficiency of individual pharmacies.

Traditionally, distributors have survived in a cost-conscious market by their ability to run highly efficient distribution operations. Their distribution operations have grown from 47 percent of the market for prescription drugs in 1970 to over 90 percent of the market today. Higher profit margins were attained several years ago with the practice of forward buying, that is, the purchase of a drug product just before a price increase. However, the composite-average gross profit margin for distributors has remained fairly steady in recent years, ranging from 4.51 to 4.16 percent between 1998 and 2001. Distributors successfully maintained profit margins by lowering expenses through efficient automation of the distributing process that relies on bar coding and computer tracking of inventory.

REPACKAGING AND PREPACKAGING

The major function of repackagers is to break down bulk products into smaller, more manageable units for distribution. Repackagers distribute medications to pharmacies, hospitals, nursing homes, mail pharmacy sites, and managed care organizations. Repackagers supply quality products to the market under similar guidelines as used by distributors, and some distributors perform a dual function as repackagers. Some of the most important functions associated with repackaged products include maintaining medication stability, National Drug Code (NDC) numbers, and expiration date.

In most countries of Europe and South America and in Australia, New Zealand, and Canada patients receive their prescription medicines in unit-of-use packaging. Unit-of-use packaging refers to "a method of preparing a legend medication in an original container, sealed and labeled, pre-labeled by the manufacturer, and containing a sufficient amount of medication for one normal course of therapy."[19] Because unit-of-use packaging is not routinely available in the United States, some outlets use prepackaging. Prepackaging is the packaging of medication using either manual labor or automated dispensing systems, where larger quantities of existing inventories from a manufacturer's original commercial container or quantities of unit-dosed drugs are repackaged into smaller quantities consistent with dosing regimens commonly prescribed by authorized health care professionals. Unit-of-use and prepackaging have the potential to save time and possibly reduce error and rework in the dispensing process.

In one small study, two teams processed fifty typical prescription orders, once using unit-of-use packaging and once by transferring medication from a bulk container. Results revealed that unit-of-use packaging reduced dispensing time by 50 percent, an average time savings of more than 27 seconds per prescription.[20] Automated dispensing of medications in unit dose or single unit-of-use packaging appears to exhibit similar outcomes with respect to time, efficiency, and meeting standards of the Joint Commission on Accreditation of Healthcare Organizations (JCAHO).[21]

In an another study, individuals representing state boards of pharmacy were contacted and asked to participate in a packaging survey covering unit-of-use, repackaging, and remote pharmacy dispensing. Of the fifty states, surveys were received from seventeen, yielding a 34 percent response rate. When asked about state requirements for prepackaging medication, respondents from twelve of the states indicated that prepackaging was allowed with existing store inventory only. A majority of the respondents believe that unit-of-use packaging would reduce errors in the dispensing process, improve patient compliance, improve patient counseling, and provide pharmacists with an average gain in time of 25 percent on a scale of 1 to 100.[22] Moreover, in some states prepackaged medication is used in remote pharmacy operations, Medicaid clinics, and in centralized filling operations.

Unit-of-use dispensing and repackaging is not totally free from challenges. Some of these challenges include insurance barriers, physician prescribing habits, patient acceptance, cross-contamination of products, and staff training. In another study by Mackowiak, patient preferences were elicited comparing plastic prescription vials or unit-of-use packaging. Results revealed that 82 percent versus 18 percent ($P < 0.001$) rated "easy to open" as the most important characteristic of prescription packaging.[23]

Questions still remain about the ability of packaging to improve patient compliance and the need to balance issues of child safety and access to medications by elderly patients who may not be able to open child-resistant packaging. Nevertheless, distributors and repackagers are working with companies that specialize in package design to provide products in packages that not only improve product handling and processing but will also provide opportunities to evaluate patient compliance. With the acceptance of unit-of-use packaging for antibiotics, corticosteriods, and oral contraceptives, trends would indicate a greater reliance on unit-dose blisters, unit-of-use packaging, strip packaging, and packages with special closures designed to track medication use.

DISTRIBUTION IN LARGE COMMUNITY PHARMACIES

Chain pharmacies (four or more stores under the same ownership) are the largest component of pharmacy practice, comprising 20,500 traditional chain drug stores and an additional 14,440 pharmacies within supermarkets and mass merchant stores.[24] Overall, the retail prescription market topped $164 billion in 2001, and chain pharmacies accounted for nearly 63 percent ($102.7 billion), mail order 16.8 percent, and independent pharmacies 20.6 percent of the total.[25] The National Association of Chain Drug Stores services 196 members of the country's largest pharmacy organizations, including traditional chain pharmacies, supermarket chains, and mass merchants. Large chain stores obtain as much as 90 to 95 percent of the prescription medications from their own distribution centers or chain warehouses and purchase the remaining 5 to 10 percent from a distributor. Chain pharmacy has also embraced the use of the Internet and online sales with more than 113 home pages affiliated with chain pharmacy companies. Sixty-seven chain pharmacies had an online pharmacy with at least the option to order refills online for pickup at the pharmacy.[26]

Mass merchandisers, as the name suggests, offer lower prices to obtain faster turnover and greater sales volume. Although prescription medications are competitively priced, the channel of distribution for these products is primarily through a wholesaler. Large, company-owned, wholesale distribution centers are reserved mostly for merchandise other than prescription medications. However, mass merchandisers and large chains have the capability at their main sites to repackage and distribute medications through separate channels, including mail pharmacy services, long-term care facilities, and clinics.

OTHER DISTRIBUTION CHANNELS

As shown in Figure 12.5, alternative distribution channels exist for hospitals and independent pharmacies. Formation of these distribution channels for hospitals was spurred in part by the federal government's adoption of a prospective system based on diagnosis-related groups (DRGs). Hospital pharmacies shifted from profit centers to cost centers with the change. Group purchasing started in the early 1990s as hospital administrators actively searched for cost-containment strategies. Hospitals turned to buying groups and prime vendor purchasing systems as a strategy to centralize purchasing and reduce costs by shifting the inventory control and management functions to drug distributors. Group purchasing organizations (e.g., Novation, Premier Purchasing Partners, VHA, MAGNET) can be divided into two broad categories depending on group membership, tax status, competition, and method of operation.[27] First, group contracting is performed if the centralized operation develops contracts for use by member institutions, which then purchase directly from the vendor at the contract prices. Second, group purchasing organizations often have a centralized management group that is responsible for negotiating, purchasing, warehousing, and distributing pharmaceuticals to the owned, leased, or managed entities. However, these two categories are not mutually exclusive, in that some buying groups not only purchase but also contract with other organizations.

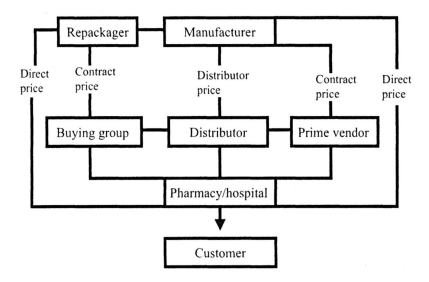

FIGURE 12.5. Alternative Distribution Channels

A prime vendor relationship is established when the hospital or other managed care organization agrees to purchase the majority of its drugs from a single source, usually a local distributor. The hospital's purchasing group uses a competitive bidding process to select the prime vendor. In pharmacy practice, group purchasing organizations may work with large chain pharmacies and independently owned pharmacies to contract for multisource and brand-name pharmaceuticals, durable medical equipment, diagnostic kits, optical, and home care products. Group purchasing in a managed care organization will be accomplished through competitive bidding for the pharmacies that provide prescription services for plan enrollees. With third parties accounting for about 80 percent of the pharmacy payments, contract negotiation is typically accomplished at the corporate level through various managed care organizations and other providers (Figure 12.6). Prescription processing is performed by pharmacy benefit management companies or PBMs (e.g., Merck-Medco Managed Care, Advance PCS, Express Scripts), which currently process over 50 percent of all community retail prescriptions in the United States.

Internet pharmacies, also known as cyberpharmacy, online pharmacy, e-pharmacy, and virtual pharmacy/drugstores, continue to increase in number as consumers seek more competitive prices and greater convenience.[28] The typical product mix includes prescription drugs, nonprescription drugs and herbal products, health and beauty aids, drug information, physician

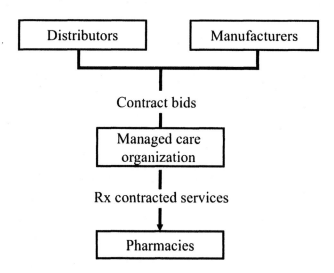

FIGURE 12.6. Distribution in a Managed Care Organization

consultation fees, consumer health information, and others.[29] Estimates of the number of Internet pharmacy sites range between 500 and 600, and consist of four major types:

1. traditional chain pharmacies with a Web presence;
2. independent community pharmacies with a Web presence;
3. stand-alone, exclusive pharmacy sites; and
4. "rogue" pharmacy sites.[30]

Internet sites offer advantages such as twenty-four-hour availability, anonymity, online access to personalized medication records, delivery services, and direct price comparisons. Alternatively, these sites may not accept all types of third-party insurance plans.[31] Concerns include the use of information and system security, medication quality and integrity, and the inability to ascertain whether licensed practitioners are dispensing drugs or providing consultations.[32] Most important, however, is the notion that some medications, including potentially dangerous substances and controlled medications, are readily available through some rogue sites. Without appropriate regulations, Internet pharmacies may undermine the safe and appropriate use of medicines because the organization and support functions usually considered necessary to quality care appear to be largely absent.[33] As these sites gain in popularity, a concerted effort is needed by national and international pharmacy leaders to address issues related to the quality, integrity, and safety of medications dispensed from online pharmacy sites.

The National Association of Boards of Pharmacy (NABP) has developed a program to certify the quality of online pharmacies—the Verified Internet Pharmacy Practice Sites (VIPPS®) Program.[34] To meet VIPPS certification standards, the pharmacy must comply with the licensing regulations of the state where it is located, as well as the states to which they dispense medications.[35] Only 22 pharmacies currently have the VIPPS seal of approval (as of October 2004), and consumers should be advised to check for this rating before using online Internet pharmacy services.

AVAILABILITY AND DISTRIBUTION OF GENERIC DRUGS

U.S. generic drugs now account for about 44 to 48 percent of the total drug market. Generics are drug products that compare to the pioneer reference drug product in dosage form, strength, route of administration, quality, and performance characteristics. Sales, estimated at approximately $11 billion in 2001, could double by 2006.[36-38] A record number of widely prescribed, brand-name drugs are expected to lose patent protection between now and 2005.[39] These blockbuster medications coming off patent generate worldwide revenues ranging from $1 billion to approximately $6 billion a year. Over the next decade, drugs with $41 billion in current sales will lose patent protection.[40] The average price of a generic drug in 2001 was about $22 compared with just over $71 for a brand-name product.[41] Generic drug use is increasing, the cost of some generics is rising by as much as 22 percent, compared to 10 percent for brand-name drugs. Yet for price-conscious and managed care customers, generics represent a dramatically better value at approximately one-third the cost of brand-name products.

Distribution channels for generic drugs follow similar pathways as previously presented; however, the pathways may be more dynamic and complex. Manufacturers may distribute drug products containing their own designated label, a private label, or a label supplied from another contracted manufacturer to a distributor who handles generics or to a manufacturer with distribution capabilities. The major distribution centers that receive products include warehousing chains, wholesalers, and smaller distributors. Other customers include independent pharmacies, hospitals, buying groups, nursing homes, the government, and repackagers.

OTHER TRENDS IN DISTRIBUTION

The U.S. health care market relies extensively on new and innovative technology to transform both the business and home environments. Broadly defined, technology in the workplace is how an organization transforms its inputs into outputs, thereby accomplishing its goals. Technology can be classified in two broad categories: those relating to the organization's operations, materials, and knowledge and those called information technologies. Operations technology includes robotics, automated dispensing systems, electronic rail systems, and pneumatic tubes.[42] For pharmacy, this process is producing dramatic revolutions in the way medications are processed and distributed from point A to point Z.

Advanced information technologies are devices that transmit, manipulate, analyze, or exploit information; digital computers that process information integral to the user's communication task of decision making; and complex computerized programs that have appeared on the market since 1970.[43] In general, four trends have been noted:

1. rapid development of software to support patient care activities,
2. increased software integration,
3. shortened computer life cycles, and
4. increased use of electronic data interchange.[44]

In pharmacy practice, these information technologies include the use of computer software for automated medication delivery systems, reminder systems, record keeping, financial analysis, inventory control, drug use control, and support of clinical services. Also included are computer-assisted communication technologies that support the growth of telemedicine and telepharmacy (e.g., electronic mail, electronic prescribing, expert systems, information retrieval systems, computer conferencing, videoconferencing, and devices used to transmit images) that establish intraorganizational and interorganizational links.[45,46]

ACHIEVING OPERATIONAL EFFICIENCY
THROUGH AUTOMATION

The ability to transform loosely coupled health care organizations into an integrated health care network of providers is contingent upon the use of technology. These technologies are likely to be used by group purchasing organizations and providers to manage the cost of medical therapy. These organizations will opt for more integrated operations with connections among many departments in a hospital or managed care setting. The major advantage of automated dispensing and monitoring systems is the ability of these systems to proactively monitor patients' medication use through advanced notification systems and through integrated networks rather than reactively waiting until the patient enters the pharmacy. Automated dispensing technologies will improve operational efficiency and increase the time available for professional interaction.[47-49]

Bar coding is spurring the adoption and use of automated dispensing technology. Hospital groups and patient-safety advocates urged the Food and Drug Administration to speed up efforts to require supermarket-style bar codes on drugs and other medical products, citing a growing body of evidence that such systems can cut medical errors in hospitals by as much as 75 percent and increase accuracy of filled orders to nearly 100 percent.[50-52] Efforts are currently underway to mandate the use of bar codes for human drug products and biological products and for unit-of-use packaging.[53,54]

There is widespread agreement that bar coding and other computer-based technologies can help; however, according to some estimates it will cost the health care industry as much as $1.5 billion to incorporate the technology.[55] Some of the barriers relate to the ability of the pharmaceutical manufacturers to change the way they package medication for hospitals; that is, to bar code medications by unit dose. Alternatively, many hospitals convert bulk medications to smaller units by repackaging and prepackaging medications for dispensing in an inpatient setting.[56] Bar coding would reduce the number of errors and ensure that medications can be verified and recorded as they are administered.

Shown in Table 12.1 are automated dispensing systems that would serve the needs of hospitals, community pharmacies, and facilities specializing in long-term care. These systems also service managed care organizations that have larger prescription volumes (e.g., mail pharmacy services, hospitals, repackagers, HMOs, and PPOs). These systems usually cost less than $400,000, and several units can be linked together to dispense larger volumes of medication. Space requirements are minimal as many of these systems occupy less than 100 square feet.[57]

CONCLUSION

Technology is influencing the integration and alignment of organizations in the managed care environment. Apropos to the issue of integration is the need for leaders in pharmacy to work with other health care providers, software companies, and companies whose function is to develop new dispensing technologies. Efforts to integrate the system for health care delivery will lead to process improvement, channel and operational efficiency, and customer satisfaction.

TABLE 12.1. Automated Systems Designed to Dispense Tablets or Capsules

Equipment	Automated for pour/ count/fill	Unit of use	No of SKUs	Estimated cost[a]
McKesson/Baker Cell	No	N/A	48	To $1,000/ month (lease only)
McKesson/APS AutoScript III	Yes	Yes	210	$350,000 to $535,000
Innovation/ PharmASSIST	No	N/A	50	$40,000
PickPoint/FlexRx	No	Yes	121	$25,000
ScriptPro/SP200	Yes	Yes	250	$200,000
ScriptPro/SPUD	No	Yes	300	$200,000
ADDS/RCDS	No	Yes	90	$55,000
Automed/Quickscript	Yes	Yes	250	$200,000
Automed/Consis 2X2	No	Yes	330	$200,000
Cardinal/Pyxis Medstations	No	Yes	200+	$70,000

[a]Prices subject to vary with respect to specific need.

NOTES

1. Huttin, C. The distribution of pharmaceuticals: An international survey. *Journal of Social and Administrative Pharmacy* 1989; 6(4): 184-196.

2. Porter, M.E. *Competitive advantages: Creating and sustaining superior performance* (New York: The Free Press, Macmillan, 1985).

3. Gronroos, C. *Service management and marketing* (Lexington, MA: Lexington Books, 1990).

4. Ozment, J. and Morash, E.A. The augmented service offering for perceived and actual service quality. *Journal of the Academy of Marketing Science* 1994; 22(4): 352-363.

5. McCarthy, J.E. and Perreault, W. *Basic marketing: A global-management approach* (Homewood, IL: Irwin, 1993).

6. Pharmaceutical Research and Manufacturers of America. *2002 Industry Profile* (Washington, DC: PhRMA, 2002).

7. National Association of Chain Drug Stores. *The Chain Pharmacy Industry Profile, 2002* (Alexandria, VA: NACDS, 2002).

8. Pharmaceutical Research and Manufacturers of America, *2002 Industry Profile.*

9. Ibid.

10. Ibid.

11. Szeinbach, S.L., Barnes, J.H., Blackwell, S.A., Horine, J.E., and Vandewalle, J. The quest for value. *Pharmaceutical Executive* 1999; 19(1): 94-100.

12. National Association of Chain Drug Stores, *The Chain Pharmacy Industry Profile, 2002.*

13. National Institutes of Health. A plan to ensure taxpayers' interests are protected. NIH response to the conference report for a plan to ensure taxpayers' interests are protected. July 2001. Available online at <http://www.nih.gov/news/070101 wyden.htm>.

14. General Accounting Office. Prescription Drugs: Drug Company Programs Help Some People Who Lack Coverage (Washington DC: GAO, 2000).

15. *2002 HDMA Industry Profile and Healthcare Factbook* (Healthcare Distribution Management Association, 2002).

16. Ibid.

17. Ibid.

18. National Institutes of Health, A plan to ensure taxpayers' interests are protected.

19. National Association of Boards of Pharmacy. *Task Force on Pharmacy Manpower Shortage, 1999-2000 committee and task force reports* (Chicago: National Association of Boards of Pharmacy, 2000).

20. Lipowski, E.E., Campbell, D.E., Brushwood, D.B., and Wilson, D. Time savings associated with dispensing unit-of-use packages. *Journal of the American Pharmaceutical Association* 2002; 42(4): 577-581.

21. Garrelts, J.C., Koehn, L., Snyder, V., Snyder, R., and Rich, D.S. Automated medication distribution systems and compliance with Joint Commission standards. *American Journal of Health-System Pharmacy* (USA) 2001; 58(December 1): 2267-2272.

22. Szeinbach, S.L., Baron, M., Guschke, T., and Torkilson, E. Survey of state requirements for unit-of-use packaging. *American Journal of Health-System Pharmacy* 2003; 60: 1863-1866.

23. Mackowiak, E.D. Unit-of-use packaging: Will it contribute to patients' therapeutic outcomes? *Journal of Managed Pharmaceutical Care* 2002; 1(3): 47-60.

24. National Association of Chain Drug Stores, *The Chain Pharmacy Industry Profile, 2002.*

25. Ibid.

26. Ibid.

27. Crawford, S.Y. Internet pharmacy: Issues of access, quality, costs, and regulation. *Journal of Medical Systems* 2003; 27(1): 57-65.

28. Ibid.

29. Lingle, V.A. Prescription drug services on the Internet. *Health Care Internet* 2001; 5(1): 39-54.

30. Ibid.

31. Landis, N.T. Virtual pharmacies boast easy access, privacy safeguards. *American Journal of Health-System Pharmacy* 1999; 56(6): 500-501.

32. Rice, B. The growing problem of online pharmacies. *Journal of Medical Economics* 2001; 78(11): 40-45.

33. Bessell, T.L., Silagy, C.A., Anderson, J.N., et al. Quality of global e-pharmacies: Can we safeguard consumers? *European Journal of Clinical Pharmacology* 2002; 58: 567-572.

34. National Association of Boards of Pharmacy. VIPPS certification process. Available online at <http://www.nabp.net/vipps/pharmacy/intro.asp>.

35. Ibid.

36. National Association of Chain Drug Stores, *The Chain Pharmacy Industry Profile, 2002.*

37. Wetrich, J.G. Group purchasing: An overview. *American Journal of Hospital Pharmacy* 1987; 44 (July): 1581-1592.

38. Buckley, B. Generic drugs are poised to take greater market share. *Drug Store News* August 20, 2001.

39. Meyer, G.F. History and regulatory issues of generic drugs. *Transplantation Proceedings* 1999; 31(Suppl 3A): 10S-12S.

40. Wetrich, Group purchasing.

41. National Association of Chain Drug Stores, *The Chain Pharmacy Industry Profile, 2002.*

42. Kirking, D.M., Ascione, F.J., Gaither, C.A, and Welage, L.S. Economics and structure of the generic pharmaceutical industry. *Journal of the American Pharmacists Association* 2001; 41: 578-584.

43. Szeinbach, S.L. Defining automation. *ComputerTalk* 1994; 14(6): 17.

44. Huber, G.P. A theory of the effects of advanced information technologies organization design, intelligence, and decision making. *Academy of Management Review* 1990; 15(1): 47-71.

45. West, D.S. and Szeinbach, S.L. Information technology and pharmaceutical care. *Journal of the American Pharmacists Association* 1997; NS37: 1-5.

46. West, D.S. and Szeinbach, S.L. Prescription technologies: Keeping pace. *Journal of the American Pharmacists Association* 2002; 42(1): 21-25.

47. Schiff, G.D. and Rucker, T.D. Computerized prescribing: Building the electronic infrastructure for better medication usage. *Journal of the American Medical Association* 1998; 279:1024-1029.

48. Carmenates, J. and Keith, M.R. Impact of automation on pharmacist interventions and medication errors in a correctional health care system. *American Journal of Health-System Pharmacy* 2001; 58(May 1): 779-783.

49. Glassman, P.A., Simon, B., Belperio, P., and Lanto, A. Improving recognition of drug interactions: Benefits and barriers to using automated drug alerts. *Medical Care* 2002; 40(12): 1161-1171.

50. Keeys, C.A., Dandurand, K., Harris, J., Gbadamosi, L., King, J., et al. Providing nighttime pharmaceutical services telepharmacy. *American Journal of Health-System Pharmacy* 2002; 59(8): 716-721.

51. Carmenates, J. and Keith, M.R., Impact of automation on pharmacist interventions and medication errors.

52. McCreadie, S.R., Stumpf, J.L., and Benner, T.D. Building a better online formulary. *American Journal of Health-System Pharmacy* 2002; 59(19): 1847-1852.

53. Marietti, C. Robots hooked on drugs: Robotic automation expands pharmacy services. 1997; 14(11): 37-38,40,42.

54. Allen, D. Bar coding unit-dose blisters. *Pharmaceutical & Medical Packaging News* 2002; (February): 22-28.

55. Landro, L. FDA is urged to hasten effort to require bar codes on drugs. *The Wall Street Journal,* online, Monday, July 29, 2002.

56. Healthcare Information and Management Systems Society (HIMSS) Fact Sheet. Bar coding for patient safety, March, 2003. <http://himss.org>.

57. Szeinbach, S.L., Taylor, T., and Gillenwater, E.L. Automated dispensing technologies: Effect on managed care. *Journal of Managed Care Pharmacy* 1995: 1(2):121-127.

Chapter 13

The Consumers of Health Care

Somnath Pal
Damary Castanheira Torres
Maria Marzella Sulli

The transition from medical care to health care during the 1990s led Americans to view a medically oriented, physician-dominated health care system to be incredibly antiquated. An imperfect relationship exists between the need for health care services and the demand for health care services. Many consumers who need health care services do not consume them, while others with little need consume a large amount. Another factor that confounds our understanding of the health care consumer relates to the existence of "third-party" entities that serve as an intermediary between the health care consumer and the point of service. To a great extent, the decision to purchase is not made by the end user (the consumer) but by a third party. Historically, this "gatekeeper" has been the physician who officially declared the individual as "sick," ordered the tests, ordered hospitalization, prescribed drugs, and scheduled follow-up visits. In a system that has been physician-dominated, this is an important consideration. Convention held that the consumer was to trust the doctor with his or her life, and this meant turning over most consumption decisions to this "gatekeeper." Recently, the physician has been joined by other decision makers, namely the third-party payers. Third-party payers, such as insurance companies, managed care programs, government health care financing agencies, and, increasingly, employers have begun taking a more active role in decision making when it comes to health care consumption. Like the physician, these decision makers take the process out of the hands of the end user.

In the twenty-first century, health is referred to as overall well-being, including physical, mental, and social elements, rather than being free from illness. Health care is no longer viewed as an exclusive territory reserved for physicians but is viewed as an effort in which patients and their families continue to be involved. As a result of this broadening notion of health care, components that were of secondary importance in the past, such as prevention, health education, and rehabilitation, continue to gain recognition. All through the 1980s, health care providers played key roles in the transition from product-centered care to patient-centered care. Health care providers started designing products with a specific market sector in mind, based on the needs and wants of consumers rather than making it "one size fits all."

THE DEFINITION OF THE HEALTH CARE CONSUMER

Since the 1970s, this country has undergone a consumer health movement. Many factors play into this movement, and the result has been patients that take a greater role in their care. This can translate into changing relationships between the providers of health care (physicians, nurses, pharmacists) and the consumers, or patients. Basically, the relationship is between someone in need of a service that involves skill and sensitivity and someone who is capable of fulfilling that need. The way in which the person in need is labeled automatically implies how they are viewed by the caregiver. Do we define these individuals as customers, patrons, clients, or patients? A customer or patron is described as a person who purchases a product or nonprofessional service such as groceries or a new suit. These two terms are used interchangeably and carry a sort of nonprofessional connotation. A client is basically described as a customer of professional services. Lawyers and accountants have "clients," essentially customers that desire professional services. "Patients" are serviced by health care providers, and are defined as individuals awaiting or under medical care or treatment. Essentially, the patient and the consumer are one and the same when one discusses the health care system. As health care professionals, we have a responsibility to meet the needs of the patient (i.e., always having the patient's best interests in mind and making decisions clinically and ethically beneficial to the patient). However, in today's health care marketplace, one also has to keep in mind the role of patients as consumers or customers, meaning that the services they need can be enhanced and marketed with services they want. The health care marketplace is growing, and more and more competition exists. In addition, the health care marketplace has changed in that there are fewer independent providers. Institutions are merging into health care conglomerates, physicians are working for these conglomerates, and managed care often dictates what services patients are eligible for and where they can go to receive them.

Because of new health care discoveries and focus on chronic illnesses, health care is experiencing a shift toward wellness. This trend provides health care professionals not just with sick "patients" but also with consumers seeking products and services to maintain health and prevent disease.

The availability of products and services for disease screening and prevention offers new options for providers and consumers. Much of the decision-making process leans on the consumer now because of the focus on prevention. Decisions about what to eat, whether to exercise, how to exercise, whether to supplement the diet with vitamins, minerals, and alternative medicine all come from the person seeking to maintain health, not necessarily from the health care professional treating them. This affects how health care professionals offer services and what services they provide. Pharmacists are focusing their services on management of medication therapy and health, because that is what the consumers are looking for. Even consumers are realizing that the more information there is out there, the more they need someone to help sort it out. Pharmacists are attempting to fill that void. Other services pharmacists are adding to meet the changing role of the consumer are the addition of health foods and a focus on supplements, as well as capitalizing on the holistic approach to health—selling candles; aromatherapy; referring patients to services such as hypnosis, physical therapy, massage; and others. Pharmacies are also providing services in the area of health screenings. In states where pharmacists are permitted under their scope of practice they are offering osteoporosis, diabetes, and cholesterol screenings and educating customers on the importance of knowledge in these areas.

One of the most important trends over the past decade has been the shift from inpatient to outpatient care, expanding the role of the patient in decision making. There are a lot more choices for outpatient services than for inpatient services and fewer restrictions placed by third-party payers. Doctors are likely to choose their patients' hospital, but the patients themselves choose the doctors, the fitness programs they join, the diet programs they use, weight-reduction programs, counseling, lifestyle management, stress management, birthing classes, and a variety of other health services that do not necessarily involve hospitals and physicians.

WHY THE SHIFT TOWARD CONSUMERISM?

Historically, patients followed doctors' orders, but the consciousnes of the right to know all about one's body has created consumers who seek information as well as care.[1] The information available to the consumer is unending, with magazines, television, books, and the Internet bursting with health-based information.

Every medical specialty has undergone phenomenal change over the past two decades, leading to the evolution of the integrated health care delivery systems, in which the hospitals have become more or less latent in comparison with other sectors of the health care economy.[2] Opportunities for innovation and entrepreneurship in health care during the twenty-first century will exceed anything we have seen in the past two decades. Most of the innovative changes have so far been among the huge number of product- and service-oriented health care companies.[3] The Internet, telehealth, and new clinical information technology will begin to drive strategy and market structure. The Internet has already changed health care practice and has begun to sway pharmaceutical consumers and providers. Sophisticated database capabilities helped to match market segments to the service mix. A possible negative side effect of this process is that health care providers will be able to carefully target the audiences they want, while avoiding the ones they do not want. This could mean that a larger number of patients will be left without easily accessible care. For the hospitals, medical groups, physician networks, pharmacies, and health plans to prosper, they must adopt a new character of novelty in their service components.[4]

Advanced Medical Technology and Health Care Consumers

Genetic research, new drugs, and medical technology will cause acceleration in both innovation and costs. Largely because of genetic research, the number of new drugs will grow rapidly; they will be effective, highly sought after by consumers, and expensive. Evidences of the impact of new technology can be seen in such inventions as laparoscopic surgery and laser eye surgery, and dozens of other technological advances are in the pipeline. The consumers will become better informed and more demanding.

The shift toward consumerism is accompanied by demands for higher-quality care, better access, and substantial improvements in service. More and more, consumers will do their homework (via the Internet, through review of direct-marketing materials, or through consumer buying groups) before they see their health care providers. In the future, the innovative health care system will come not from a single source (such as, in the past, the introduction of Diagnosis-Related Groups) but from multiple sources, including the growing role of consumers and technology. From the entrepreneur's perspective, things could not be better—the greater the number and extent of changes, the more attractive the opportunities. Consumers, for their part, will be pleased with the results. If technology dominates and consumers take charge, many health care leaders and their organizations will be compelled—if they are to survive and prosper—to make quick changes to keep pace with the dynamic, ever-changing health care marketplace of the future. All these factors suggest that change is taking shape, driven by the increasing power of consumers.[5] Cost-containment pressures will coexist with growth pressures.

Changes in Consumers' Perception of Health Care

As a society, Americans have been reevaluating many standards that relate to health care. The increasing involvement of consumers in the health care they and their families receive is in part due to a change in their perception. Studies have revealed that the Americans dislike managed care but are pleased with the services of the health care providers, especially the physicians and the pharmacists.[6] The role of health care consumer implies greater asymmetry and power differential in the relationship with a health professional. The role of health care provider implies certain obligations and privileges based on the requirements of becoming a member of a health profession. Due to the extensive education and training period necessary to gain the specialized knowledge required to practice a profession, society grants a great deal of autonomy and self-regulation to the professions. Health care consumers in turn expect the professional practitioner to act ethically.[7] Specifically, the professional must act in a manner that places the patient's welfare above any self-interest or benefit, that will do no harm to the patient (nonmaleficence), and that will help the patient to meet his or her needs (beneficence). The professional is also expected to treat patients in a fair and equitable manner (justice), be truthful with patients in providing information about their health status and treatment (veracity), and respect the confidentiality of each patient. In exchange for meeting these obligations of practice, the professional is granted the authority (cultural and social) necessary to care for patients.

Americans do not hesitate to express their discontent at the spiraling costs of health care. They have come to consider health care as a right but at the same time have become more realistic about their ability to pay for it. These health care consumers realize that no matter what, they have to pay more, and so in return look forward to having control over the choice of their own health plans, physicians, hospitals, and pharmacists.[8] Many have become somewhat disenchanted with technology and, in terms of health care, are looking for a little less high tech and a little more high touch. This goes to show that health care consumers are progressively demanding greater freedom of choice primarily due to the changes in their perceptions of health care.[9]

Consumers' Perception Leading to Incongruities

Incongruity was created when consumers were not willing to pay for health care services for which the provider encumbered cost. So, some entrepreneurs aggressively acted to fill the void between reality and the perception of consumers by venturing into the creation of the health maintenance organizations (HMOs). On one hand, health care consumers resist HMOs for restricting their freedom of choice, but on the other hand, when the plans give them an option to go outside the network for differential copay, an overwhelming number of consumers do not exercise that option. Health care administrators and the employers (who are paying the premiums for health care coverage for their employees) are attempting to contain cost by monitoring drug/service utilization. Without relying on giving incentives to the providers, some elements of motivation need to be incorporated into the health plans so that the consumers will demonstrate more cost-effective behavior.

Another incongruity is that, even as employers try to reduce their costs of health care coverage for employees and their families, many consumers are willing to pay significantly more for what they regard as better coverage and more user-friendly care. Thus, the next wave of health care change may well include "premium-priced packages"—offerings of very comprehensive coverage (after high deductibles) matched with accessible and attentive customer service and high-quality providers.

WHERE DO CONSUMERS MOST OFTEN GET THEIR HEALTH INFORMATION?

Direct-to-Consumer Advertising

Since the Food and Drug Administration published guidelines for direct-to-consumer (DTC) broadcast advertising in 1997, consumers have been exposed to advertisements for prescription medications in newspapers, magazines, billboards, and television. Spending on DTC advertising rose from $17 million in 1985 to $2.5 billion in 2000.[10] However, the consumer cannot purchase prescription medications without authorization of a prescriber; in most cases, a physician. So, in addition to detailing physicians on the benefits of their products, manufacturers hope that by informing the general public about the products available they will prompt sales. Money is spent on advertising a product that people would have to convince a physician or other health care provider to prescribe for them, or identify the presence of a condition they have never been diagnosed with based on an advertisement. This can cause deterioration in the patient-provider relationship, as clinicians become annoyed with answering questions from patients derived from DTC advertising.[11]

DTC ads are also used to dispel myths about a condition and minimize the embarrassment associated with certain conditions through information sharing and destigmatization. This can benefit patients who might otherwise be intimidated to share embarrassing symptoms with their health care provider.

Overall, DTC has changed the way patients feel about health care. It has created a more informed consumer, empowering patients to play more of a role in the choice of medication they use.[12]

Use of the Internet by Health Care Consumers

The Internet is another modern means of patient/consumer empowerment. It provides a wealth of information to consumers in an easily accessible format. It increases the consumer's ability to self-treat conditions, by offering information on symptoms and illness, and the ability to purchase products through Internet pharmacies. The disadvantage to this plethora of readily available information is the likelihood that the information is incorrect, misleading, biased, medically unproven, or even dangerous. It has been reported that Web sites failed to mention major safety warnings of medications listed on their sites in over 30 percent of cases.[13] As health care providers, pharmacists need to be aware of reputable medical Web sites so they can guide their patients toward them when they are seeking information. The most widely trusted sites are those that are published by the government, national organizations, or medical universities.[14]

To accurately assess how the Internet affects consumerism in health care, we need to understand who is using the Internet for health care information and what type of information they are searching for. To examine how patients with chronic illnesses use the Internet, Millard and Fintak conducted a survey of over 10,000 Americans.[15] The questions were how the use of the Internet replaced or supplemented health care contacts, how online behaviors varied by disease state and demographics, and which sources of information were most valued and reputable. The conditions that most often spurred searches were allergies, arthritis, and hypertension. Patients in poorer health were more likely to spend more time on the Internet looking for health information, as were the uninsured. These results are not surprising considering that patients may go to the Internet when they are frustrated with their current care for chronic illness and access to care is difficult because of a rural location or lack of insurance coverage.

The Internet also serves as a tremendous resource for providers, enabling information sharing from all over the world, remote access to references and databases, and providing the opportunity for telemedicine and tele-pharmacy. Telemedicine has been defined as the use of electronic informa-tion and communications technologies to provide and support health care when distance separates the participants.[16] Technically, pharmacists have been providing telemedicine services for years, by answering questions and communicating with physicians via telephone and fax. With the Internet, pharmacists are able to receive prescriptions electronically, communicate with patients in a more efficient manner, and have information at their fin-gertips with the click of a mouse. This all serves to streamline the process of delivering pharmaceutical services, something that is highly necessary in this era of increasing prescription volume and shortage of pharmacists. A limitation of using the Internet to provide telemedicine is that patients may be reluctant to share information due to questionable security and confiden-tiality practices.[17]

In conclusion, the Internet has empowered consumers to learn more about the illnesses they have, the treatments that are available, and the pro-viders from which they can choose. We have only begun to appreciate how large an effect the Internet will have on our practice as pharmacists, with more and more innovations reaching us daily.

CHANGING DEMOGRAPHICS
OF HEALTH CARE CONSUMERS

The demographic change distressing the American health care system has been the noteworthy increase in the health care expenditures among those over sixty-five years of age.[18]

The aging of the population is greatly affecting home health care, hospi-tals, and long-term care organizations (including assisted living facilities and nursing homes). In turn, this provides an opportunity for the health care providers to be innovative in repackaging their products and/or services to meet the specific needs and expectations of the specific subgroups.[19] One such subgroup could be the elderly with high income and significant accumulated wealth.

Impact of Aging

Human development is a continuous transition from one state to the next. Age is a key variable in categorizing life stages when transition into a differ-ent stage occurs. [20] To better comprehend the reasons why people behave in a certain way when it comes to health care, we must understand the theories of aging. These theories provide the background information for observed patterns of perceptions and compliance behaviors. Since more than one explanation is probable, more than one theory can be used to explain age-related multifactorial health care behavior. Each person ages in a different way and so one person's behavior cannot be explained the same way as another person's behavior just because they happen to have matching age, analogous experiences, or the same disease. So, in order to study health care behavior one must be familiar with individual differences in aging, that is, *chronological, psychological,* and *social.* [21]

Chronological Aging

Chronological aging refers to the changes in the ability to function due to changes in cells and tissues, causing wear and tear of the biological system and its subsystems and propensity to morbidity and mortality. Thus, chronological aging can be attributed to natural changes and/or outcome of a disease.[22] Chronological aging is also likely to bring variation to the health care needs of the individual. This in turn can impinge on health care behavior, predominantly in later life.[23,24] For example, with increasing age, consumers may encounter difficulty reading the fine print on drug labels and/or opening medication bottles.[25]

Health care providers need to repackage or develop products or services to compensate for the effects of chronological aging. For example, dispense medications in non-child-resistant capped bottles, encourage the use of "pill-boxes" to serve as reminders to take the medications, set up an automated system to mail out reminder cards for refills as they fall due, or change the pharmacy store layout to make it easier for the elderly to identify and remove products from the shelves.[26] Several other aspects of health care consumption in later life can be examined from a biological or geriatric point of view. For example, preferences for certain services and health care products (e.g., disposable underwear for those who suffer from incontinence, dietary foods for those who suffer from diabetes) can be predicted rather accurately from health statistics on the aged population.

Psychological Aging

Psychological aging refers to constant change in cognition (ability to think and reason, i.e., mental activities) and personality. Comprehending changes in the cognitive abilities of the consumer would help the health care providers to better understand the people's capability to process information and their responsiveness to persuasion.[27] The processing-resource theorists have concluded that our mental activities require varying amounts of cognitive resources, which show a wide individual variation. Such resource variations principally depend on the stage of life an individual is in.[28] However, longitudinal studies suggest that it is possible to continuously improve existing cognitive skills and acquire compensatory and new cognitive skills throughout life.[29,30]

Such improvements may be through higher education, increased societal roles, or enhancement in the level of intellectual stimulation in one's setting (e.g., learning to use a digital sphygmomanometer or home diagnostic devices). Factors such as lifestyle and familiarity and interest in technological products have been found to be good predictors of the older person's embracing of such innovations.[31]

The cognitive personality theory defines personality as the interaction of the environment and the individual's perceptions of reality within social constraints.[32] Thus, it may be said that personality is the outcome of the individual's coping strategies, the features of the environment, and social competence or incompetence. Because the theory is concerned with the individual's way of perceiving reality and responding in a manner consistent with his or her own perceptions, this theory comes closest to explaining behaviors of health care consumers than other personality theories of aging.

For example, the motive toward achieving consistency within one's overall conceptualization of self can be traced to the publications on self-concept. Rosenberg suggests that the persistence of the self-consistency motive is so strong that it gets in the way of the change of self-views developed in early life, even though such views are not considered acceptable by others, such as thinking young and not "acting one's age."[33] This self-consistency motive explains the propensity to use products and services (such as antiaging skin creams, health spas, and cosmetic surgery) aimed at helping the aging person maintain his or her youthful image. The self-consistency motive can also be held responsible for the failure of products such as Affinity shampoo (created in the early 1980s to deal with the problems of over-forty hair) and Kellogg's 40+ cereal. Examples of implications of the self-consistency motive cited by Dychtwald and Flower include: packaging of products and/or services to segments defined by cognitive age rather than by chronological age. Such packaging of health care products and/or services can be developed without having to deal with consumers' psychological acceptance or rejection of their chronological age. Furthermore, consumer researchers could identify health care products that are associated with older age as well as products and brand names that are age-irrelevant and promote positive self-image. Such research could help marketers better position their products and services to appeal to the aging population. [34]

What if mental decline did not have to be a natural consequence of aging? What if part of the secret to staying sharp lies in the foods we eat? Emerging evidence suggests that getting enough of certain nutrients—namely iron, zinc, and B vitamins—may help stave off the cognitive decline seen with aging, possibly even Alzheimer's and dementia.

To predict health care consumer behavior, other doctrines of the cognitive personality theory could also be used. For example, perceived decline in social competence due to physiological changes may create the need to remain independent. The motive to remain independent as well as other psychological motives (e.g., security) could be used to explain health care behavior. Schewe shows how such information could benefit marketers and advertisers and gives several examples of product positioning and advertising appeals that could be developed for the older health care consumer market.[35]

Social Aging

Social aging refers to

1. changes in social relationships that define social status within a society (e.g., married versus single) and
2. various roles people are expected to play at various stages in life (e.g., children, couples, parents, grandparents).

Such changes are likely to affect a wide range of health care consumers, including buying role in later life and normative expectations (e.g., acceptance of senior discounts).

Interrelationship of the Concepts of Aging

The three concepts of aging (namely, chronological, psychological, and social aging) are independent of one another and therefore useful not only in directly addressing various aspects of health care behavior in later life but also in helping us understand the indirect impact of a given type of aging on health care behavior via its effects on other forms of aging. Chronological aging can affect both psychological as well as social aging. It may limit psychological growth (although there is no evidence of universal age-related decline of cognition, or disintegration of the emotional system or structure of personality) and could cause early retirement and social withdrawal, contributing to the person's social aging.[36-39]

Psychological aging can affect both chronological and social aging; for example, depression can lead to poor eating habits, which affect the person's biological system and its ability to fight disease.[40] Depression can also lead to withdrawal and social isolation, that is, social detachment. Finally, social aging has implications for chronological and psychological aging. For example, social isolation can alter food-consumption habits, directly affecting nutrition, which relates to disease, and indirectly affecting the person's psychological state.[41]

In summary, the three aging processes are relevant to the study of health care behavior because they produce certain changes that are either directly related to health care behavior, such as ability to process information, or they relate to factors such as personality and self-concept, which influence consumer behavior. Thus, it can be concluded that a model of aging and health care behavior should take into account not only the various perspectives on aging but also how the various types of aging relate to health care behavior, directly or indirectly.

BEHAVIORAL MODELS
IN THE PATIENT-PRACTITIONER RELATIONSHIP

Sociologists, psychologists, and other social scientists have been interested in the client- or patient-professional relationship for many years, particularly the doctor-patient interaction.[42-47] Three basic, generic models of the patient-provider relationship can be placed along a continuum of responsibility for health-related decisions (see Figure 13.1).

In the oldest, the paternalistic model, the health professional is viewed as the expert in medical (and often times nonmedical and moral) matters. The paternalistic health professional knows what is best for the patient. This model assumes that the health care provider will make all major decisions for the patient, and the patient is expected to rely on the wisdom and beneficence of the expert, much as a young child depends on his or her parents. Proponents of this model can often be detected by such phrases as, "speaking as your pharmacist (nurse, physician), I believe you should . . ."

Expert model	**Social contract model**	**Engineering model**
Practitioner makes decisions	Mutual participation in decision making	Patient makes informed decisions

FIGURE 13.1. Continuum of Decision-Making Responsibility in the Patient-Practitioner Relationship

The engineering model is located at the other end of the continuum from the expert/paternalistic model. The health professional takes no responsibility for the final health-related decisions of his or her patients.[48] Francoeur notes health providers provide patients with the responsibility of dealing with their own illnesses. The provders thus sacrifice personal responsibility in favor of providing patients with control over their ultimate health decisions. [49] This model has its roots in the image of the scientist (and physician) as an objective seeker of the truth. Health professionals who subscribe to this model view themselves primarily as scientists applying the benefits of scientific research and truth and believe that they must ignore all issues related to personal values and deal only with the facts. Above all else, the provider must remain impartial and objective. The goal is to present all the facts to the patients so that they can make their own decisions about the best course of action to take. The health professional then carries out the patient's decision, whatever that may be (e.g., to have surgery, to discontinue treatment, to select a less costly but less efficacious option, to modify the . drug regimen). In this model, the professional's personal values do not enter into the delivery of health care, and the major responsibility of the health care provider is to give the patient all the information necessary for him or her to make an informed decision.

The social contract model lies midway between the two extremes of the continuum and focuses on the need for genuine human interaction in the patient-practitioner relationship. This model assumes that an implied contract comes into existence when any person seeks the advice and help of another person who acknowledges and accepts the appeal for help. Whether the details of such a contract are verbalized or not, the help seeker and the helper enter a contract with each other.[50] Implicitly, they accept mutual obligations and rights. This model recognizes that the relationship is a pure person-to-person one between practitioner and patient. In many cases, the relationship itself is therapeutic.

Early studies of the practitioner-patient interaction have primarily focused on its conceptualization as an asymmetrical relationship in which the physician was completely dominant and the patient was expected to comply with medical advice and treatment. Very few of the early studies looked at the relationship of patients with other health care providers or the relationships of health providers with one another. Only recently have the researchers become interested in assessing the effects of increasing numbers of women health professionals on the practitioner-patient relationship.[51]

Fiduciary Relationship Behavioral Model

Two of the early pioneers in conceptualizing the doctor-patient relationship were Thomas Szasz and Mark Hollender.[52] They presented a threefold typology of the doctor-patient relationship based on the patient's level of functioning (see Table 13.1).

They suggested that each of the three basic models of the doctor-patient relationship is appropriate and necessary under various conditions and circumstances related to patient competence and health status.

In the activity-passivity model, the social prototype is one of parent to infant. The health professional's role is to take charge and make decisions necessary for the optimal care of the patient. Treatment of the patient takes place regardless of the patient's contribution or wishes, and the patient is expected to remain dependent and passive. Often the patient is not fully aware of what is happening to him or her, and is unable to participate in the decision-making process. Generally this model comes into play only when the patient is incompetent to make his or her own decisions (e.g., patient is under anesthesia, comatose, has acute life-threatening trauma or severe bleeding, is in a diabetic coma, delirium, has had a stroke, or is in other such states). This model corresponds to the expert/paternalistic end of the decision-making continuum discussed previously.

The guidance-cooperation model parallels the relationship of parent to older child or adolescent. The professional's role is as expert telling the patient what to do. The patient is expected to cooperate and comply with the advice. The patient is aware of what is going on and is capable of following directions and of exercising some judgment. The patient is expected to assume that "the physician knows what is best for me." The clinical applica-

TABLE 13.1. Three Basic Models of the Physician-Patient Relationship

Model	Physician's role	Patient's role	Clinical application of model	Prototype of model
Activity-passivity	Does something to the patient	Recipient (unable to respond)	Anesthesia, acute trauma, coma, delirium	Parent-infant
Guidance cooperation	Tells the patient what to do	Cooperator (obeys)	Acute infections, other acute illnesses	Parent-child, parent-adolescent
Mutual participation	Helps the patient help himself (uses expert help)	Participant in partnership	Most chronic illnesses, psychotherapy	Adult-adult

tion of this model is most appropriate for patients with acute medical problems, infections, broken bones, or other non-life-threatening trauma, as well as during the postsurgical recovery period and early stages of diagnosis of chronic diseases.

The third model, mutual participation, corresponds to the midpoint of the decision-making responsibility continuum and is based on the social contract model of adult-to-adult interaction. The practitioner's role is to use his or her expertise to help patients to help themselves. The patient's task is to use the expert help offered and to fully participate in partnership with the practitioner to resolve or minimize morbidity from health-related problems. The day-to-day treatment of illness is carried out by the patient, with only occasional consultation with the physician; the patient takes on much of the responsibility for his or her own welfare. This model of the relationship is most appropriate for management of patients with chronic illnesses (e.g., diabetes, arthritis, hypertension, heart disease); rehabilitation patients (post-acute trauma or stroke); and patients with psychological problems who are being treated by counseling.

Problems in the doctor-patient relationship may arise if both parties do not hold the same conceptualization of the relationship or if circumstances change such that a different model is more appropriate and one party or the other resists making the change. Definitions of "good" and "bad" patients and "good" and "bad" doctors (or pharmacists, nurses, counselors, dentists) may reflect the mismatch in expectations concerning appropriate role-playing behavior.

To illustrate this point, consider the patient who presents at an emergency room with symptoms of an acute myocardial infarction. At that point, the physician must rather quickly determine the patient's status. Certainly the activity-passivity model of interaction is appropriate. During the patient's recovery period in the hospital, a shift to a guidance-cooperation pattern of interaction would be expected. Patients who refuse to give up the passive dependency state and want all decisions to be made for them will be encouraged or persuaded by the hospital staff to give up some of this dependency and become more cooperative and take more responsibility for personal care. However, if the physician continues to act in an authoritative manner and insists on complete control with little or no input from the patient, the patient may become dissatisfied and resistant in some way. After discharge from the hospital, the patient is expected to become much more active in decision making concerning treatment, use of medications, and making changes in lifestyle (e.g., diet, exercise, smoking cessation, stress reduction). If either the patient or the physician resists moving to a mutual-participation style of interaction, dissatisfaction is likely to ensue.

Sick Role Behavioral Model

Talcott Parsons proposed a model of the sick role as a way to understand the social and psychological dynamics of the patient-physician relationship.[53] This model was based on the premise that illness is disruptive in a society. He further suggested that a truly sick person should be temporarily relieved from some of his or her obligations and responsibilities while recovering from an illness. However, without some official labeling of who is sick and who is well, any member of society could use illness as an excuse to avoid work or other responsibilities. Therefore, society requires experts who can decide who is sick and who is well. The health professions, in particular medicine, have been given the authority to diagnose and treat individuals who are physically or psychologically unable to perform their social roles. When an individual has defined himself or herself as ill and initiates contact with a health care provider, control of the interaction is immediately shifted to the health care professional. The diagnosis serves to legitimize or validate the illness perceived by the patient and to initiate adoption of the sick role.

The sick role, as proposed by Parsons, imposes on the patient two obligations and grants two privileges (see Table 13.2).

TABLE 13.2. Parson's Model of the Doctor-Patient Sick-Role System

Patient's status: Sick role	Doctor's status: Professional role
Obligations	*Responsibilities*
• To be motivated to get well	• To act for the welfare of the patient (orientation toward the collective versus self)
• To seek technically competent help	
• To trust the physician and accept the asymmetry of the relationship (the competence/knowledge gap)	• To be guided by the rules of professional behavior (universalism versus particularism)
	• To apply a high degree of achieved skill and knowledge in solving problems of illness
	• To be objective and emotionally detached (affective neutrality)
	• Professional self-regulation (to monitor competence and ethical behavior)
Privileges	*Rights*
• Exemption from performance of normal social role obligations	• Access to physical and personal intimacy necessary for diagnosis and treatment
• Exemption from responsibility for one's own state of illness	• Professional autonomy
	• Professional dominance

First, the patient is expected to seek technically competent help to deal with the illness. The patient is also expected to trust the health care provider and accept the power differential resulting from the competence gap in the relationship. Second, the patient is expected to do everything that is necessary to get well. In return, the patient is exempt from being held responsible for becoming ill and is temporarily exempt from performing some or all of his or her normal social role responsibilities.

The model of the sick role is the most traditional one and closely parallels the activity-passivity and guidance-cooperation models proposed by Szasz and Hollender.[54] Parson's model is applicable primarily for patients with acute and short-term illnesses that are easily diagnosed and readily treated. This model has been criticized because it is not really appropriate for understanding the behavior of patients with chronic illnesses, permanent disabilities, psychiatric illness, or such conditions as alcoholism and drug abuse. It would not be functional for a society to grant long-term or permanent exemption from social role obligations to its members suffering from a chronic condition. In addition, there appears to be a major shift in this country in attitudes toward individuals assuming more responsibility for chronic illnesses and conditions that are related to lifestyle decisions.[55,56]

Individual Consumer Behavior: A Five-Stage Model

A five-stage model of the consumer decision-making process from a marketing perspective is presented by Kotler and Clarke (see Figure 13.2).

This model can be used to increase our understanding of the process a consumer uses in determining which health-related product or service he or she wants to purchase to meet an identified need. This model may also be used to increase our understanding of what type of pharmacy setting and which pharmacy services consumers prefer. The five steps of this model and the questions to be addressed at each stage are as follows:

1. *Need arousal:* What needs or wants are identified by the individual that may give rise to interest in searching for a product or service?
2. *Information gathering:* How does the individual gather information relevant to determining what product or service to select?
3. *Decision evaluation:* How does the individual evaluate the alternative under consideration?
4. *Decision execution:* What action does the individual take after the best alternative is selected?
5. *Postdecision assessment:* How does the individual's post-purchase experience affect his or her subsequent attitude and behavior toward the product or service provider?

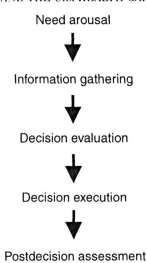

Need arousal

Information gathering

Decision evaluation

Decision execution

Postdecision assessment

FIGURE 13.2. Five-Stage Model of Consumer Buying Process (*Source:* Adapted from Kotler, P. and Clarke, R. N. *Consumer Analysis: Marketing for Health Care Organizations* [Englewood Cliffs, NJ: Prentice-Hall, 1987], pp. 256-288.)

Need arousal is concerned with the initial triggering factors or cues that signal the arousal of a particular need or want that is not being adequately met. The cue may be internal or external. An internal cue is related to a change in feeling state, attitude, physiological state; appearance of a symptom; or other such stimulus that indicates a need to take action. An external cue is a stimulus coming from another person or other sources of information (e.g., a newspaper article, an advertisement, a special program on television, a self-help medical book) that signals the need to take action. The types of specific needs or wants that are identified as being unmet vary from basic physiological needs related to maintenance of homeostasis of the body, to psychological needs related to connection and support or to higher-level needs related to self-development and creative activity.[57]

Maslow conceptualized a five-level, hierarchical model of human needs, which includes (from lowest to highest levels): Level I—physiological needs (e.g., hunger, thirst, warmth); Level II—safety needs (e.g., security, protection); Level III—social needs (e.g., sense of belonging, being loved and cared for); Level IV—esteem needs (e.g., self-esteem, recognition, status); and Level V—self-actualization needs (e.g., self-development, creativity, realization of goals). Maslow proposed that people work to satisfy the lower, basic level needs first before devoting energy toward meeting higher-level needs. As each level of needs is satisfied, it no longer serves as a motivator for action. Thus as a hungry person is satiated, and if he or she senses no cues that safety needs are unmet, then the social needs would become salient and motivate the person to seek out interaction with others. Kotler and Clarke, in commenting on the applicability of Maslow's hierarchy of needs, suggested:

> It is easy to see Maslow's hierarchy of needs at work in the health care field. The very poor, for example, will not undertake self-actualizing health activities, like jogging or exercise, until their basic needs for food and shelter are met. We see that certain health care and social services cater to physiological needs, like the Meals on Wheels programs for the elderly, while others, like sports medicine clinics and psychological counseling, appeal to the higher social, esteem, and self-actualization needs.[58]

Needs are rather generalized conditions or states requiring relief or remedy. *Wants,* on the other hand, are rather specific objectives that may be expected to meet identified needs, For example, when a person senses internal cues that indicate hunger, the hunger can be remedied by the intake of food. What food to consume to relieve this need is a matter of want—an ice cream cone, a broiled steak, a carton of yogurt, or a bag of potato chips will all relieve hunger. What product does a patient want to relieve a headache—aspirin, acetaminophen, or ibuprofen? What type of pharmacy should services be sought from—a busy chain store located in a supermarket, one located in a medical building, an apothecary shop, or the corner drugstore? Exposure to advertisements, consumer information, investigative news reports on television, or advice from professional caregivers and members of a person's social network all influence the selection of alternatives (i.e., creation of wants) to meet identified needs.

During the information-gathering stage, a person seeks information from many sources to increase the number of options from which to choose. The amount of information sought depends on several factors, including the intensity of need, the amount of information generally available, the complexity or level of risk associated with the choices, and individual variation in information neediness.

Ray has proposed three models of decision making based on the need for information and the amount of information perceived to be available.[59] For some decisions the choices are relatively clear, risk-free, and all the information necessary to make an informed decision is readily available. General first aid and home remedy decisions for minor ailments appear to fall into the category of low-involvement decision making. For more serious and/or high-risk decisions, generally, a learning model of decision making is followed. The person experiences a fairly high level of desire for information and perceives that sufficient information is available to evaluate the choices. A patient discussing with a pharmacist the side effects experienced with a new medication may seek information on the seriousness and permanence of the symptoms, whether or not the symptoms will go away with continued consumption of the medication, what will happen if the dose is reduced or the medication discontinued, and if there are other, similar medications that could be prescribed that would not have the same side effects. Ultimately, the patient must decide whether to talk to the pharmacist, to return to the physician for modification of treatment regimen, to try to self-regulate the medication to reduce the bothersome symptom(s), to just tolerate it, to stop taking the drug, to find another doctor, or to seek out alternative therapy. Without adequate, readily available information, the patient might not select the best option and might jeopardize his or her health status.

What happens when the desire for information is great and the level of information available is perceived to be low? A dissonance-attribution model applies in this situation. Kotler and Clarke have discussed the dilemma faced by a person who views a decision to be made as high-risk or important and, at the same time, does not perceive that adequate information is available to distinguish among the alternatives.[60] Thus, the person's resulting behavior appears at times to be irrational or irresponsible. The patient, faced with an important decision and no usable information on which to base that decision, arbitrarily decides on a course of action. Selecting a pharmacist, primary physician, or a specialist to care for you often is difficult. Kotler and Clarke illustrated this process with an example:

> Many people, for example, pick a primary care physician out of the Yellow Pages. The Yellow Pages listing gives no information other than the physician's specialty, address, and telephone number. Given the importance of having a competent patient-physician relationship, this decision process seems irrational. However, it is based on two factors: (1) there is very little information available on physicians; (2) the information that is available does not allow meaningful distinctions between physicians. . . . Some people try to gather information that will distinguish among physicians by speaking to friends and neighbors. Assuming these information sources are not themselves medical professionals, they will be unable to judge the medical competence of various physicians.[61]

Consider an older man newly diagnosed as having prostate cancer. His physician recommends immediate surgery. What information does he want? Where does he go to get this information? He may wonder: *Is my doctor's diagnosis correct? Will surgery save my life? Is my doctor a good surgeon? Are there other alternative treatments? What will happen if I do not have the surgery? Should I get a second opinion? What will be my level of incapacity after surgery?* Depending on the patient's age, socioeconomic status, education, cultural background, general level of health knowledge, and a host of other factors, he may or may not ask these questions of his physician. He may go to the library and try to find information on prostate cancer; he may talk with friends and family or seek out other men who have had similar surgery to learn what to expect. He may not be able to find the information he seeks. His physician may not recognize subtle cues that indicate he needs information but is afraid to ask. The patient may feel helpless in seeking information and simply trust his physician's judgment and go along with whatever he or she recommends.

Once a person has developed a list of alternatives to choose from based on the information gathered, the process of choice narrowing occurs (decision evaluation stage). For example, assume that an elderly husband feels he can no longer properly take care of his wife, who has been diagnosed as suffering from Alzheimer's disease. Her behavior has become more unpredictable and her husband is concerned about keeping her safe; he is also exhausted from caring for her, as well as from his own failing health. In talking with his children, his wife's physician, his neighbors, and a home care nurse, he perceives his options to be as follows:

1. Move his wife into a nursing home
2. Move her into their daughter's home
3. Make alterations in the home environment to make it safer for her (e.g., remove the knobs from the stove, put a fence around the property with a locked gate to keep her from wandering)
4. Arrange for respite care once a month so he can get a break from his caregiving chores
5. Ask the physician to order home health care services to assist him in the personal care of his wife on a regular basis
6. Arrange for a live-in helper

There are probably other alternatives he did not think of in making this list. How does he make a choice among the set of alternatives he has under consideration? His original list of six options is fairly generic. Initially, he may select several of these to narrow the choices. He may outright reject choices one and two, which involve moving his wife out of the home and having someone else care for her; he believes he and his wife should stay together as long as possible. That leaves him with four options. Depending on his income, he may also have to reject option six, hiring someone to help him. At the decision execution stage, he decides to talk with his wife's physician to see if he can get home care services for her such as Meals on Wheels or housekeeping help, since his health is poor as well. Also, he asks his son-in-law to help make the house safer, and to install a fence around the perimeter of the yard. His physician recommends that he try day care for his wife several times a week to give him a chance to get out of the house, run errands, or visit friends. These choices are all much more specific and are made based on personal values, cues from others, knowledge about the specific choice attributes, and perceptions concerning the utility of each alternative in meeting the identified need.

Once some action has been taken, the person continues to evaluate in order to determine if the option(s) selected has adequately addressed the original need (postdecision assessment stage). If the person's expectations, in general, have been met, then he or she will be satisfied. If dissatisfied with the decision made, the individual will then try to reduce the dissatisfaction by changing the focus (look at the positives, ignore the negatives) or reconsider some of the earlier alternatives previously rejected. If the man in the previous example is not satisfied with the result of the options selected or if he is unable to cope with his dissatisfaction, he may reconsider options one, two, or six, or continue to gather information to develop other alternatives not previously considered.

Consumer Behavior in Health and Sickness

Studies that have examined the health-related beliefs and behaviors of the American public have revealed a high level of misinformation regarding the value of taking extra vitamins, the necessity of having daily bowel movements, appropriateness of home remedies, and of self-diagnosis and self-care.[62,63]

Becker has noted that nearly 16 million Americans reported self-diagnosis for arthritis, asthma, allergies, hemorrhoids, heart trouble, high blood pressure, or diabetes. Investigators consistently reported relatively poor public participation in health screenings, immunization clinics, and other preventive health programs.[64]

Compliance with medical advice and medication regimens is notoriously poor. Mass health education programs that focus on cessation of smoking, prevention of sexually transmitted diseases, drug and alcohol abuse, seat belt use, and childhood immunizations often have minimal impact on altering behavior. As a result, legislation has been enacted to force public health-related behavioral changes on the population (e.g., seat belt laws, child-restraint laws, requirement of immunizations to begin school, warnings on tobacco and alcohol products, and random drug testing in the workplace). These findings reveal a rather discouraging range of diverse and complex health-related attitudes and behaviors among the public that frequently appear to be irrational, erroneous, and relatively resistant to change.

In addition to reducing the risk of injury and disease, the authors of the report believed that receiving adequate health information could increase the ability of individuals to make safe and effective health-related choices in a "changing and increasingly complex health care environment."[65] When a person decides to seek medical advice or care, and some may delay doing so for a variety of reasons, he or she brings to the encounter a variety of expectations, some realistic and some irrational. In addition to the technical expertise that a person seeks from the health care provider, sympathy, empathy, understanding, compassion, and consideration are expected as well. · For many patients these latter needs are the most important, and satisfaction with the interaction may hinge on having these needs addressed. The quality of this interaction is reflected in the patient's satisfaction with the encounter and resolution of the problem. If the patient deems the practitioner-patient relationship to be unsatisfactory, then it is likely that he or she will attempt to fulfill relationship needs elsewhere (e.g., find another physician or pharmacist, experiment with alternative or nontraditional treatments and practitioners, or fall prey to the sellers of useless or dangerous products). It is crucial that health care providers recognize that these covert needs exist and convey to their patients respect, concern, and caring.[66,67]

HEALTH, ILLNESS, AND SICK-ROLE BEHAVIOR

Three categories of behavior are related to health care, including pharmaceutical care, which are important in understanding and motivating patient interaction within the health care system. Health behavior is defined as any activity undertaken by an individual who believes him or herself to be healthy, for the purpose of preventing illness or detecting disease in the asymptomatic stage. This would include such activities as beginning an exercise program, weight reduction, stress reduction, making an appointment for a yearly Pap smear, regular self-examination for breast or testicular cancer, following good dental hygiene practices, or altering one's diet to decrease fat and cholesterol consumption.

Illness behavior is any activity undertaken by a person who believes he or she may be ill for the purpose of defining his or her state of health and discovering a suitable treatment or remedy for the problem. Discussing a health problem with a family member, friend, or pharmacist; making an appointment to see a physician or other health care provider; reading relevant self-help medical books; self-testing to determine one's blood pressure, blood sugar level, or if pregnant; or experimenting with over-the-counter (OTC) or leftover prescription medications all are examples of illness behavior.

Sick-role behavior is defined as activity undertaken by individuals who consider themselves to be ill, or who have been diagnosed by a health professional as being ill, for the purpose of getting well. Examples of this type of activity include following medical advice, taking medications as prescribed, selecting an appropriate OTC product, or staying home from work or school to rest and recuperate.

Health Behavior

Of all health-related behavior, the most difficult to predict is that of healthy individuals. Although the person has no clear-cut symptoms to prompt the taking of preventive and protective action, the effort and money spent on this type of activity are potentially the most beneficial, cost-effective, and productive of those expended on other types of health care activity.[68]

The health belief model (HBM) was first proposed by Rosenstock and later modified by Becker and others to explain individual health behavior (see Figure 13.3).[69,70]

As indicated in the model, the authors have hypothesized that people generally do not engage in preventive health care practices or participate in health detection and screening programs unless they possess a minimal level of relevant health motivation and knowledge, view themselves as vulnerable and the condition as threatening, are convinced of the efficacy of the intervention or activity under consideration, and perceive few difficulties or barriers to undertaking the appropriate action. Specifically, the HBM includes the following elements:

- The individual's readiness to take action as determined by both his or her perceived likelihood of susceptibility to a particular illness and assessment of the probable severity of its consequences (physiological, psychological, and economic)

- The individual's evaluation of the benefits versus the costs associated with taking the proposed action, that is, weighing of the feasibility and efficaciousness of the advocated health behavior against perceptions of the physical, psychological, social, and financial costs or barriers involved in taking the action
- The presence of a cue to action that would trigger the person to engage in the appropriate health behavior; this cue can be either internal (e.g., a symptom or change in feeling state) or external (e.g., interpersonal interaction, mass media campaign, or professional advice)

Although a range of demographic, personality, cultural, social, and structural factors are assumed to affect a person's health motivations and perceptions, in this model these factors are not viewed as direct causes of health action; rather, they are seen as influencing the belief dimensions of the model, which in turn directly determine health behavior.

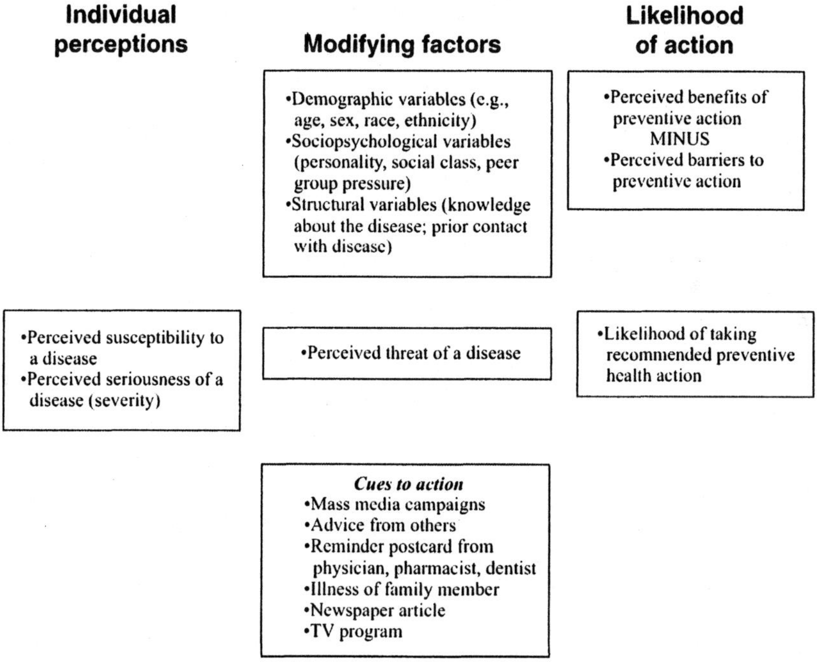

Individual perceptions	Modifying factors	Likelihood of action
	•Demographic variables (e.g., age, sex, race, ethnicity) •Sociopsychological variables (personality, social class, peer group pressure) •Structural variables (knowledge about the disease; prior contact with disease)	•Perceived benefits of preventive action MINUS •Perceived barriers to preventive action
•Perceived susceptibility to a disease •Perceived seriousness of a disease (severity)	•Perceived threat of a disease	•Likelihood of taking recommended preventive health action
	Cues to action •Mass media campaigns •Advice from others •Reminder postcard from physician, pharmacist, dentist •Illness of family member •Newspaper article •TV program	

FIGURE 13.3. The Health Belief Model As a Predictor of Preventive Health Behavior

Illness and Sick-Role Behavior

The HBM has been modified somewhat for use in predicting the likelihood of a person engaging in illness behavior and in sick-role behavior (see Figures 13.4 and 13.5). Understanding the behavior of people when they perceive themselves to be ill can be enhanced by viewing this behavior as a sickness career. The sickness career begins with a state of wellness. Wellness means different things to different people, but a variety of studies have shown that the general criteria by which people define themselves as being well include a feeling of well-being, the absence of symptoms, or the ability to perform normal personal and work functions and activities. Most people, even those who feel well, are able to identify the presence of some symptoms at any time. Often these symptoms will be viewed as normal, minor inconveniences. These symptoms may trigger a desire for further information, however, when they persist or affect functioning.

Ultimately, a decision must be made about the meaning and significance of symptoms that persist, change, or become bothersome to the person. Twaddle and Hessler have discussed a variety of factors that go into deter-

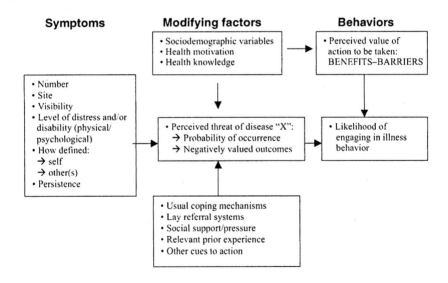

FIGURE 13.4. The Health Belief Model Modified to Explain Illness Behavior (*Source:* Becker, M. H. Psychological Aspects of Health-Related Behavior. In Freeman, H. E., Levine, S., and Reeder, L. G. (eds.), *Handbook of Medical Sociology,* Third Edition [Englewood Cliffs, NJ: Prentice-Hall, 1979], pp. 253-274.)

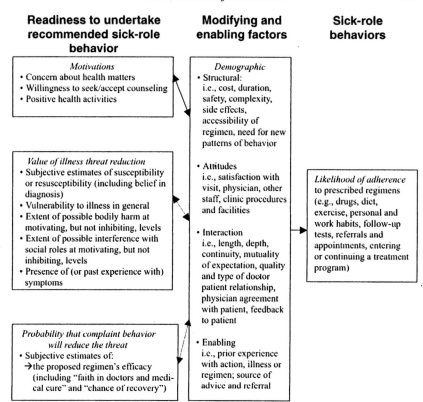

Readiness to undertake recommended sick-role behavior

Motivations
• Concern about health matters
• Willingness to seek/accept counseling
• Positive health activities

Value of illness threat reduction
• Subjective estimates of susceptibility or resusceptibility (including belief in diagnosis)
• Vulnerability to illness in general
• Extent of possible bodily harm at motivating, but not inhibiting, levels
• Extent of possible interference with social roles at motivating, but not inhibiting, levels
• Presence of (or past experience with) symptoms

Probability that complaint behavior will reduce the threat
• Subjective estimates of:
→the proposed regimen's efficacy (including "faith in doctors and medical cure" and "chance of recovery")

Modifying and enabling factors

Demographic
• Structural:
i.e., cost, duration, safety, complexity, side effects, accessibility of regimen, need for new patterns of behavior

• Attitudes
i.e., satisfaction with visit, physician, other staff, clinic procedures and facilities

• Interaction
i.e., length, depth, continuity, mutuality of expectation, quality and type of doctor patient relationship, physician agreement with patient, feedback to patient

• Enabling
i.e., prior experience with action, illness or regimen; source of advice and referral

Sick-role behaviors

Likelihood of adherence to prescribed regimens (e.g., drugs, diet, exercise, personal and work habits, follow-up tests, referrals and appointments, entering or continuing a treatment program)

FIGURE 13.5. The Health Belief Model Modified to Explain Sick-Role Behavior (*Source:* Becker, M. H. Psychological Aspects of Health-Related Behavior. In Freeman, H. E., Levine, S., and Reeder, L. G. (eds.), *Handbook of Medical Sociology,* Third Edition [Englewood Cliffs, NJ: Prentice-Hall, 1979], pp. 253-274.)

mining if a change in health status is significant.[71] They reported that people may define themselves as ill based on one or more of the following criteria:

• Interference with normal activities and functions (e.g., change in bowel habits, loss of strength, reduced ability to work, or loss of enjoyment of leisure activities)
• Clarity of symptoms (e.g., sharp pain, unexplained bleeding, fever, productive cough, other symptoms that are visible to family and friends, or symptoms the person considers to be serious)

- Tolerance threshold exceeded (some people can tolerate more pain or functional incapacity than others, either because of personal characteristics, cultural factors, or the nature of their work activities)
- Familiarity with symptoms (common symptoms a person has experienced previously and recovered from are likely to be viewed as less serious than those with which a person has no previous experience or knows to be serious)
- Assumptions about the cause of symptoms (e.g., in the case of chest pain, it may be viewed as indigestion, muscle strain, or a heart attack)
- Assumptions about prognosis of the suspected disease state (if long-term incapacity or possible death is associated with the cause of the symptoms, they are likely to be viewed as serious. A headache assumed to be caused by a brain tumor is viewed more seriously than a migraine or tension headache)
- Interpersonal influences (reference groups and lay-referral network)
- Other concurrent life events and crises (in some cases, symptoms that might be viewed as normal or only a nuisance can attain greater attention and significance in the face of other problems in a person's life; a person's coping ability may be compromised by too many demands at one time)

The process whereby a person evaluates the significance of changes in health status is quite complex and involves several steps, including consultation with others (support network or lay-referral system). Once a set of symptoms is defined by the person as being important and potentially serious, a decision must be made as to the best course of action. Is medical help needed, and if so, what kind of help? Self-treatment is often the first method of treatment.

Lay-Referral System

The vast majority of health care decisions made by individuals in response to symptoms are made without contact with a health care professional. Most people depend on advice from family and friends in deciding whether or not to seek professional help, and if so, what kind of professional to go to. Freidson has defined this process, whereby a person concerned about the meaning of a set of symptoms or other health problem consults with family and friends as a lay-referral network or system. According to Freidson, using the lay-referral system involves a series of steps, each likely to include diagnosis, prescription, and referral.

The lay-referral system has been found to be highly developed and a significant pathway to the health care delivery system for lower socioeconomic groups, certain cultural groups, and the elderly. It is important not to discount the influence of the lay-referral system in determining who will seek health care, from whom (traditional or alternative providers), and how treatment recommendations will be followed. It has been suggested, for example, that elderly arthritis sufferers often decide on the amount of a prescribed anti-inflammatory drug to take, the frequency with which to take it, and the point at which to cease taking it by soliciting opinions from fellow arthritis sufferers who have taken the same medication.[72] In addition, information often is shared about other drugs or treatments that may have been effective, but which the person's doctor has not prescribed. Whether the neighborhood pharmacist is part of the lay-referral system has yet to be studied effectively. However, this certainly seems to be an appropriate role responsibility for pharmacists to assume.

Self-Diagnosis and Treatment

Self-care has always been the predominant way in which people have dealt with health problems since the beginning of time.[73] In *The Hidden Health Care System,* Levin and Idler describe the essential components of self-care activities and suggest that the amount of self-care practiced in the United States far exceeds the care delivered by health care professionals.[74] Levin and Idler have noted:

Self-medication is certainly the most researched aspect of self-care for minor illness and injury, but the wide range of other such activities deserves mention and further study: first aid for minor injuries, cuts, scrapes, bruises, and burns; vaporizers and bed rest for colds and flu; ointments, compresses, and astringents for skin problems; home surgery for blisters and splinters; kisses and Band-Aids for imaginary "boo-boos"; massage and hot baths for sore muscles; chicken noodle soup and "a nice hot cup of tea" for anything; hot water bottles and heating pads for menstrual cramps; ice packs for swellings; vinegar douches and yogurt for vaginal infections; hydrogen peroxide for ear wax; salt water gargles—the list could go on and on. In addition to these treatments, certain diagnostic and monitoring equipment are increasingly found in home use, such as, thermometers, sphygmomanometers (to measure blood pressure), otoscopes, home throat culture and urine-testing kits, and home pregnancy tests.[75]

What is perhaps most interesting about self-care is its sheer magnitude. Roghmann and Haggerty reported that over 90 percent of health-related actions taken by 500 families in one study were based on self-decisions.[76] Demers and his co-workers reported that only 10 to 20 percent of the health problems identified by people received professional attention.[77] Reissman has suggested that from 65 to 85 percent of medical care is provided by nonprofessionals, and he concluded that the ratio of nonprofessional to professional health care for all health problems is about 7:1.[78] Self-care is prevalent in all cultures, and the rate of self-care does not appear to vary significantly in countries with national health programs that remove the economic barriers to seeking care.[79] Schwartz and Biederman have suggested that self-care is likely to increase dramatically as the number of persons suffering from chronic illnesses increases. With the rapid aging of the U.S. population, there will be more people suffering from such diseases as diabetes, arthritis, heart disease, and cancer.

Care of the Sick

A brief examination of the history of care of the sick reveals that treatment of the sick person, both medical and social, has changed drastically with the level of civilization and ascription of disease causation. So too have the expectations for helpers and patients. At the most primitive level of civilization, the sick were left to fend for themselves or to die and there was no obligation placed on family or social group members to help. As civilization advanced, illness was ascribed frequently to evil spirits and methods of assistance were limited to incantations and sometimes magic potions to drive away the disease-causing spirits. At the time the Old Testament was being written, illness was placed in a religious context as punishment for one's own or the family's sins and transgressions. The period of the New Testament in Western civilization brought about a sharp change in attitudes, even to the point of allocating grace to those who associated with or aided the sick. By the eighteenth century, secular authority had gained influence in health care and, as it became obvious that providing care to keep the population healthy contributed to the common good, care of the sick became important. New advances in understanding disease causation removed blame from the individual for his or her plight.[80]

In spite of the progress we have made in understanding disease processes, vestiges of the old attitudes remain. Many people still have difficulty adopting a wholesome attitude toward individuals suffering from a psychiatric illness or those who are severely handicapped, for example, and still others lean toward a punishment-for-transgressions attitude regarding people with acquired immunodeficiency syndrome (AIDS). Many of these old attitudes are present in other cultures as well. Understanding the behavior patterns that a society expects of those who have officially been sanctioned as sick is important for all health professionals. This prescribed behavior varies by culture, of course, and depends on the severity and type of disease state present.

DIVERSITY IN THE U.S. CONSUMER

The landscape of the American consumer has undergone significant changes in the past thirty years and predictions are that these changes will continue. The largest minority group in the United States is Latinos, and by 2040 they will be the largest ethnic group in this country. Asian-Americans also represent a large population in the United States. At the same time, other ethnic groups have been immigrating to the United States, including Eastern Europeans and people from Western Asia and the Caribbean. The foreign-born population increased by 3 percent, or 1 million, to 33.5 million in 2003 and approximately one-half of these entered illegally. In many minority groups, the mean age is younger and 48 percent of all children in the United States are racial and ethnic minorities. As these children reach adulthood, the face of the American consumer will be very different and the power of the minority consumer will be far greater than it is now.[81]

The effect these new ethnic groups will have on the United States is still to be determined, but they introduce new challenges for those who deal with consumers. These challenges include language barriers, lack of formalized or legal immigration status and expectations of the health care system from their own cultural background. Challenges to the consumer include navigating the new and often poorly understood health care system in light of these barriers.

Several explanatory models of disease causation exist. Humoral medicine, which focuses on maintaining balance between opposite forces, is the most common model. In the Latino culture these forces are referred to as "hot" and "cold" and in Asian cultures these forces are referred to as "yin" and "yang." Other cultures also embrace this explanation for illness, including India, Northern Africa, and Native Americans. Hot and cold do not refer to actual temperatures in the body but to abstract qualities of the body state, herbs, foods, and other treatments. The treatment prescribed is meant to bring the body back into balance, usually by treating the hot diseases with cold treatments and vice versa. Hot diseases such as fever, infection, diarrhea, constipation, skin problems, sore throat, liver problems, or kidney problems are treated with cold remedies and foods, including tropical fruits, fresh vegetables, dairy, chicken, fish, honey, raisins, sage, milk of magnesia, and bicarbonate of soda. Cold diseases may include cancer, pneumonia, malaria, menstrual difficulties, tooth pain, earache, rheumatism, cold, tuberculosis, headache, and stomach cramps and can be treated with hot food and herbs such as temperate-zone fruits, chocolate, cheese, eggs, hard liquor, oils, beef, lamb, cereal grains, chili peppers, penicillin, tobacco, ginger, garlic, cinnamon, anise, vitamins, iron, cod liver oil, and castor oil. Many of these treatments are often used alongside Western medicine to complement the physician's recommendation. Consumers may not be aware of possible detrimental interactions that some of these combinations may have. When Western medicine practitioners try to force an explanation of signs and symptoms onto a patient, trust and compliance may be compromised and therefore compliance with the prescribed regimen may be quite poor.[82-89]

Appropriate medical roles and responsibilities vary from culture to culture. Many Eastern European immigrants are accustomed to an authoritarian style, in which the physician directs medical care and asking questions is considered disrespectful. Some Asian immigrants expect the health care provider to assist in the cure, not take over. In some Asian cultures, eye contact with an elder, or someone in that role, is not polite and so patients may bow their head in deference and nod in acceptance, which a Western health care provider may assume to be understanding when in fact such understanding of the directions does not exist. In the United States, independence and the right to make independent decisions about medical care and other aspects of life are highly valued. Complete disclosure of health information is also valued in the U.S. culture. This disclosure allows patients to make informed decisions about their health. In Latino culture, the family unit is often involved in decision making. Therefore, it is important for health care providers not to exclude the family unit, which may alienate the patient and possibly affect compliance. In many cultures around the world, including, Latino, Asian, Indian subcontinent, and some European cultures, informing patients of fatal illnesses is not the norm. Sensitivity to this issue when dealing with the family is also important.[90,91]

Race discordance between the health care provider and the patient contributes to the difficulties often encountered. Besides language barriers, patients may feel white health care providers do not share their perception of their symptoms and disease. Many health care providers may be dismissive of holistic medicine used by their patients, thereby alienating the patient further. Many patients do not admit to their provider that they are using some form of alternative medicine. Patients often initially turn to the traditional cultural healer, or when they feel Western medicine is not working. An encompassing approach that allows the patient to use the holistic healer and Western medicine may be best. Gender discordance may also be important, particularly for cultures where modesty in women is highly valued, including many Muslim cultures. Race discordance does not appear to be improving for some ethnic groups. According to the American Association of Colleges of Pharmacy, only 14 percent of pharmacy graduates are racial or ethnic minorities, in contrast with the 25 percent of the overall population that falls into this group.[92,93]

A difference in response to drugs has been identified among patients with different ethnic backgrounds and between men and women. Differences in metabolism rates of several compounds have been identified. Many Asian patients are slow acetylators and so levels of drugs that require this pathway for metabolism may be higher in Asian versus white patients, which may lead to increased toxicity. Also, African Americans have a different clinical response to some antihypertensive drugs as compared to white patients. As the body of knowledge of pharmacogenomics grows and more information is available about these genetic racial differences, therapeutic regimens will be more individualized.[94] Minority patients are markedly affected by health care conditions as compared with white patients for many reasons. Some of these include: lower socioeconomic status, poor health behaviors, lack of access to health care, poor living and/or working environment, discrimination, lack of health insurance, overdependence on public health facilities, geographical location with few health care providers, insufficient or cumbersome transportation, and cost.[95]

Indian Subcontinent and Middle Eastern Population

Emmigration from Western Asia and the Middle East has increased. These consumers may be escaping political turmoil or religious persecution, or seeking opportunities in the United States. The family unit is usually very strong and cultural differences can be pronounced between this population and Americans. Regarding health care beliefs, this population often has religious explanations of disease. Many Indians believe in karma, an idea that every action a person takes has consequences that depend on not only the action but also the person's motivation. Thus, an Indian may ascribe his or her illness primarily as a result of past action. Susceptibility based on gender is also a common belief. These populations utilize and rely on health care providers and are accepting of suggestions for change to improve signs and symptoms.[96]

Eastern European Population

After the collapse of the USSR and due to regional conflicts that ensued, a significant increase in the number of Eastern European and Russian immigrants was seen. Searight published a study of twelve interviews with recent Bosnian immigrants. These consumers expressed dissatisfaction with the U.S. health care system for several reasons. These included confusion with insurance coverage, lack of personalization of care and access to specialty care, and an opinion of the U.S. health care system as bureaucratic.[97] The U.S. health care system differs significantly from the socialized medicine most of the consumers were used to in the countries of origin. The cost associated with health care and the myriad insurance possibilities are also confusing, particularly for patients who do not speak English. Many are well-educated and discerning health care consumers who may find themselves in a very different socioeconomic class in the United States.

Latinos

Between 1990 and 2000, the Latino population increased by 57.9 percent and now represents 12.5 percent (35,305,818) of the total population in the United States. Latinos are diverse in origin, customs, beliefs, and health care utilization.[98] Latinos are the fastest-growing minority in the United States and yet to group them all together is to miss the many differences in this group. Some Latinos, such as Cubans and Puerto-Ricans, have been in the United States for several generations and behave quite differently as consumers than recent immigrants from other countries in Central and South America. Cubans and Puerto-Ricans are more likely to behave as white Americans do, with the possible exception of more recent immigrants from these countries. Among recent immigrants, the diversity in their country of origin cannot be overlooked when attempting to explain consumer behavior.

Mexicans are one of the largest Latino groups (at about 10 million) in the Unitied States. Many are in the United States illegally and often work in jobs where health care benefits are not offered. They are often reluctant to use the other federally sponsored options due to fear of deportation. In addition, the use of the "curandero" or healer is commonplace for them and other Latino immigrants. The curandero is from the same country, shares the beliefs and attitudes of the patient, and is interested in all aspects of the patient's life. Often these patients will turn to these folk healers initially and present to the physician and pharmacist only with more advanced disease. Patients often expect a rapid response with therapy, and if this response is not seen they may end the relationship with the health care provider. These patients may also feel that health care providers are cold and indifferent and do not want to spend time to diagnose and treat them properly as compared to the curandero. Many feel that use of the curandero is acceptable for minor complaints or to treat complaints that were unsatisfactorily treated with modern medicine.[99] South and Central Americans are one of the fastest-growing immigrant groups within the Latino immigrant population. They often have religious or indigenous worldviews, and these views may extend to health. Ignoring these views and explanations may compromise the trusting relationship needed to care for these patients.[100]

Health care beliefs can affect mortality. Scarinci and colleagues surveyed native and immigrant Latino women in a clinic regarding knowledge and use of the Pap smear for cervical cancer screening, an intervention with evidence to support decrease in mortality from cervical cancer. They found that Latino immigrant women were less likely to have a Pap smear and had less knowledge of cervical cancer. Their cultural beliefs and disease explanations influenced their knowledge and willingness to get a Pap smear.[101] Latino-Americans have higher incidence and mortality rates from diabetes, obesity, and hypertension and they are less likely than white patients to receive some interventions such as cardiac bypass surgery.[102] Taken together, these behaviors, beliefs, and risk factors can all contribute to health disparities between Latino and white patients.

Asians

Asians account for 3.6 percent (10,123,169) of the population in the United States and this group is one of the fastest-growing minority groups in the United States, with a growth rate of 74.3 percent between 1990 and 2000. Pacific Islanders are also immigrating to the United States in record numbers. The growth rate for Pacific Islanders and native Hawaiians was the highest of all groups at 130 percent between 1990 and 2000.[103] Although the overall numbers in this group remain small in comparison to other minority groups, they will become a driving force in the future if these immigration rates are sustained. These patients come from China, the Philippines, Cambodia, Laos, Korea, Vietnam, Japan, Taiwan, and Thailand, among others. There is significant diversity among all these consumers in language, religion, worldview, background, literacy, education, and rural versus urban origin.

Many Asian-Americans subscribe to the hot-cold disease explanatory model. They often expect a rapid response to therapy and may discontinue medication if they do not achieve that response. Asians tend to have a healthier diet and are less likely to have heart disease, diabetes, and some cancers such as breast or prostate cancer. However, they are more likely to have hepatitis, tuberculosis, cervical cancer (especially Vietnamese women), liver cancer, and stomach cancers.[104]

African Americans and Blacks

Blacks and African Americans currently represent 12.3 percent (33,947,837) of the U.S. population. They were the slowest-growing minority, with a growth rate of 21 percent. The mean age was younger than other races (thirty years of age versus thirty-seven for whites).[105] A telephone survey of white and black non-Hispanic consumers showed that black respondents were less trustful of physicians and more concerned about privacy and unsanctioned harmful experimentation than white respondents.[106]

Many African Americans have been in the United States for generations and do not face language barriers; however, they may still have problems accessing and utilizing the U.S. health care system. There are many health disparities between African-American and Caucasian patients. African Americans have worse outcomes for many diseases, including breast, prostate, lung, and colorectal cancers; heart disease; diabetes; and many others. These disparities are only partly explained by late diagnosis. Further research into the cause and resolution of this issue is warranted.[107]

There has been an increased immigration to the United States from Caribbean and African nations. This group of consumers is quite different than the African Americans who have been in the United States for generations. Some may be escaping poverty or political turmoil in their own countries, where the health care system was poorly coordinated and difficult to access. Many have relied on traditional healers to help with medical problems and may be distrustful of the regimented U.S. health care system. A study of South African blacks by Farrand found that most patients preferred a combination approach to medical needs that incorporated traditional healers and Western medicine.[108] In another study conducted in South Africa, 70 percent of patients interviewed consulted traditional healers first, even for potentially life-threatening conditions.[109] Incorporation of an understanding of traditional practices into Western medicine may improve the health of these consumers and increase utilization of Western medicine.

The Role of Gender

Women are more frequent consumers of health care than men, and traditionally they are the primary health care providers and decision makers for the family by scheduling and taking the children to the doctor, visiting the pharmacy, and administering medications. Women also utilize more health care resources, both during the childbearing years and as elderly consumers, since women are more likely to outlive men and so will live longer with chronic illnesses.[110] Women use the Internet for health care information more commonly than men. Many of the direct-to-consumer advertisements are also directed at women.

The concept of women's health was conceived in the 1980s, and this focus of medicine has expanded tremendously since.[111] OTC products and vitamins are targeted to women, such as One-A-Day Women's with extra iron, folate and calcium. Women increasingly work outside of the home, and in the fall of 2003, women outnumbered men in many freshman classes countrywide. These political, social, and financial advances have given women more and more power as consumers. Also, as the large "baby boom" population born in the 1940s and 1950s reaches sixty-five years of age, older women will also wield more power than the current older generation. The implications of these changes on consumerism in the United States remain to be seen.

Elderly

It has been well documented that the elderly population is growing at a dramatic pace and is poised to become one of the largest consumer groups in the United States. This population explosion is due to several reasons. Citizens of the United States enjoy an unprecedented growth in health care advances, which began in the twentieth century and continues to gain momentum. Many of these advances serve to prolong life, whereas 100 years ago, most people would have died at a much earlier age without the surgical and medical advances that are so commonplace now. In addition, we are now seeing the "baby-boomer" post–World War II generation entering their sixth decade of life. It is projected that in 2003 the over-sixty-five population will exceed 50 million and account for 22 percent of the population in the United States. Not only is this a very large population but also they have grown up during a time when consumerism was a driving force in which they actively participated. The impact of these changes in U.S. society remains to be seen, but the elderly will likely be an unprecedented driving force in the marketplace.

Currently, the elderly population has different expectations. They commonly expect the health care provider to tell them what to do and often hesitate to ask questions or challenge the provider. They often get their health information from one another. Since many elderly people on Medicare lack prescription coverage benefits, they may share medications and attempt to stretch medications by taking them only half as often. Compliance rates may also be a problem, with only 50 to 67 percent of elderly patients complying with the prescribed regimens.[112]

Medication usage is high in elderly patients compared to younger patients. They usually have at least one chronic disease and take an average of fourteen prescriptions annually. They are usually on more than one drug; the average ranges from three to twelve concomitant drugs. In addition, 70 percent also take OTC medications. The large number of drugs and complicated regimens may lead to drug interactions that may put them at risk for serious complications and poor compliance.[113]

Within the over-sixty-five age group, the three subgroups are commonly referred to as the young-old (sixty-five to seventy-four years old), the middle-old (seventy-five to eighty-four years old), and the old-old (eighty-five years old and over). With improved technology and prolongation of life, people are now often living to their eighties and nineties. The average lifespan of a child born today is seventy-six years, versus forty-nine years at the turn of the nineteenth century. With this new longevity, the old-old demographic group has emerged. This is the fastest-growing segment of the population, and the oldest baby boomers will hit this age in 2030. They are often high-utilization consumers of health care and they represent a diverse group. Some may still live independently, others are in skilled nursing facilities, and yet others are in assisted living homes. This diversity makes it difficult to pigeonhole this group. Utilization of nursing home beds by this age group is about 23 percent, or 1.5 million beds. This will increase significantly to 4.5 million beds when the baby-boomers reach this life stage. It is expected that as baby-boomers enter this age demographic the utilization of many resources will skyrocket, and many have questioned the preparedness of the U.S. health care system to handle this surge.[114]

CONCLUSION

Many changes in consumers and providers of health care occurred in the twentieth century. The provision of health care has adapted to changes in consumers' expectations and demands and changes to consumers themselves. The health care system and the providers must continue to adapt to the needs and demands of the consumers while maintaining the integrity of the care provided.

NOTES

1. Friedson, E. *Professional powers: A study of the institutionalization of formal knowledge* (Chicago: University of Chicago Press, 1986).
2. Bellandi, D. Searching for better bait: Systems struggling to lure docs, trustees to integration. *Modern Healthcare* 1988; 28-30.
3. Coddington, D.C., Moore, K.D., and Fischer, E.A. *Integrated health care: Reorganizing the physician, hospital and health plan relationship* (Englewood, CO: Center for Research in Ambulatory Health Care Administration, 1994).
4. Coddington, D.C., Ackerman, F.K., Fischer, E.A., and Moore, K.D. *The changing dynamics of integrated health care: Success factors for the future* (Englewood, CO: Medical Group Management Association, 2001).
5. Howgill, M.W.C. Health care consumerism, the information explosion, and branding: Why 'tis better to be the cowboy than the cow. *Managed Care Quarterly* 1998; fall: 33-43.
6. Huber, R. Managed care gets a bum rap. *Business Week* 1999; 25: 12.
7. Beauchamp, T.L. and Childress, J.F. *Principles of biomedical ethics,* Fourth edition (New York: Oxford University Press, 1994).
8. Kane, L. Collect premium fees for premium care? *Medical Economics* 1999 January 11; 76(1): 127-128, 130.
9. Miller, K. Health care intentions: Seeing demand as consumers do. *Health care Strategist* 1999 February; 3(2): 7-10.
10. Vogel, R.J., Ramachandran, S., and Zachry, W.M. A 3-stage model for assessing the probable economic effects of direct-to-consumer advertising of pharmaceuticals. *Clinical Therapeutics* 2003; January; 25(1): 309-329.
11. Zachry, W.M. III, Dalen, J.E., and Jackson, T.R. Clinicians' responses to direct-to-consumer advertising of prescription medications. *Archives of Internal Medicine* 2003; 163(15): 1808-1812.
12. Department of Economics and School of Law, Emory University, Atlanta, Georgia. Pharmaceutical advertising as a consumer empowerment device. *Journal of Biolaw and Business* 2001; 4(4): 59-65.
13. Tatsioni, A., Gerasi, E., Charitidou, E., Simou, N., et al. Important drug safety information on the Internet: Assessing its accuracy and reliability. *Drug Safety* 2003; 26(7): 519-527.
14. Dutta-Bergman, M. Trusted online sources of health information: Differences in demographics, health beliefs, and health-information orientation. *Journal of Medical Internet Research* 2003; 5(3): e21.
15. Millard, R.W. and Fintak, P.A. Use of the Internet by patients with chronic illness. *Disease Management & Health Outcomes* 2002; 10(3): 187-194.
16. Angaran, D.M. Telemedicine and telepharmacy: Current status and future implications. *American Journal of Health-System Pharmacy* 1999; 56: 1405-1426.
17. Pennbridge, J., Moya, R., and Rodrigues, L. Questionnaire survey of California consumers' use and rating sources of health care information including the Internet. *Western Journal of Medicine* 1999; 171(5-6): 302-305.
18. Administration on Aging. Average health care expenditures among Medicare beneficiaries age 65 or older. Available online at <www.agingstats.gov/chartbook 2000/15>.

19. Austin, M. Schonbrun's back, and he's thinking ahead. *Denver Business Journal* 1999; May 21-27: A12.

20. Pol, L.G., May, M.G., and Hartranft, F.R. Eight stages of aging. *American Demographics* 1992; August: 54-57.

21. Moody, H.R. Toward a critical gerontology: The contribution of the humanities to theories of aging. In James E. Birren and Vern L. Bengtson (eds.), *Emergent theories of aging* (New York: Springer, 1988), pp. 9-40.

22. Cristofalo, V.J. An overview of the theories of biological aging. In James E. Birren and Vern L. Bengtson (eds.), *Emergent theories of aging* (New York: Springer, 1988), pp. 118-127.

23. MacNeil, R.D. and Teague, M.L. *Aging and leisure: Vitality in later life* (Englewood Cliffs, NJ: Prentice-Hall, 1987).

24. Schewe, C.D. Marketing to our aging population: Responding to psychological changes. *Journal of Consumer Marketing* 1988; 15(summer): 61-73.

25. Moschis, G.P. *Marketing to older consumers* (Westport, CT: Quorum Books, 1992).

26. Pirki, J.R. and Babic, A.L. *Guidelines and strategies for designing transgenerational products* (Acton, MA: Copley Publishing Company, 1988).

27. Philips, L.W. and Sternthal, B. Age differences in information processing: A perspective on the aged consumer. *Journal of Marketing Research* 1977; 14: 444-457.

28. Light, L.L. Language and aging: Competence versus performance. In James E. Birren and Vern L. Bengtson (eds.), *Emergent theories of aging* (New York: Springer, 1988), pp. 177-213.

29. Perlmutter, M. Cognitive potential throughout life. In James E. Birren and Vern L. Bengtson (eds.), *Emergent theories of aging* (New York: Springer, 1988), pp. 247-268.

30. Willis, S. and Schaie, K.W. Gender differences in spatial ability in old age: Longitudinal and intervention findings. *Sex Roles* 1988; 18(3/4): 189-203.

31. Moschis, G.P. and Sachdev, H. *Age-related differences in acceptance of technological innovations* (Atlanta: Georgia State University, Center of Mature Consumer Studies, 1991).

32. Thomas, H. Theory of aging and cognitive theory of personality. *Human Development* 1970; 13: 1-16.

33. Rosenberg, M. *Conceiving the self* (New York: Basic Books, 1979).

34. Dychtwald, K. and Flower, J. *Age wave* (New York: St. Martin's, 1989).

35. Schewe, C. Strategically positioning your way into the aging marketplace. *Business Horizons* 1991; May-June: 59-66.

36. Perlmutter, Cognitive potential throughout life.

37. Wood, J.J. *Relational communication: Continuity and change in personal relationships* (Second edition) (Belmont, CA: Wadsworth Publishing Company, 1987).

38. Smedley, L.T. The patterns of early retirement. AFL-CIO American Federationist. 1975.

39. Herzog, R.A. et al. Urinary incontinence and psychological distress among older adults. *Psychology and Aging* 1988; 392: 115-121.

40. Letsou, A.P. and Price, L.S. Health, aging, and nutrition. *Clinics in Geriatric Medicine* 1987; 3(2): 253-260.

41. MacNeil and Teague, *Aging and leisure.*

42. Freidson, E. *Patients' view of medical practice* (New York: Russell Sage Foundation, 1961).

43. Bloom, S. *The doctor and his patient* (New York: Russell Sage Foundation, 1963).

44. Reeder, L.G. The patient-client as a consumer: Some observations on the changing professional-client relationship. *Journal of Health and Social Behavior* 1972; 13: 406-412.

45. Wilson, R. and Bloom, S. Patient-practitioner relationships. In Freeman, H.E., Levine, S., and Reeder, L.G. (eds.), *Handbook of medical sociology* (Englewood Cliffs, NJ: Prentice-Hall, 1972), pp. 315-339.

46. Kaplan, S.H., Greenfield, S.S., and Ware, J.E. Assessing the effects of physician-patient interactions on the outcomes of chronic disease. *Medical Care* 1989; 27(Suppl): S110-S127.

47. Greenfield, S.S., Kaplan, S.H., and Ware, J.E. Expanding involvement in care: Effect on patient outcomes. *Annals of Internal Medicine* 1985; 102: 520-528.

48. Veatch, R.M. Models for ethical medicine in a revolutionary age. *Hastings Center Report* 1972; 2: 5-7.

49. Francoeur, R.T. *Biomedical ethics: A guide to decision making* (New York: John-Wiley and Sons, 1983).

50. Ibid.

51. Sherwin, S. *No longer patient: Feminist ethics and health care* (Philadelphia: Temple University Press, 1992).

52. Szasz, T.S. and Hollender, M.H. A contribution to the philosophy of medicine: The basic models of the doctor-patient relationship. *Archives of Internal Medicine* 1956; 97: 585-592.

53. Parsons, T. *The social system* (Glencoe, IL: The Free Press, 1951).

54. Szasz and Hollender, A contribution to the philosophy of medicine.

55. Crawford, R. Individual responsibility and health politics. In Conrad, P. and Kern, R. (eds.), *The sociology of health and illness: Critical perspectives,* Third edition (New York: St. Martin's Press, 1990), pp. 387-395.

56. Knowles, J.H. The responsibility of the individual. In Conrad, P. and Kern, R. (eds.), *The sociology of health and illness: Critical perspectives,* Third edition (New York: St. Martin's Press, 1990), pp. 376-386.

57. Maslow, A.H. *Motivation and personality* (New York: Harper & Row, 1954), pp. 80-106.

58. Kotler, P. and Clarke, R.N. *Consumer analysis: Marketing for health care organizations* (Englewood Cliffs, NJ: Prentice-Hall, Inc., 1987), pp. 256-288.

59. Ray, M.L. *Marketing communication and the hierarchy of effects* (Cambridge: Marketing Science Institute, 1973).

60. Ibid.

61. Kotler and Clarke, *Consumer analysis.*

62. Anonymous. *A study of health practices and opinions.* Public Health Service Publication PB-210 978 (Washington, DC: GPO, 1972).

63. Becker, M.H. Psychological aspects of health-related behavior. In Freeman, H.E., Levine, S., Reeder, L.G. (eds.), *Handbook of medical sociology,* Third edition (Englewood Cliffs, NJ: Prentice Hall, 1979), pp. 253-274.

64. Ibid.

65. Hirt, E.J. (ed.). *The health policy agenda for the American people* (Chicago: American Medical Association, 1987), pp. 82-85, p. 83.

66. Berger, B. Building an effective therapeutic alliance: Competence, trustworthiness, and caring. *American Journal of Hospital Pharmacy* 1993; 50: 2399-2403.

67. Manasse, H.R. The CARE in pharmaceutical care. *Journal of Pharmacy Technology* 1992; 3: 39-52.

68. Smith, M.C. and Knapp, D.A. *Pharmacy, drugs and medical care,* Third edition (Baltimore: Williams and Wilkins, 1981).

69. Rosenstock, I.M. Historical origins of the health belief model. *Health Education Monographs* 1974; 2: 328-335.

70. Ley, P. *Communicating with patients* (London: Croom Helm, 1988); cited in Knowlton, C.H. and Penna, R.P. *Pharmaceutical care* (New York: Chapman and Hall, 1996), p. 225.

71. Twaddle, A.C. and Hessler, R.M. *A sociology of health* (Saint Louis: Mosby, 1977).

72. Arluke, A. Judging drugs: Patients' conceptions of therapeutic efficacy in the treatment of arthritis. *Human Organization* 1980; 39: 84-88.

73. DeFreise, G. and Woodmert, A. The policy implications of self-care in the study of health and illness behavior. *Social Policy* 1982; 13: 55-58.

74. Levin, L.S. and Idler, E.L. *The hidden health care system: Mediating structures and medicine* (Cambridge: Ballinger, 1981), p. 75.

75. Ibid.

76. Roghmann, K.J. and Haggerty, R.J. The diary as a research instrument in the study of health and illness behavior: Experiences with a random sample of young families. *Medical Care* 1972; 10: 143-163.

77. Demers, R.Y., Altmore, R., Mustin, H., Kleinman, A., and Leonardo, D. An exploration of the dimensions of illness behavior. *Journal of Family Practice* 1980; 11: 1085-1092.

78. Reissman, F. The self-help ethos. *Social Policy* 1982; 13: 42-45.

79. Kronenfeld, J.J. Self-care as a panacea for the ills of the health care system: An assessment. *Social Science and Medicine* 1979; 13A: 263-267.

80. Conrad, P. and Schneider, J.W. Professionalization, monopoly, and the structure of medical practice. In Conrad, P. and Kern, R. (eds.), *The sociology of health and illness: Critical perspectives,* Third edition (New York: St. Martin's Press, 1990), pp. 141-147.

81. U.S. Census Bureau. *Statistical abstract of the United States* (Washington, DC: U.S. Department of Commerce, 2000).

82. Anderson, E.N. Why is humoral medicine so popular? *Social Science and Medicine* 1987; 25: 331-338.

83. Kendall, L. Cold wombs in balmy Honolulu: Ethnogynecology among Korean immigrants. *Social Science and Medicine* 1987; 25: 367-376.

84. Koo, L.C. Concepts of disease causation, treatment and prevention among Hong Kong Chinese: Diversity and eclecticism. *Social Science and Medicine* 1987; 25: 405-418.

85. Laderman, C. Destructive heat and cooling prayer: Malay humoralism in pregnancy, childbirth and the postpartum period. *Social Science and Medicine* 1987; 25: 357-366.

86. Maduro, R. Curanderismo and Latino views of disease and curing. *Western Journal of Medicine* 1983; 139: 868-874.

87. Manderson, L. Hot-cold food and medical theories: Overview and introduction. *Social Science and Medicine* 1987; 25: 329-330.

88. Pool, R. Hot and cold as an explanatory model: The example of Bharach district in Gujarat, India. *Social Science and Medicine* 1987; 25: 389-400.

89. Sukkary-Stolba, S. Food classification and the diets of young children in rural Egypt. *Social Science and Medicine* 1987; 25: 401-404.

90. Lock, M. Japanese responses to social change—Making the strange familiar. *Western Journal of Medicine* 1983; 139: 829-834.

91. Wheat, M.E., Browenstein, H., and Kvitash, V. Aspects of medical care of Soviet Jewish émigrés. *Western Journal of Medicine* 1983; 139: 900-904.

92. American Association of Colleges of Pharmacy. Profile of pharmacy students, fall 2003. Available online at <http://www.aacp.org/Docs/MainNavigation/InstitutionalData/5876_highlights.pdf>.

93. Baldwin, D. Disparities in health and health care: Focusing efforts to eliminate unequal burdens. *Online Journal of Issues in Nursing* 2003; 8(1): Manuscript 1. Available online at <http://nursingworld.org/ojin/topic20/tpc20_1.htm>.

94. Levy, R.A. *Ethnic and racial differences in responses to medicines* (Reston, VA: National Pharmaceutical Council, 1993).

95. Baldwin, Disparities in health and health care.

96. Kulwicki, A. An ethnographic study of illness perceptions and practices of Yemeni-Arabs in Michigan. *Journal of Cultural Diversity* 1996; 3: 80-89.

97. Searight, H.R. Bosnian immigrants' perceptions of the United States health care system: A qualitative interview study. *Journal of Immigrant Health* 2003; 5: 87-94.

98. U.S. Census Bureau, *Statistical abstract of the United States*.

99. Applewhite, S.L. Curanderismo: Demystifying the health beliefs and practice of elderly Mexican Americans. *Health Social Work* 1995; 20: 247-253.

100. Murguia, A., Peterson, R.A., and Zea, M.C. Use and implications of ethnomedical health care approaches among Central American immigrants. *Health Social Work* 2003; 28: 43-51.

101. Scarinci, I.C. et al. An examination of sociocultural factors associated with cervical cancer screening among low-income Latina immigrants of reproductive age. *Journal of Immigrant Health* 2003; 5: 119-128.

102. Baldwin, Disparities in health and health care.

103. U.S. Census Bureau, *Statistical abstract of the United States*.

104. Baldwin, Disparities in health and health care.

105. U.S. Census Bureau, *Statistical abstract of the United States*.

106. Bouware, L.E. et al. Race and trust in the health care system. *Public Health Reports* 2003; 118: 358-365.

107. Baldwin, Disparities in health and health care.

108. Farrand, D. Is a combined Western and traditional health service for black patients desirable? *South African Medical Journal* 1984; 66: 779-780.

109. Puckree, T. et al. African traditional healers: What health care professionals need to know. *International Journal of Rehabilitation Research* 2002; 25(4): 247-251.

110. Rothert, M.L. and O'Connor, A.M. Health decisions and decision support for women. *Annual Review of Nursing Research* 2001; 19: 307-324.

111. Anonymous. Women's health: Marketing challenges for the 21st century: The future of women's health care reflects demographic, social and economic trends. *Marketing Health Services* 2000; 20: 4-11.

112. Fincham, J.E. and Wertheimer, A.I. Initial drug noncompliance in the elderly. *Journal of Geriatric Drug Therapy* 1986; 1: 29-33.

113. Raetzman, S.O. Older Americans and prescription drugs: Utilization, expenditures, and coverage. *AARP Public Policy Institute Brief* 1991; 9: 1-15.

114. Randall, T. Demographers ponder the aging of the aged and await unprecedented looming elder boom. *JAMA* 1993; 269: 2331-2332.

Chapter 14

The Drug-Use Process

Jack E. Fincham

INTRODUCTION

The purpose of this chapter is to provide information regarding the drug-use process as influenced by patient behavior, patient compliance, and other variables. Methods utilized to diagnose and avert patient noncompliance are presented and discussed. Potential points of impact by a pharmacist are evaluated for use in numerous settings where pharmacists practice.

The use of drugs as a form of medical treatment in the United States is an enormously complex process. Individuals can purchase medications through numerous outlets. Over-the-counter (OTC) medications can be purchased in pharmacies, grocery stores, supermarkets, convenience stores, via the Internet, and through any number of additional outlets. Prescriptions can be purchased through traditional channels (community chain and independent pharmacies), from mail-service pharmacies, through the Internet, from physicians, from health care institutions, and elsewhere. The monitoring of the positive and negative outcomes of the use of these drugs, both prescription and OTC, can be disjointed and incomplete.

It is important to realize that although pharmacists are the gatekeepers for patients to obtain prescription drugs, patients can obtain prescription medications from other pharmacies and/or physicians. Patients may also borrow from friends, relatives, or even casual acquaintances. In addition, patients obtain OTC medications from physicians through prescriptions, on advice from pharmacists, through self-selection, or through the recommendations of friends or acquaintances. Through all of this, it must be recognized that there is a formal (structural) and informal (word of mouth) component at play. Pharmacists or physicians may or may not be consulted regarding the use of medications. However, in some cases, health professionals are unaware of the drugs patients are taking. In addition, herbal remedies or health supplements may be taken without the knowledge or input of a health professional.

As an example, consider the patient medication profiling capability of most pharmacists. Computerization of patient medication records is commonplace in pharmacy. This computerization allows for ease in billing third-party prescription programs, maintenance of drug allergy information, allows for drug-use review, notification of drug interactions, and aids in the meeting of OBRA '90 requirements. Thus, computerization permits drug-related information to be easily entered, retained, and retrieved. However, OTC medications are rarely entered into such records (one exception may be OTC drugs prescribed by physicians and dispensed through a prescription by pharmacists). This exclusion of a whole class of drugs from the monitoring programs of pharmacy may have a profound affect on the ability of pharmacists to monitor the drug therapies of their patients. If the patient purchases the OTC medication in the pharmacy, the pharmacist may have an idea of the drugs consumed. However, if the OTC drugs are purchased in a nonpharmacy outlet, the pharmacist is completely in the dark concerning the drugs a patient may be taking. Patients may also utilize numerous pharmacies for varying prescription products; in this case there is no one record repository for all medications patients may be taking.

External variables may greatly influence patients and their drug-taking behaviors. Coverage for prescribed drugs allows those with coverage to obtain medications with varying cost-sharing requirements. However, many do not have insurance coverage for drugs or other health-related needs. It has been estimated that for the two-year period between 2001 and 2002, 74.7 million individuals (30.1 percent of the population) under the age of sixty-five were without health insurance for all or part of this period.[1] Certainly, these considerations have huge ramifications for how and when consumers obtain prescribed and OTC medications. Those who do have health insurance have recently seen premiums drastically rise, 8.4 percent in 2000, and 11 percent in 2001.[2] Miller notes that employees are not just being asked to pay more for health insurance, but to pay it all.[3]

SELF-CARE

When examining the utilization of health care, the possibility exists that an individual strives to obtain an optimal state of health but yet does not look to health care providers for advice regarding a health problem. Ory, DeFriese, and Duncker have suggested that self-care: "has evolved in usage to identify a particular role for laypersons in shaping both the processes and outcomes of the care they receive from professionals, a role extending to the self-management of chronic conditions."[4] These authors also indicate that self-care involved actions persons take to self-diagnose and prevent or treat common conditions, both acute and chronic.[5]

Through self-care, an individual might enter the health care system only so far, perhaps to obtain a diagnosis, but will not rely on a physician for treatment of the diagnosed condition. Self-help or self-care may be utilized to try to treat the condition. Appropriateness of self-care lies in the ability of patients to interpret symptoms and understand the symptom experience and what it means.[6] Dean describes four components of self-directed care:

1. Individual self-care
2. Family care
3. Care from extended social network
4. Mutual aid responses to health problems, self-help groups[7]

Self-care can have tangible benefits for many involved in health care delivery. An active orientation toward health care can serve to foster a partnership between physician and patient. Self-limiting conditions could be treated by the individual as well as providers other than the physician, namely a pharmacist. Self-care could save the patient time and expense, and the need for more costly care could be averted.

Self-care or self-help may be one of the unrecognized causes or contributors to noncompliance with prescribed medical and therapeutic regiment. The individual patient may feel that, in the case of drugs, a certain medication may not be needed to treat a certain condition, or that a different medication other than the one prescribed would be more appropriate.

SELF-MEDICATION

Self-medication can be broadly defined as a decision made by a patient to consume a drug with or without the approval or direction of a health professional. The self-medication activities of patients have increased dramatically in the late twentieth century. Many current impacts upon patients have continued to fuel this increase. There are ever-increasing locations from which to purchase OTC medications. There have been many prescription items switched to OTC classification in the past fifty years. In addition, patients are increasingly becoming comfortable with self-diagnosing and self-selection of OTC remedies. The number of switched products is dramatically and significantly fueling the rapid expansion of OTC drug usage.[8,9] Dean notes that in many studies, self-medication with nonprescribed therapies exceeds the use of prescription medications.[10]

These factors influencing self-medication in turn affect pharmacists. Certainly economically, as more OTC products are available for purchase and more places sell them, pharmacists are affected. As self-diagnosis and self-selection of products occurs, pharmacists may not be fully aware of all drugs patients are taking.

Patients' use of self-selected products can have the potential for enormous benefits for patients, as well as others.[11] Through the rational use of drugs, patients may avoid more costly therapies or professional services. Self-limiting conditions on even some chronic health conditions (allergies, dermatological conditions, etc.), if appropriately treated through patient self-medication, allow the patient to have a degree of autonomy in health care decisions.

Advocates of self-medication have suggested that patients who are properly educated to self-medicate are more likely to be independent, knowledgeable, and compliant.[12] Elsewhere, it has been suggested that patient self-medication is a form of patient education.[13]

OTCs are widely used by all age groups. In a large cohort of preschool-age children, 53.7 percent of children had been given some type of OTC medication in the past thirty days.[14] The efficacy and effectiveness of OTC use in children has been challenged. In a critical review of clinical trials over a forty-year period in preschool children, Smith and Feldman concluded that "no good evidence has demonstrated the effectiveness of OTC remedies."[15] Elsewhere, Weiland points to the risks in which patients may be placed by OTC use.[16]

The prominence of OTC usage will continue for several reasons. Manufacturers leverage OTCs when prescription-only products are more suitably made available for patient self-use and when patent protection is lost on products that are generally safe for patients. Retailers appreciate the profitability of OTC products in their sales mix. Patients favor products easily purchased as OTCs, because they do not need to be seen by a physician and receive a prescription for their use in a self-medication situation. Pharmacists should not forget about this important classification of drugs when assessing patient profiles and examining appropriateness of other products consumed by patients, whether they be by prescription or OTC.

PATIENT COMPLIANCE

Definitions of Compliance

The definitions used to categorize patients as compliant or noncompliant have varied tremendously. This variance in defining compliance has been seen as problematic.[17] Compliance is certainly not an "either or" patient behavior, thus the definitions of compliance behavior must be varied to reflect eclectic patient behaviors. See Exhibit 14.1 for several definitions of varying types of compliance. Patients can certainly progress from one of these types of compliance to another. See Figure 14.1 for a depiction of a continuum of compliance activities.[18,19] However, patients who are taking multiple therapies may actually be in several of these categories at the same time depending on how many medications they are consuming.

Noncompliance is not a new construct, it has been referred to for a long time.[20] Mention of the problem of noncompliance has been made numerous times in the medical, pharmacy, and nursing literature. The topic has also been noted in the lay press, where noncompliance has been described as risky.[21]

The consequences and ramifications of patient noncompliance with medication regimens pervade all aspects of the delivery of health care. Noncompliance has the potential to deleteriously affect pharmaceutical manufacturers, prescribers, dispensers, patients, and society as a whole.

EXHIBIT 14.1. Definitions of Varying Forms of Compliance

initial compliance: The patient receives a written prescription and transfers it to a pharmacy or has the prescription phoned to a pharmacy, but does not wait or return to pick up the filled prescription. Patients who do not present written prescriptions for filling could be included in this group.

partial compliance: The process of taking a prescribed and dispensed medication at less than the level the prescriber or dispenser intended.

compliance: The process of complying with a prescribed and dispensed regimen precisely as the prescriber or dispenser intended. Compliance may also refer to a therapeutic endpoint, such as normotension for hypertensive patients.

hypercompliance: The situation whereby a patient takes a prescribed and dispensed medication at a level over the recommended and intended dosing interval.

Initial compliance ⟶ Partial compliance ⟶ Compliance ⟶ Hypercompliance

FIGURE 14.1. The Compliance Continuum

Although not all factors affecting patient noncompliance have been quantified, a growing body of research and knowledge has been accumulating to shed light on the noncompliance problem. Potential effects on medication nonadherence have been formulated, instituted, and evaluated. Despite the steady increase of advances regarding the knowledge of noncompliance, much work remains to be done.

Drug manufacturers, patients, and providers have come to the realization that the problem of medication noncompliance does not rest with one segment of the health care system. Just as the problem pervades all aspects of health care delivery, the responsibility for finding a solution to the understanding and reversal of patient noncompliance (where it is appropriate to do so) must also be shared. Pharmaceutical manufacturers must strive to formulate pharmaceuticals that help to facilitate medication consumption. Manufacturers must follow up the prescribing and dispensing of pharmaceuticals to ascertain if in fact the formulation, packaging, or dosage form design of a product enhances patient compliance with that compound. Physicians most certainly must share in the responsibility for patient compliance. Postprescribing follow-up of patients should be undertaken to ascertain proper drug selection for individual patient needs, both in the therapeutic- and compliance-related sense of medication requirements. Certainly the writing of a prescription must not signal the end of physician involvement in medication compliance considerations of patients. Patients must be given responsibility for, and input into, the medication regimens they are required to take. The patient could be the individual most responsible for the final compliance decision. If aspects of a medication regimen are unacceptable, patients must inform physicians and pharmacists of their wishes, desires, problems, or concerns.

Before patients reach the stage of noncompliance with drug therapies, they initially enter the health care system at varying entry points. They may see a physician, a pharmacist, or perhaps both. They may also bypass the professions entirely and self-medicate with drugs obtained from others. Before examining self-medication or noncompliance any further, an examination of why patients enter the health care system must be examined. Patients enter the health care system with varying intents and a multiplicity of purposes. Pharmacists may see patients at the beginning, midpoint, or end of their entry into the health system. Pharmacists should seek a firm understanding of why patients enter the formal health care system and what they seek to obtain.

Whose Problem Is It?

Whose problem is noncompliance? Some have questioned the treatments many patients receive and ask if cooperation with or control of patients is a goal.[22] Others argue about the term to use—compliance or adherence.[23] Elliot has noted that adherence with medication parallels adherence with appointments.[24] Some patients are accidentally noncompliant and simply are not aware of their noncompliant behavior.[25]

Noncompliance: Negative Connotations

Regardless of the setting studied or the terms used to describe noncompliance, the connotations are certainly negative. The cooperative patient is stated to be compliant, undemanding, or accepting. The uncooperative patient is referred to as difficult, recalcitrant, unreasonable, or demanding.[26] Assigning such a negatively charged label to a patient does no good if there is not a corresponding effort to understand actions, either by the patient or · health professionals, which may lead a patient into noncompliance.

Role of the Pharmacist

Pharmacists can significantly affect patient noncompliance. It is not possible to entirely control patients' usage of drugs; since drugs can be obtained from so many sources, the pharmacist is often unable to be fully aware of all locations where a patient obtains medications. However, pharmacists can play a major, active role in ensuring proper patient compliance. The role of the pharmacist as an optimizer of patient compliance cannot be overstated.[27] Therapeutic benefits to patients, economic rewards to pharmacists, and more appropriate usage of health resources will all be enhanced through appropriate patient compliance monitoring by pharmacists.

How Can Pharmacists Affect Noncompliance?

The roles pharmacists can play in resolving the problem of noncompliance are varied. Home visits by pharmacists have been suggested by some.[28] A more complete integration into the traditional primary health care team has been proposed elsewhere.[29] Pegrum has proposed the delivery of "seamless care" by and between community and hospital pharmacists through enhanced communication and interaction and sharing of information between the two practice sites.[30] Consumers themselves are expecting more from pharmacists as well.[31] More and more patients expect advice, explanation, and information to enhance patient understanding. Where does the pharmacist enter the compliance milieu? The potential for pharmacists to affect medication noncompliance is both enormous and rewarding. The pharmacist is the focal professional with regard to patient medication consumption. All points lead to the pharmacist, so to speak. The convergence of the marketing, prescribing, obtaining, and provision of product centers around the pharmacist. This convergence applies in all health care settings, whether ambulatory or institutional. Physicians who dispense medications to patients exclude pharmacists from the dispensing process; however, in the vast majority of dispensing situations pharmacists are the medication dispensers, and the potential for impact by the pharmacist may be the untapped answer for many of the problems of medication noncompliance. The provision of pharmaceutical care entails the dispensing of knowledge as well. Proper use of a drug may not occur without proper delivery of drug knowledge to the patient.

No professional is in a better position to first detect and inform others of the noncompliant patient. Often, the pharmacist has a special relationship with both physician and patient. Because of this relationship, the pharmacist may "bridge the gap" between the wishes of the physician and the special problems and/or concerns of the patient. Considering the role of the pharmacist in the provision of pharmaceuticals to patients, the pharmacist also may be the professional to depend upon with regard to strategic, mechanical, or behavioral attempts to affect the noncompliant patient.

Noncompliance As an Alternative

Noncompliance may seem to some patients a viable alternative to complying with drug therapy regimens, especially when a patient may have definite opposing viewpoints to those of a physician. Weintraub referred to patients purposely not complying with medication regimens, stating that patients' reasons for not complying seem to be valid in some cases.[32] Elsewhere, noncompliance with mood-altering drugs may a response by patients asserting their independence from psychiatric treatment.[33]

The late Ivan Illich perhaps stated it best: "To take a drug, no matter which and for what reason—is a last chance [for the patient] to assert control over himself, to interfere on his own with his own body rather than let others interfere."[34]

Estimation of Noncompliance Rates

Various authors have estimated the rate of compliance to be between 30 and 80 percent.[35] Rates for estimated compliance can vary as much as the differences between the samples studied, as well as the therapeutic focus of interest in the study designs. Investigators from fifty years ago narrowed their investigation of noncompliance to specific diseases that are treated by very narrow ranges of drug therapies. In a study of noncompliance with penicillin regimens to treat streptococcal infections, 34.3 percent of a sample was found to have taken less than the prescribed course of therapy.[36] Whether the effort is general or specific with regard to estimating noncompliance, Blackwell pointed out that there is neither a typical drug defaulter nor a single, simple solution to the puzzle of noncompliance.[37]

The Consequences of Noncompliance

One of the inherent assumptions in many of the studies of noncompliance is that benefits in treatment outcomes will follow good patient compliance. Almost no studies have been done relating patient outcomes to noncompliance. Various authors have commented on the lack of a positive, definitive linking of noncompliance to deleterious effects in patient outcomes.

Ramifications of Noncompliance

The ramifications of noncompliance can possibly affect the prescription drugs available for use as well as the assessed utility of drugs currently in use. Goetghebeur and Shapiro question the validity of clinical trials for new therapies, especially when substantial variation in dosing intervals is expected.[38] They suggest using a repeated-outcome-measures approach and also incorporating a diary approach for patients to record dosing information. Pocock and Abdalla have questioned the accuracy of pill counts in measurement of compliance in clinical drug trials.[39] Pullar and Feeley suggest that confirmation of noncompliance may be assessed in clinical trials, but that compliance is harder to quantify.[40]

Noncompliance and Emergency Room Visits and Hospitalization

In a study examining the revolving door admission-readmission phenomenon in a sample of chronically ill mental patients, alcohol and drug problems and noncompliance were identified as major factors related to mental facility readmissions.[41] Prince, Goetz, Rihn, and Olsky have chronicled drug-related emergency room visits and hospitalizations in relation to noncompliance.[42] A total of 2 percent of HMO emergency room visits were due to medication misadventures.[43] In this study, underuse was the most common problem identified for adolescent patients, and overuse the most common problem of elderly patients. In another analysis of emergency room admissions, 58 percent of 565 visits were due to patient noncompliance.[44] The reality is we barely recognize the significant influence of noncompliance on emergency room and hospital admission and readmission rates.

Measurement of Compliance

Recently, novel methods of compliance measurement have been designed and evaluated. Because no "gold standard" for compliance measurement exists, innovative technologies have been applied with positive results.[45] One such method, continuous dosage monitoring, records the time of bottle opening. In one study, this electronic assessment of compliance provided evidence of seizure-related noncompliance not evident by examining history, drug serum concentrations, or total pill counts.

Methods to Detect Compliance

Several methods have been utilized to detect compliance. These methods include interrogation of the patient, tablet estimates,* markers,† drug detection in serum, or failure to dispense.[46] Of these five methods, failure to dispense is the most accurate method of measuring noncompliance.

In an evaluation of the various methods available for the detection of compliance, Rapoff and Christophersen have rank ordered the measures of compliance according to their objectivity.[47] Their rating of compliance measures listed from most to least objective is as follows:

Assay (blood, urine, feces, saliva)
Observational methods
Pill counts
Treatment outcome
Physician estimates (overestimate compliance)
Patient reports

---

*This could also include capsules or liquid: the balance of the remaining drug is compared with what was dispensed to determine if the appropriate amount was taken for a specified period of time.

†When either the patient's urine or feces are examined, it is possible to see the marker, usually a chemical, in the material excreted.

Rapoff and Christophersen concluded their assessment of compliance measures by stating, "One reason for the failure of investigators to specify the definition of acceptable compliance is the lack of a clearly objective or universal method for classifying patients as compliant or noncompliant."[48]

Physicians' Estimates of Their Patients' Compliance

Several compliance investigators have researched the ability of physicians to estimate their patients' compliance. Some have questioned whether a physician even considers the possibility of noncompliance in a patient population.[49] It may be wise to exercise caution in considering physicians and their ability to make judgments of their patients' compliance behavior.

Hayes and Lucas have also questioned physician compliance.[50] These researchers noted that only 59 percent of eligible patients receive angiotensin-converting enzyme (ACE) inhibitors and only two-thirds receive thrombolysis or angioplasty.

Factors Affecting Compliance

Despite the compilation of factors (illness related and/or patient specific), noncompliance still is a pervasive problem in many patients.[51] Drug compliance is therefore an individual specific response by patients that is variable and often unable to be predicted in any number of differing patients and/or diseases. Over 250 separate and distinct factors have been found to be related to compliance.[52] The factors to be discussed in this section make up a portion, but not the total, of these over 250 factors.

Haynes, after a review of compliance studies, assessed various factors with respect to influencing compliance either positively or negatively.[53] The factors were separated into categories related to the disease, referral process, clinic, and treatment. The factors and their effect upon compliance are shown in Table 14.1.

Individual studies that have included factors shown to affect compliance will now be presented.

Satisfaction with Care

Physician communication style and patient satisfaction with care are both positively correlated with higher rates of patient compliance.[54] The more the care can be provided in a patient-centered approach, the more likely the patient will be satisfied with care and compliant with recommendations.[55]

TABLE 14.1. Categories of Compliance Factors and Their Effects

Factors in Compliance	Effect on Compliance
Disease (mental illness, schizophrenia, paranoia, personality disorders)	Negative
Symptoms present	Negative
Disability	Positive
Referral process	
Time from referral to appointment (long)	Negative
The clinic	
Waiting time (long)	Negative
Individual appointment time (as opposed to cues)	Positive
Patient making own appointments as opposed to physician making appointment	Positive
The treatment	
Parenteral (refers to injections, either intravenous, intramuscular, or subcutaneous)	Positive
Duration (long)	Negative
Number of medications	Negative
Treatment prescribed	Negative
Cost (increased)	Negative
Safety containers (lock top, child-resistant containers)	Negative
Erring pharmacist	Negative

Source: Haynes, R. B. Determinants of Compliance: The Disease and Mechanics of Treatment. In Haynes, R. B., Taylor, D. W., and Sacketter, D. L. (eds.), *Compliance in Health Care* (Baltimore: Johns Hopkins University Press, 1979).

Age

The age of a patient has been shown to positively affect, negatively affect, or have no effect upon compliance. The vast majority of studies have shown no significant correlation between age and compliance.[56] It is fruitless to examine compliance and age and assume that there is a causal link.

Gender

Gender has not been shown to be a reliable predictor of compliance. The ratio of studies showing no relationship to those with a positive relationship regarding gender and compliance is over 2 to 1.[57] It is discriminatory to assume one gender is more or less compliant than the other. In one study, women have been shown to suffer death from myocardial infarctions if noncompliant with medications.[58] Compliance is a major problem for all, however, regardless of gender.

Cost

Patient compliance has been shown to be deleteriously affected by the cost of prescription drugs.[59] As coverage for prescription drugs in insurance plans is diminished, compliance can be expected to diminish as well. Compliance diminishes with economic stress regardless of whether the condition is reflux disorder, respiratory infections, depressive disorders, or general infectious disease.[60-64]

Knowledge of the Disease

Knowledge of a particular disease (causation, prognosis, cure possibility) has been shown to be positively related to compliance with cardiovascular disease and specific lipid disorders.[65-67]

Work Disruption

Work disruption, as measured by the effort required to seek care and wait for services while taking time off from work, has been shown to be negatively related to compliance.[68] Many patients are paid on an hourly basis and not reimbursed or excused for time away from work to visit the clinic.

Income

Income has been shown to have a direct relationship with patient compliance; however, there are inherent problems in generalizing from these studies to other study populations. Often, there has not been enough of a range in income in the groups studied to allow for a definite link to be established between income and compliance. For example, if the patient compliance in a population studied is low, and the income range of the group is narrow (as is the case in many compliance studies), a low income will automatically be correlated with poor patient compliance due to the economic status of the study population and the study design of the experiment. A similar spurious result could occur if both the range of incomes and reported compliance were high. Generalization from these samples to a broader population would yield an erroneous result.

Continuity of the Physician-Patient Relationship

The presence of a continuous physician-patient relationship has been shown to have a positive influence on patient compliance.[69]

Medication Errors

Medication errors have a devastating effect upon patients, families, and certainly compliance. Medication errors increase emergency room visits and affect patients upon dismissal.[70] Data is difficult to quantify on this important compliance impediment.[71] Confusion and errors only enhance patient drug-taking problems.[72]

Noncompliance can result when prescribers change the dosage of previously prescribed therapies but pharmacists are not notified of the adjusted dosage. Also, if patients are not adequately informed by the physician of such changes, they would certainly be in a position to be noncompliant through no fault of their own.

Disease States and Compliance

Tuberculosis

Noncompliance with tuberculosis chemotherapy has hastened the presence of drug-resistant strains.[73-75] Noncompliance and HIV infection are special issues in the treatment of tuberculosis.[76] Pediatric patients with tuberculosis are affected as well.[77] Overuse and misuse of antibiotics has led to the emergence of resistant nosocomial bacteria.

Asthma

Noncompliance with asthma therapies is a common cause of treatment failure.[78] An indication of the complexity of compliance was found in one study, in which the same patients were more significantly compliant with oral theophylline medications than with inhaled anti-inflammatory medications.[79]

HIV

HIV patients are at risk for noncompliance.[80] In addition, HIV patients with depression suffer many more symptoms due to noncompliance.[81-83]

Contraception

Long-acting contraceptives, such as Norplant and Depo-Provera, have been discontinued because of patients' suffering adverse drug reactions (ADRs).[84] Health professionals need to help patients make a transition to another form of contraception if adverse effects force a patient to be noncompliant.

Helicobacter Pylori

Recent treatment advances to treat the bacterial cause of peptic ulcer disease only work if patients are compliant.[85]

Mental Health

Chronic mental health patients exhibit poor compliance.[86]

Cardiovascular Disease

Compliance with antihypertensive medications may be worse than originally thought. It has also been estimated that only two-thirds of hypertension patients who are at least partially compliant take enough medication to adequately control their disease.[87-89] Compliance with congestive heart failure (CHF) medications is poor, and this is a major factor in hospital readmissions in the elderly.[90] Compliance with antihypertensive medications has been mentioned earlier; it is worth stressing that the major cause of morbidity and mortality in the United States is cardiovascular disease, and noncompliance with cardiovascular medications is certainly one causative factor.[91-93]

Seizure Disorders

Noncompliance with antiepileptic therapies places patients at risk for increased seizure activity.[94]

Cerebrovascular

Noncompliance with prescribed therapy places the 500,000 stroke patients (per year in the United States) at risk for additional strokes or temporary ischemic attacks (TIAs).[95,96]

Ophthalmic

Ophthalmalogic patients need help in understanding the disease, the prescribed therapy, and the proper use of dose-delivery devices.[97-99]

Dosing

Simple, well-designed dosage schedules are necessary to avoid tolerance and rebound phenomenon and to improve compliance with oral nitrates to treat angina pectoris.[100] Once-a-day dosing offers advantages of improved compliance, however more dose-free days may also be a result of once-daily dosage forms.[101] One has to balance whether partial compliance with multiple-interval dosing is more advantageous than missing an entire day of therapy when a day's dose is entirely omitted.[102,103] There may be other advantages to once-daily therapies. In a study of arthritis patients, O'Connor, Anderson, Lennox, and Muldoon found that compliance increased with a once-daily regimen of ibuprofen.[104] Patient symptoms also improved, even though the total daily dose of ibuprofen was reduced. Adverse effects also decreased with the long-acting ibuprofen formulation.

Devices to Aid Patient Compliance

Many devices have been used in an effort to improve patient compliance. These range from prescriber order entry by physicians with the goal of decreasing prescription processing time and increasing the opportunities for pharmacists to work with patients.[105] Computer-generated reminder charts for patients and various caps and counter devices have also been tried.[106]

Technology alone will not solve the vexing problem of noncompliance, in fact in some cases it may diminish compliance. In a study examining the combination of two inhaled asthma preparations in one inhaler (budesonide plus terbutaline sulfate) as a tool to increase compliance, the results were just the opposite.[107] Only 15 percent of patients were compliant more than 80 percent of the time. The use of a tablet splitter to enable economic savings by dividing a higher-dose tablet into two smaller doses was found to discourage patients from complying because of confusion.[108] The use of a notched, clicking cap for prescription medications has been shown to increase compliance.[109] Caps imbedded with electronic devices that can then download information to track compliance have been used as compliance-detecting and -recording tools.[110,111] Other electronic devices can measure removal compliance from blister-packaged doses.[112] Blister packaging and compliance packaging have been used to enhance compliance.[113] Unit-of-use blister packaging has been advocated for use in the United States.[114] Blister packaging and unit-of-use materials are extensively used for prescription medications elsewhere in the world.[115] However, unit-of-use packaging is not without controversy, it has in fact been criticized for lack of standardization between products and manufacturers, which can confuse patients.[116]

THE USE OF MODELS
TO PREDICT HEALTH CARE UTILIZATION

Predictive models of patient behavior have been useful in assessing the impacts of patient drug-taking behavior. DiMatteo and Dinicola pointed out that many of these models are not models in a technical sense, but are lists of relevant variables.[117] These models have been utilized to predict an individual's behavior with regard to specific aspects of health care utilization. Factors have been identified which have been shown to be predictive of drug-taking activities of patients. In a general sense, it is always beneficial to know how certain attributes affect varying patient populations in different fashions. However, there is no typical patient nor is there a model of drug-taking behavior applicable to all patients. Patients are individuals whose responses to drugs, as well as to drug-taking activities, are individual specific.

It is unfair to patients to assume that, because a certain attribute is possessed, a predictable drug-taking behavior will occur. If the compliance studies which utilized a predictive model have told us one thing, it is that there is no typical patient or typical drug-taking behavior. Nothing in the health care system is absolute, including the prediction of drug-taking activities. The most crucial consideration to keep in mind with regard to patient compliance is that strategies with noncompliant patients must be individualized. What works for one patient may or may not be useful for someone else.

Noncompliance Interventions

Of the varying noncompliance interventions: organizational, educational, or behavioral, organizational interventions have been shown to be the easiest to implement, followed by educational and behavioral.[118] Organizational interventions include providing consistent care and the use of reminders for enhancing compliance (e.g., post cards, reminder phone calls).[119]

Educational interventions include written package inserts, labeling, verbal instruction, written instruction, and slide/tape presentations.[120] Behavioral interventions include tailoring of regimens, self-monitoring, reinforcement, or graduated regimen implementation.

When designing written materials for patients, it must be noted that the readability of materials is a vital factor to consider.[121] In addition, illiteracy or marginal literacy is an unfortunate factor negatively influencing some patients' abilities to read, comprehend, and thus respond to cues for enhancing compliance through written materials.[122]

Concerning the provision of counseling materials as a method of enhancing patient compliance, it should be noted that although either verbal or written counseling can enhance compliance, the best way to enhance compliance is through a combination of verbal and written counseling.[123] This provision of counseling should also be individualized, because the ability to comprehend or even read varies tremendously from patient to patient. The combination of written and verbal counseling is crucial in that it allows for reinforcement of other educational formats and repetition in the messages, and patients prefer the combination.[124]

Various packaging aids or "pill taking" reminders are available from various sources. Some patients respond to these materials better than others. For some patients, the introduction of these packaging aids provides an order to their drug taking and thus can be very useful.

The lack of adequate information that patients receive concerning the drugs they take has prompted the federal government to become involved in mandating the provision of information to patients. The OBRA '90 guidelines stipulate that certain information must be offered to patients, among other tenets. Some pharmacy systems are deficient in enabling pharmacists to provide this information.[125] Yet there has been a virtual explosion in the information available to patients and providers alike.[126]

These governmental efforts are not for lack of cause; patients simply do not understand enough about the drugs they take. Efforts to institute mandated patient package inserts (PPIs) in the 1970s and 1980s were aimed at the lack of patient drug knowledge. However, written information alone is not the answer. Individualized assessment and interventions must be aimed at particular and specific patient needs.

Communication

Regardless of form, communication must be seen as the key component for increasing compliance. DiMatteo and colleagues have suggested the use of communication with patients to engender informed choices that in turn lead to enhanced communication.[127] Lambert and Lee have noted that both content and design are crucial to success.[128] Labeling techniques influence as well.[129] Roter promotes the use of a collaborative process when compliance difficulties arise.[130]

Manufacturers

Many manufacturers are succeeding in developing a personal relationship with patients. Increased name recognition, brand loyalty, establishing communication conduits, therapeutic switches, and potentials for increased product usage are but a few of the reasons for doing so. Pharmacists' responses to such manufacturer outreach programs vary. In a national study, Smith and Basara found that most pharmacists believed that pharmacists should not be compensated for switching patients therapies.[131] An interesting finding was that respondents did not feel patient compliance was a major problem. Elsewhere, Smith and Basara have noted that most pharmacists in the study felt that although the manufacturers' programs did benefit and improve compliance, the manufacturer should not be involved in patient education and compliance monitoring.[132] They conclude that pharmacist-manufacturer relations may improve by incorporating pharmacists into the programs.

The Elderly As a Special Class of Patients Affected by Noncompliance

Compliance in elderly populations is a complex issue.[133] In a qualitative analysis of elderly drug taking, Thompson suggested numerous opportunities to promote the quality use of medicine, including

- accurate and specific labeling of prescription medications,
- providing adequate drug information, and
- monitoring for adverse affects.[134]

These suggestions have been seconded by Corby and O'Donovan.[135]

One thing is clear, the elderly are no more noncompliant than other age groups because of their age.[136] However, many attributes predispose the elderly to noncompliance, including

- social isolation,
- chronic diseases,
- multiple drug regimens,
- complex drug regimens, and
- severity of disease.

However, even these factors may not apply to all groups of elderly patients.[137] Alzheimer's disease is devastating and has many effects, including a worsening of problems with noncompliance.[138] Community-based compliance education has been suggested by Buerger as a potential way of influencing elderly noncompliance.[139] Specific places the elderly find themselves in, such as hospices, are ideal sites to examine the specific medication needs of the elderly.[140]

The results of elderly noncompliance are devastating. Bero, Lipton, and Bird found that 35 percent of elderly patients are readmitted to hospitals with drug-related problems within six months of initial discharge.[141] Drug-related factors were a major reason, rather than a contributing reason, for 50 percent of the readmissions.

SUMMARY

Both self-medication and patient compliance behaviors are exceedingly complex. McDonald, Garg, and Haynes point out that patient interventions to affect compliance are complex, labor intensive, and not particularly effective.[142] These authors further suggest that more convenient care, reminders, self-monitoring by patients, reinforcement, family therapy, and additional attention may need to be in play for compliance improvement to occur. Meredith notes that a focus on the individual, rather than a general approach, is more likely to be successful.[143] Others have called for more efficient and more effective approaches to enhance compliance.[144]

For the most part, with regard to compliance-enhancing strategies, the more things that are done the better the chances of success. Enhancing compliance is more art than science, and more trial and error than smooth precision. Success may be frustratingly difficult to achieve, but enhanced and suitable patient compliance should be the ultimate goal of the prescribing, dispensing, and therapeutic monitoring process. Pharmacists can have no more rewarding, yet vexing, experience than successfully helping patients comply with treatment and reach therapeutic goals.

NOTES

1. Stoll, K. *Going without health insurance: Nearly one in three non-elderly Americans* (Washington, DC: Families USA, 2003). Publication No. 03-103.

2. Miller, J.L. *A perfect storm: The confluence of forces affecting health care coverage* (Washington, DC: National Coalition on Health Care, 2001).

3. Ibid.

4. Ory, M.G., DeFriese, G.H., and Duncker, A.P. Introduction. In M.G. Ory and G.H. DeFriese (eds.), *Self-care in later life* (New York: Springer Publishing Company, 1998), p. xv.

5. Ibid, pp. xvi-xvii.

6. Stoller, E.P., Forster, L.E., and Portugal, P. Self-care response to symptoms by older people: A health diary study of illness behavior. *Medical Care* 1993; 31(1): 24-42.

7. Dean, K. Lay care in illness. *Social Science and Medicine* 1986; 22(2): 275-284.

8. Gannon, K. Switched drugs lend vitality to surging OTC market. *Drug Topics* 1991; 135(May 20): 32, 36.

9. Janoff, B. Making the switch. *Progressive Grocer* 1999; 78(5): 135-136.

10. Dean, Lay care in illness.

11. Catford, J. Health promotion in the marketplace: Constraints and opportunities. *Health Promotion International* 1995; 10(1): 41-50.

12. Kelly, J.M. Implementing a patient self-medication program. *Rehabilitation Nursing* 1994; 19(2); 87-90.

13. Barry, K. Patient self-medication: An innovative approach to medication teaching. *Journal of Nursing Care Quality* 1993; 8: 75-82.

14. Kogan, M.D., Pappas, G., Yu, S.M., et al. Over-the-counter medication use among U.S preschool-age children. *JAMA* 1994; 272: 1025-1030.

15. Smith, M.B. and Feldman, W. Over-the-counter cold medication: Critical review of clinical trials between 1950 and 1991. *JAMA* 1993; 269: 2258-2263, p. 2260.

16. Weiland, J. Are patients at risk in their attempts to self-medicate with OTC products? *Maryland Pharmacist* 1996; 72(March-April): 26-28.

17. Dunbar-Jacobs, J., Dwyer, K., and Dunning, E.J. Compliance with antihypertensive regimen: A review of research in the 1980s. *Annals of Behavioral Medicine* 1991; 13(1): 31-39.

18. Fincham, J.E. and Wertheimer, A.I. Elderly patient initial noncompliance: The drugs and the reasons. *Journal of Geriatric Drug Therapy* 1988; 2(4): 53-62.

19. Fincham, J.E. Medication compliance and the elderly. *Journal of Pharmacoepidemiology* 1995; 4(2): 7-14.

20. Sbarbaro, J.A. and Steiner, J.F. Noncompliance with medications: Vintage wine in new (pill) bottles. *Annals of Allergy* 1991; 66: 273-275.

21. Kjellgren, K.I., Ahlner, J., and Saljo, R. Taking hypertensive medication—Controlling or co-operating with patients? *International Journal of Cardiology* 1995; 47(3): 257-268.

22. Ibid.

23. Fawcett, J. Compliance: Definitions and key issues. *The Journal of Clinical Psychiatry* 1995; 56(Suppl. 1): 4-8.

24. Elliott, W.J. Compliance strategies. *Current Opinion in Nephrology and Hypertension* 1994; 3(3): 271-278.

25. Isaac, L.M. and Tamblyn, R.M. Compliance and cognitive function: A methodological approach to measuring unintentional errors in medication compliance in the elderly. *Gerontologist* 1993; 33: 772-781.

26. Powers, M.J. and Ford, L.C. The best kept secret: Consumer power and nursing potential. In Lasagna, L. (ed.), *Patient compliance* (Mt. Kisco, NY: Futura Publishing Co., 1976).

27. Bruzek, R. Community pharmacist: delivering quality care and lower costs. *Journal of the American Association of Preferred Provider Organizations* 1994; 4(November-December): 32, 35-36.

28. Schneider, J. and Barber, N. Provision of a domiciliary service by community pharmacists. *International Journal of Pharmacy Practice* 1996; 4(March); 19-24.

29. Bond, C.M., Sinclair, H.K., Taylor, R.J., et al. Pharmacists: Resource for general practice? *International Journal of Pharmacy Practice* 1995; 3(March): 85-90.

30. Pegrum, S. Seamless care: Need for communication between hospital and community pharmacists. *Pharmaceutical Journal* 1995; 254(April 1): 445-446.

31. Morrow, N., Hargie, O., and Woodman, C. Consumer perceptions of and attitudes to the advice-giving role of community pharmacists. *Pharmaceutical Journal* 1993; 251(July 3): 25-27.

32. Weintraub, M. Intelligent noncompliance and capricious compliance. In Lasagna, L. (ed.), *Patient compliance* (Mt. Kisco, NY: Futura Publishing Company, 1976).

33. Kaplan, E.M. Antidepressant noncompliance as a factor in the discontinuation syndrome. *Journal of Clinical Psychiatry* 1997; 58(Suppl. 7): 31-36.

34. Illich, I. *Medical nemesis* (New York: Bantam Books, 1976).

35. Haynes, R.B., McDonald, H.P., and Garg, A.X. Helping patients follow prescribed treatment. *JAMA* 2002; 288(22): 2880-2883.

36. Mohler, D.N., Wallin, D.G., and Dreyfus, E.G. Studies in the home treatment of streptococcal disease, failure of patients to take penicillin by mouth as prescribed. *New England Journal of Medicine* 1955; 252: 1116-1118.

37. Blackwell, B. Patient compliance. *New England Journal of Medicine* 1973; 289: 249-252.

38. Goetghebeur, E.J.T. and Shapiro, S. Analysing non-compliance in clinical trials: Ethical imperative or mission impossible? *Statistics in Medicine* 1996; 15: 2813-2826.

39. Pocock, S. and Abdalla, M. The hope and hazards of using compliance data in randomized controlled trials. *Statistics in Medicine* 1998; 17: 303-317.

40. Pullar, T. and Feeley, M.P. Reporting compliance in clinical trials. *Lancet* 1990; 336: 1253-1254.

41. Haywood, T.W., Kravitz, H.M., Grossman, L.S., et al. Predicting the "revolving door" phenomenon among patients with schizophrenic, schizoaffective, and affective disorders. *American Journal of Psychiatry* 1995; 152(6): 856-861.

42. Prince, B.S., Goetz, C.M., Rihn, T.L., and Olsky, M. Drug-related emergency department visits and hospital admissions. *American Journal of Hospital Pharmacy* 1992; 49: 1696-1700.

43. Schneitman McIntire, O., Farnen, T.A., Gordon, N., et al. Medication misadventures resulting in emergency department visits at an HMO medical center. *American Journal of Health System Pharmacy* 1996; 53(June 15): 1416-1422.

44. Dennehy, C.E., Kishi, D.T., and Louie, C. Drug-related illness in emergency department patients. *American Journal of Health-System Pharmacy* 1996; 53(June 15): 1422-1426.

45. Von Renteln Kruse, W. Recording methods in regard to patient compliance in medical practice: Clinical trials and consequences. *PZ-Prisma* 1997; 4(October): 189-194.

46. Ibid.

47. Rapoff, M.A. and Christophersen, E.R. Compliance of pediatric patients. In Stuart, R.B. (ed.), *Adherence, compliance and generalization in behavioral medicine* (New York: Brunner-Mazel, 1982).

48. Ibid, p. 92.

49. Stoeckle, J.D. *Encounters between patients and doctors: An anthology* (Cambridge, MA: The MIT Press, 1987).

50. Hayes, G. and Lucas, B. Tools for improving compliance. *Patient Care* 1999; 33(15): 15-16.

51. Ibid.

52. Haynes, R.B., Taylor, D.W., and Sackett, D.L. (eds.), *Compliance in health care* (Baltimore: Johns Hopkins University Press, 1979).

53. Haynes, R.B. Determinants of compliance: The disease and mechanics of treatment. In Haynes, R.B., Taylor, D.W., and Sackett, D.L. (eds.), *Compliance in health care* (Baltimore: Johns Hopkins University Press, 1979).

54. Bultman, D.C. and Svarstad, B.L. Effects of physician communication style on client medication beliefs and adherence with antidepressant treatment. *Social Science and Medicine* 2000; 40: 173-185.

55. Stevenson, F., Barry, C., Britten, N., et al. Doctor-patient communication about drugs: The evidence for shared decision making. *Social Science and Medicine* 2000; 50: 829-840.

56. Haynes, Taylor, and Sackett (eds.), *Compliance in health care.*

57. Ibid.

58. Gallagher, E.J., Viscoli, C.M., and Horwitz, R. The relationship of treatment adherence to the risk of death after myocardial infarction in women. *JAMA* 1993; 270: 742-744.

59. Andrade, S. Compliance in the real world. *Value in Health* 1998; 1(3): 171-173.

60. Bloom, B.S. Cost and quality effects of treating erosive esophagitis: Re-evaluation. *PharmacoEconomics* 1995; 8(August): 139-146.

61. Kuti, J.L. Cost-effective approaches to the treatment of community-acquired pneumonia in the era of resistance. *PharmacoEconomics* 2002; 20(8): 513-528.

62. Van Barlingen, H.J. Model to evaluate the cost-effectiveness of different antibiotics in the management of acute bacterial exacerbations of chronic bronchitis in Germany. *Journal of Medical Economics* 1998; 1: 201-218.

63. Revicki, DA. Modeling the cost effectiveness of antidepressant treatment in primary care. *PharmacoEconomics* 1995; 8(December): 524-540.

64. Verghese, A. Use of oral antibiotics in daily clinical practice. *Drugs* 1991; 42(Suppl. 4): 1-5.

65. McCann, B.S., Bovbjerg, V.E., Curry, S.J., et al. Predicting participation in a dietary intervention to lower cholesterol among individuals with hyperlipidemia. *Health Psychology* 1996; (1): 61-64.

66. McCann, B.S., Bovbjerg, V.E., Brief, D.J., et al. Relationship of self-efficacy to cholesterol lowering and dietary change in hyperlipidemia. *Annals of Behavioral Medicine* 1995; 17(3): 221-226.

67. McCann, B.S., Retzlaff, B.M., Walden, C.E., and Knopp, R.H. Dietary intervention for coronary heart disease. In Shumaker, S.A., Schron, E.B., et al. (eds.), *The handbook of health behavioral change* (New York: Springer Publishing Co., 1998), pp. 191-215.

68. Nutt, D. Treatment of depression and concomitant anxiety. *European Neuropsychopharmacology* 2000; 10(Suppl. 4): S433-S437.

69. Stevenson et al., Doctor-patient communication about drugs.

70. Naylor, D.M. Assessing the need for a domiciliary pharmaceutical service for elderly patients using a coding system to record and quantify data. *Pharmaceutical Journal* 1996; 258(April 5): 479-484.

71. Garrard, J. Management and prevention of medication errors in managed care organizations. *Preventive Medicine in Managed Care* 2001; 2(2): 61-73.

72. Dennehy, C.E., Kishi, D.T., and Louie, C. Drug-related illness in emergency department patients. *American Journal of Health-System Pharmacy* 1996; 53(12): 1422-1426.

73. Houston, S. and Fanning, A. Current and potential treatment of tuberculosis. *Drugs* 1994; 48(November): 689-708.

74. Bloch, A.B., Simone, P.M., McCray, E., and Castro, K.G. Preventing multidrug-resistance tuberculosis. *JAMA* 1996; 275(February 14): 487-489.

75. Davidson, P.T. and Le, H.Q. Drug treatment of tuberculosis. *Drugs* 1992; 43: 651-673.

76. Humma, L.M. Prevention and treatment of drug-resistant tuberculosis. *American Journal of Health-System Pharmacy* 1996; 53(October 1): 2291-2298, 2335-2337.

77. Starke, J.R. Tuberculosis in children. *Primary Care* 1996; 23(4): 861-881.

78. Weinstein, A.G. Clinical management strategies to maintain drug compliance in asthmatic children. *Annals of Allergy, Asthma & Immunology* 1995; 74: 304-310.

79. Kelloway, J.S., Wyatt, R.A., and Adlis, S.A. Comparison of patients' compliance with prescribed oral and inhaled asthma medications. *Archives of Internal Medicine* 1994; 154(12): 1349-1352.

80. Morse, E.V., Simon, P.M., Coburn, M., et al. Determinance of subject compliance within an experimental anti-HIV drug protocol. *Social Science Medicine* 1991; 32: 1161-1167.

81. Puzantian, T. and Dopheide, J.A. Major depression in patients with HIV infection and AIDS. *California Pharmacist* 1995; 42(February): 27-32.

82. Morse et al. Determinance of subject compliance.

83. Puzantian and Dopheide. Major depression in patients with HIV infection and AIDS.

84. Harel, Z., Biro, F.M., Kollar, L.M., et al. Adolescents' reasons for and experience after discontinuation of the long-acting contraceptives Depo-Provera and Norplant. *Journal of Adolescent Health* 1996; 19(2): 118-123.

85. Barbezat, G.O. Treatment of *H. pylori:* Who does what, and to whom? *New Ethicals* 1995; 32(May): 11-12, 14-16.

86. Kelly, G.R. and Scott, J.E. Medication compliance and health education among outpatients with chronic mental disorders. *Medical Care* 1990; 28: 1181-1197.

87. Urquhart, J. Partial compliance in cardiovascular disease: Risk implications. *British Journal of Clinical Practice* Supplement 1994; 73: 2-12.

88. Rudd, P., Ramesh, J., Bryant-Kosling, C., and Guerrero, D. Gaps in cardiovascular medication taking: The tip of the iceberg. *Journal of General Internal Medicine* 1993; 8: 659-666.

89. Eraker, S.A., Kirsch, J.P., and Becker, M.H. Understanding and improving patient compliance. *Annals of Internal Medicine* 1984; 100: 258-268.

90. Monane, M., Bohn, R.L., Gurwitz, J.H., et al. Noncompliance with congestive heart failure therapy in the elderly. *Archives of Internal Medicine* 1994; 154 (February 28): 433-437.

91. Richardson, M.A., Simons-Morton, B., Annegers, J.F. Effect of perceived barriers on compliance with antihypertensive medication. *Health Education Quarterly* 1993; 20: 489-503.

92. Rudd, P. Partial compliance in the treatment of hypertension: Issues and strategies. *Primary Cardiology* Supplement 1992; 1: 17-23.

93. Petri, H. and Urquhart, J. Patient compliance with beta-blocker medication in general practice. *Pharmacoepidemiology and Drug Safety* 1994; 3(5): 251-256.

94. Chadwick, D. Do anticonvulsants alter the natural course of epilepsy? Case for early treatment is not established. *British Medical Journal* 1995; 310(January 21): 177-178.

95. Pecini, M. Pharmacist-managed ticlopidine clinic. *American Journal of Health-System Pharmacy* 1995; 52(September 15): 2030-2031.

96. Schmidt, B.A. and Jue, S.G. Detecting potential medication adherence problems in stroke patients: Implications for pharmacists' interventions. *ASHP Annual Meeting* 1994; 51(June): P-86(D).

97. Claydon, B.E. Non-compliance in general health care. *Ophthalmic and Physiological Optics* 1994; 14(3): 257-264.

98. Kass, M. A., Gordon, M., and Meltzer, D. Can opthamologists correctly identify patients defaulting from pilocarpine therapy? *American Journal of Opthamology* 101, 524-530.

99. Gowan, J. and Roller, L. Prescription problems. *Australian Journal of Pharmacy* 1995; 76(February); 172-173.

100. Held, P. and Olsson, G. The rationale for nitrates in angina pectoris. *The Canadian Journal of Cardiology* 1995; 11 (Suppl. B): 11B-13B.

101. Waeber, B., Erne, P., Saxenhofer, H., et al. Use of drugs with more than a twenty-four hour duration of action. *Journal of Hypertension* Supplement 1994; 12(8): S67-S71.

102. Eisen, S.A., Miller, D.K., Woodward, R.S. et al. The effect of prescribed daily dose frequency on patient medication compliance. *Archives of Internal Medicine* 1990; 150: 1881-1884.

103. Garrett, S.S. Deciding between once- and twice-daily dosing. *American Journal of Health-System Pharmacy* 1996; 53(April 1): 730-731.

104. O' Connor, T.P., Anderson, A.M., Lennox, B., and Muldoon, C. Novel sustained-release formulation of ibuprofen provides effective once-daily therapy in the treatment of rheumatoid arthritis and osteoarthritis. *British Journal of Clinical Practice* 1993; 47(1): 10-13.

105. Segarra, J., DeStefano, J.J., and Davis, R.H. Streamlining outpatient prescription dispensing utilizing prescriber order entry. *ASHP Midyear Clinical Meeting* 1991; 26(December): P-425D.

106. Forcinio, H. Packaging solutions that help patient compliance. *Pharmaceutical Technology* 1993; 17(March); 44, 46, 48, 50.

107. Bosley, C.M., Parry, D.T., and Cochrane, G.M. Patient compliance with inhaled medication: Does combining beta-agonists with corticosteroids improve compliance? *European Respiratory Journal* 1994; 7(3): 504-509.

108. Carr Lopez, S.M., Mallett, M.S., and Morse, T. Tablet splitter: Barrier to compliance or cost-saving instrument? *American Journal of Health-System Pharmacy* 1995; 52(December 1): 2707-2708.

109. Perri, M., Martin, B.C., and Pritchard, F.L. Improving medication compliance: A practical intervention. *Journal of Pharmacy Technology* 1995; 11(July-August): 167-172.

110. Urquhart, J. When outpatient drug treatment fails: Identifying noncompliers as a cost-containment tool. *Medical Interface* 1993; 6(April): 65-67, 71-73.

111. Cramer, J.A. Microelectronic systems for monitoring and enhancing patient compliance with medication regimens. *Drugs* 1995; 49(March): 321-327.

112. Wingender, W. and Kuppers, J. Bayer compliance device. *Drug Information Journal* 1993; 27(4): 1103-1106.

113. Tiano, F.J. Compliant packaging. *Clinical Research Practices and Drug Regulatory Affairs* 1994; 11(1): 39-46.

114. Beagley, K.G. Will unit-of-use take off? *Pharmaceutical & Medical Packaging News* 1996; 4(6): 20-21, 24, 28.

115. Forcinio, H. Packaging solutions that help patient compliance.

116. Rigby, M. Pharmaceutical packaging can induce confusion. *British Medical Journal* 2002; 324: 679.

117. DiMatteo, M.R. and Dinicola, D.O. *Achieving patient compliance* (New York: Pengamon, 1982).

118. Haynes, Taylor, and Sackett (eds.), *Compliance in health care.*

119. Dunbar, J.M., Marshall, G.D., and Hovell, M.F. Behavioral strategies for improving compliance. In Haynes, R.B., Taylor, D.W., and Sackett, D.L. (eds.), *Compliance in health care* (Baltimore, MD: The Johns Hopkins University Press, 1979).

120. Ibid.

121. Riche, J.M., Reid, J.C., Robinson, R.D., and Kardash, C.A.M. Text and reader characteristics affecting the readability of patient literature. *Reading Improvement* 1991: 28: 287-292.

122. Ellis, W.M. Marginal literacy in the adult world: Implications for pharmacists. *ASHP Annual Meeting* 1995; 52(June): PI-20.

123. Raynor, D.K. The influence of verbal and written information on patient knowledge and adherence to treatment. In L.B. Myers and K. Midence (eds.), *Adherence to treatment in medical conditions* (Amsteldijk, the Netherlands: Overseas Publishing Association, 1998), pp. 83-111.

124. Ibid.

125. Cataldo, R. OBRA '90 pharmacy system survey results. *American Pharmacy* 1994; NS34(6): 18-19.

126. Wechsler, J. Information explosion. *Pharmaceutical Executive* 1995; 15 (July): 16, 18, 20.

127. Dimatteo, M.R., Reiter, R.C., and Gambone, J.C. Enhancing medication adherence through communication and informed collaborative choice. *Health Communication* 1994; 5: 253-266.

128. Lambert, B.L. and Lee, J.Y. Patient perceptions of pharmacy students' hypertension compliance gaining messages: Effects of message design logic and content themes. *Health Communication* 1994; 6(4): 311-326.

129. Morrell, R.W., Park, D.C., and Poon, L.W. Effects of labeling techniques on memory and comprehension of prescription information in young and old adults. *Journal of Gerontology* 1990; 45: 166-172.

130. Roter, D. Advancing the physician's contribution to enhancing compliance. *Journal of Pharmacoepidemiology* 1995; 3(2): 37-48.

131. Smith, M. and Basara, L. Pharmacists' opinions about manufacturers' outreach programs. *Journal of the American Pharmacists Association* 1996; NS36(August): 497-502.

132. Basara, L.R. and Smith, M.C. Pharmacist perspectives on patient programs. *Pharmaceutical Executive* 1995; 15(November): 83-86.

133. Herrier, R.N. Medication compliance in the elderly. *Journal of Pharmacy Practice* 1995; 8(October): 232-244.

134. Thompson, S. Opinions and prescription medication use practices among the non-institutionalised elderly. Doctoral thesis, Victorian College of Pharmacy, Monash University, Melbourne, Victoria, Australia, 1996.

135. Corby, D. and O' Donovan, D. Can the community pharmacist improve geriatric compliance? *Irish Pharmacy Journal* 1995; 73(March): 74, 76-77, 79, 82.

136. Lorence, L. and Branthwaite, A. Are older adults less compliant with prescribed medication than younger adults? *British Journal of Clinical Psychology* 1993; 32: 485-492.

137. Coons, S.J., Sheahan, S.L., Martin, S.S., et al. Predictors of medication noncompliance in a sample of older adults. *Clinical Therapeutics* 1994; 16(1): 110-117.

138. Philpot, M. and Puranik, A. Psychotropic drugs and community care. *New Ethicals* 1995; 32(October): 23-24, 26-28.

139. Buerger, D. How to start a community-based education program. *Consultant Pharmacist* 1995; 10(August): 852, 849.

140. Burch, P.L. and Hunter, K.A. Pharmaceutical care applied to the hospice setting; a cancer pain model. *Hospice Journal* 1996; 11(3): 56-59.

141. Bero, L.A., Lipton, H.L., and Bird, J.A. Characterization of geriatric drug-related hospital readmissions. *Medical Care* 1991; 29(October): 989-1003.

142. McDonald, H.P., Garg, A.X., and Haynes, R.B. Interventions to enhance patient adherence to medication prescriptions. *JAMA* 2002; 288(22): 2868-2879.

143. Meredith, P.A. Enhancing patients' compliance. *British Medical Journal* 1998; 316: 393-394.

144. Haynes, McDonald, and Garg, Helping patients follow prescribed treatment.

Chapter 15

Provisions of Care to Subpopulations: A Cultural Perspective

Eucharia E. Nnadi

INTRODUCTION

Diversity in the workplace and the health care industry is becoming an important issue as our country becomes more diverse. Achieving and maintaining workforce diversity should be a priority and concern for health organizations. Diversity can make a difference between a health care organization that is merely sufficient and one that is highly effective and successful. Corporate America recognizes the value and importance of diversity. In fact, some Fortune 500 companies provide incentives for their executives to deal successfully with workforce diversity.[1]

Having a diverse workforce means having people with different demographic, cultural, aptitude, and personality differences, and the ability to work together to achieve organizational goals. The key to successfully managing a diverse workforce is respecting individual differences and talents while avoiding stereotyping and discrimination in the work place. Diversity provides a heterogeneous workforce, thus providing a wide variety of talents in handling challenges and issues in the workplace.

A diverse group enhances the performance of an organization. Individuals are more likely to use the services of a pharmacy where the pharmacist or other employees are seen as having characteristics in common with them. Diversity, if not managed well, can also create problems for an organization. The key to success is to take full advantage of diversity without the potential disadvantages.

According to the U.S. Bureau of Census, the overall resident population is expected to increase at a rate of about 1.1 percent per year. There has been a steady increase since 1970. Between 1970 and 1980, the minority population increased 3.2 percent per year; between 1980 and 1990, it rose 2.8 percent per year. The minority population is expected to continue to increase. Minority groups (African American [blacks], Hispanic, and Asians) make up an increasing percentage of the U.S. resident population each year. In 1970, the minority population was 16.5 percent and increased to 24.4 percent in the year 1990 (see Table 15.1).[2] In the year 2000, African Americans comprised of 12.3 percent of the population, Hispanics 12.5 percent, Asians 3.6 percent, American Indians and Alaska Natives 0.9 percent, Native Hawaiian and other Pacific Islanders 0.1 percent, and two or more (mixed) races were 2.4 percent. Therefore, about 30 percent of the population in the year 2000 were minorities (see Table 15.2).[3] The population of minorities is expected to continue to increase.

The United States is therefore going through major demographic changes as a result of heightened immigration and higher birth rates among minorities. In some U.S. cities, no clear racial majorities exist anymore, and in some cities racial minorities are becoming the majority. Managing diversity is therefore more important than ever. Recent projections suggest that while the white population may stop growing or decline, the minority population will double within the next decade. Racial, economic, ethnic, and demographic changes are occurring in both urban and suburban communities.

MINORITIES: DIVERSITY IN THE HEALTH CARE FIELDS

Given the changes in our population, the health care industries of which pharmacy is an integral part must also diversify. To manage diversity, one must understand diversity. Diversity, as stated earlier, includes the employer's ability to accept and appreciate differences among individuals. By

TABLE 15.1. Estimated U.S. Resident Population by Racial/Ethnic Category: Understanding Census Years 1970-2010 (Projection)—Percentage Enrollment in Health Professions

Year	Minority[a] population	Underrep.[b] minorities	Black	Hispanic	Indians	Asian	White
1970	16.5	15.8	10.9	4.5	0.4	0.8	83.5
1980	20.3	18.7	11.5	6.5	0.6	1.6	79.7
1990	24.4	21.5	11.8	9.0	0.7	2.8	75.6

Sources: U.S. Bureau of Census, Current Population Reports, Series P-25, Nos. 917, 952, 995, 1095, and 1104; U.S. Bureau of Census, U.S. Population Estimates by Age, Sex, Race, and Hispanic Origin: January 1990 to September 1993. *Note:* Minorities: Underrepresented minorities (black, Hispanic, American Indian, includes Alaskan Natives) and Asians (includes Pacific Islanders).
[a]Includes black Americans, Hispanic Americans, American Indians, and Asians.
[b]Includes black Americans, Hispanic Americans, and American Indians.

TABLE 15.2. Profile of General Demographic Characteristics for the United States: 2000

Subject	Number	Percent
Total population	281,421,906	100.0
Sex and age		
Male	138,053,563	49.1
Female	143,368,343	50.9
Under 5 years	19,175,798	6.8
5 to 9 years	20,549,505	7.3
10 to 14 years	20,528,072	7.3
15 to 19 years	20,219,890	7.2
20 to 24 years	18,964,001	6.7
25 to 34 years	39,891,724	14.2
35 to 44 years	45,148,527	16.0
45 to 54 years	37,677,952	13.4
55 to 59 years	13,469,237	4.8
60 to 64 years	10,805,447	3.8
65 to 74 years	18,390,986	6.5
75 to 84 years	12,361,180	4.4
85 years and over	4,239,587	1.5
Median age (years)	35.3	(X)
18 years and over	209,128,094	74.3
Male	100,994,367	35.9
Female	108,133,727	38.4
21 years and over	196,899,193	70.0
62 years and over	41,256,029	14.7
65 years and over	34,991,753	12.4
Male	14,409,625	5.1
Female	20,582,128	7.3
Race		
One race	274,595,678	97.6
White	211,460,626	75.1
Black or African American	34,658,190	12.3
American Indian and Alaska Native	2,475,956	0.9
Asian	10,242,998	3.6
Asian Indian	1,678,765	0.6

TABLE 15.2 *(continued)*

Subject	Number	Percent
Chinese	2,432,585	0.9
Filipino	1,850,314	0.7
Japanese	796,700	0.3
Korean	1,076,872	0.4
Vietnamese	1,122,528	0.4
Other Asian[1]	1,285,234	0.5
Native Hawaiian and Other Pacific Islander	398,835	0.1
Native Hawaiian	140,652	–
Guamanian or Chamorro	58,240	–
Samoan	91,029	–
Other Pacific Islander[2]	108,914	–
Some other race	15,359,073	5.5
Two or more races	6,826,228	2.4
Race alone or in combination with one or more other races:[3]		
White	216,930,975	77.1
Black or African American	36,419,434	12.9
American Indian and Alaska Native	4,119,301	1.5
Asian	11,898,828	4.2
Native Hawaiian and Other Pacific Islander	874,414	0.3
Some other race	18,521,486	6.6
Hispanic or Latino and race		
Total population	281,421,906	100.0
Hispanic or Latino (of any race)	35,305,818	12.5
Mexican	20,640,711	7.3
Puerto Rican	3,406,178	1.2
Cuban	1,241,685	0.4
Other Hispanic or Latino	10,017,244	3.6
Not Hispanic or Latino	246,116,088	87.5
White alone	194,552,774	69.1
Relationship		
Total population	281,421,906	100.0
In households	273,643,273	97.2
Householder	105,480,101	37.5

Subject	Number	Percent
Spouse	54,493,232	19.4
Child	83,393,392	29.6
Own child under 18 years	64,494,637	22.9
Other relatives	15,684,318	5.6
Under 18 years	6,042,435	2.1
Nonrelatives	14,592,230	5.2
Unmarried partner	5,475,768	1.9
In group quarters	7,778,633	2.8
Institutionalized population	4,059,039	1.4
Noninstitutionalized population	3,719,594	1.3
Households by type		
Total households	105,480,101	100.0
Family households (families)	71,787,347	68.1
With own children under 18 years	34,588,368	32.8
Married-couple family	54,493,232	51.7
With own children under 18 years	24,835,505	23.5
Female householder, no husband present	12,900,103	12.2
With own children under 18 years	7,561,874	7.2
Nonfamily households	33,692,754	31.9
Householder living alone	27,230,075	25.8
Householder 65 years and over	9,722,857	9.2
Households with individuals under 18 years	38,022,115	36.0
Households with individuals 65 years and over	24,672,708	23.4
Average household size	2.59	(X)
Average family size	3.14	(X)
Housing occupancy		
Total housing units	115,904,641	100.0
Occupied housing units	105,480,101	91.0
Vacant housing units	10,424,540	9.0
For seasonal, recreational, or occasional use	3,578,718	3.1
Homeowner vacancy rate (percent)	1.7	(X)
Rental vacancy rate (percent)	6.8	(X)

TABLE 15.2 *(continued)*

Subject	Number	Percent
Housing tenure		
Occupied housing units	105,480,101	100.0
Owner-occupied housing units	69,815,753	66.2
Renter-occupied housing units	35,664,348	33.8
Average houshold size of owner-occupied units	2.69	(X)
Average household size of renter-occupied units	2.40	(X)

Source: U.S. Census Bureau, Census 2000.
– Represents zero or rounds to zero. (X) Not applicable.
[1]Other Asian alone, or two or more Asian categories.
[2]Other Pacific Islander alone, or two or more Native Hawaiian and Other Pacific Islander categories.
[3]In combination with one or more of the other races listed. The following six numbers may add to more than the total population and the six percentages may add to more than 100 percent because individuals may report more than one race.

understanding diversity, the employer is better able to provide a work environment that encourages employees to reach their full potential regardless of the employees' ethnic identities, in the interest of achieving overall organizational objectives.

Definitions of racial minority sometimes vary from one publication to another. Universally accepted definitions of racial and ethnic categories have not yet been established. Although the Office of Management and Budget (OMB) in 1975 issued definitions for use by federal agencies, they are subject to multiple interpretations in their use. Sometimes professional associations and academic institutions adopt their own definition of racial/ethnic categories for their data collection on racial and ethnic identities of individuals. For the purpose of this chapter, minorities include the following racial groups: African American (blacks), Hispanic, American Indian (includes Alaskan Natives), and Asian (includes Pacific Islanders).

The issues of availability and accessibility to health care continues to be of concern. Although health care services may be available, it may not necessarily be accessible to all members of society. One of the concerns in the provision of health services is access to these services by minority populations. For those who do not have health insurance coverage, health services are often inaccessible. Inaccessibility to health services often leads to higher morbidity and mortality among minority populations. The more representative the mix of minorities in the health care work force as health care providers, the more responsive our health care system will be to meeting the health care needs of our ever-growing diverse population. It is therefore important to examine minorities' access into the health profession's programs.

Examining the status of minorities in the health fields often poses interpretation problems because of difficulties in getting comparable and commensurable data for several health occupations. Detailed and reliable demographic data for minorities in health professions and occupations are often difficult to secure. However, since professional education is a prerequisite for entry into the health fields, educational data provide insight into the admissions of minorities into the health occupations (see Tables 15.3 and 15.4).

Over the past few years, there has been a gradual increase in the number of minorities enrolled in health professional schools; however, this increase for the most part has not kept up with the increase in the minority population, except for the Asian population. The enrollment of the Asian population in 1992-1993 year has either kept up or exceeded the percentage in the population, except for veterinary medicine. The enrollment data in the Doctor of Pharmacy as the first professional degree program for the 1993 to 1994 school year showed that 13.1 percent were African American, 3.4 percent were Hispanics, 24.4 percent were Asians, and only 0.3 percent were Indians.[4]

The enrollment of minorities in health profession schools in 1999-2000 has not kept pace with percentage of minorities in the general population, except for Asians. The enrollment for Asians has continued to exceed their percentage in the general population (see Tables 15.5 and 15.6). Although enrollment into a health professional school does not guarantee graduation from the school and practicing the profession, it is the first and perhaps the most critical step in the process of becoming a health professional. One cannot become a health care professional without enrolling into a health professional school. Enrollment trends, therefore, provide insight into the expected number of minorities in the profession.

In 1993 to 1994 professional baccalaureate degrees in pharmacy were awarded to only 4.9 percent African Americans, 3.7 percent Hispanics, 0.3 percent American Indians, and 10.3 percent Asian Americans. In the same year, PharmD degrees were also awarded, of which only 6.2 percent were awarded to African Americans, 2.9 percent to Hispanics, 0.4 percent to American Indians, and 25 percent to Asian Americans. Of all the MS degrees in pharmaceutical sciences awarded in 1993 to 1994, only 2.3 percent were to African Americans, and 3.7 percent were to Hispanics. No American Indians received a degree, while 9.6 percent of recipients were Asians. Only 1.9 percent of the PhD degrees were awarded to African Americans,

TABLE 15.3. Total Enrollment in Selected Health Professions Schools in the United States by Racial/Ethnic Category: Recent Years

A. Number of students

Health Profession	Academic year	Total enroll.	Minor. enroll.	Underrep. minor.[a]	Racial/ethnic category				
					Black	Hispanic	Amer. Indian	Asian	Other
Allopathic medicine (MD)	1993-94	66,629	20,002	9,250	4,900	3,986	364	10,752	853
Osteopathic medicine (DO)	1992-93	7,375[b]	1,312	569	231	293	45	743	na
Dentistry	1992-93	15,980	4,794	2,144	944	1,152	48	2,650	na
Optometry	1991-92	4,864[c]	1,110	458	141	295	22	643	na
Pharmacy	1992-93	31,519	na	3,524	2,340	1,088	96	4,135	na
Podiatric medicine	1992-93	2,438	669	397	226	162	9	246	26
Veterinary medicine	1992-93	8,628	656	503	183	270	50	139	14
Registered nursing (RN)	1992[d]	257,983	39,805	31,499	22,147	7,667	1,685	8,306	21,816[f]
Baccalaureate		102,128	16,679	12,713	9,154	2,896	663	3,966	85,442
Associate		132,603	20,227	16,540	11,327	4,237	976	3,687	112,366
Diploma		23,252	2,899	2,246	1,666	534	46	653	20,353[f]
Public health	1992-93[e]	11,088	2,433	1,754	790	871	93	679	8,655[f]
Allied health	1991-92[g]	108,084	22,675	18,650	11,453	6,700	497	4,025	85,409
Chiropractic	1992-93[h]	6,411	596	302	110	168	24	294	5,061

B. Percent of students

Health profession	Academic year	Total enroll.	Minor. enroll.	Underrep. minor.[a]	Racial/ethnic category				
					Black	Hispanic	Amer. Indian	Asian	Other
Allopathic medicine (MD)	1993-94	100.0	30.0	13.9	7.4	6.0	0.5	16.1	1.3
Osteopathic medicine (DO)	1992-93	100.0[b]	17.8	7.7	3.1	4.0	0.6	10.1	na
Dentistry	1992-93	100.0	30.0	13.4	5.9	7.2	0.3	16.6	na
Optometry	1991-92	100.0[c]	22.8	9.4	2.9	6.1	0.5	13.2	0.2
Pharmacy	1992-93	100.0	na	11.2	7.4	3.5	0.3	13.1	na
Podiatric medicine	1992-93	100.0	27.4	16.3	9.3	6.6	0.4	10.1	1.1
Veterinary medicine	1992-93	100.0	7.6	5.8	2.1	3.1	0.6	1.6	0.2
Registered nursing (RN)	1992[d]	100.0	15.4	12.2	8.6	3.0	0.7	3.2	84.6[f]
Baccalaureate		100.0	16.3	12.4	9.0	2.8	0.6	3.9	83.7[f]
Associate		100.0	15.3	12.5	8.5	3.2	0.7	2.8	84.7[f]
Diploma		100.0	12.5	9.7	7.2	2.3	0.2	2.8	87.5[f]

333

TABLE 15.3 (continued)

Health profession	Academic year	Total enroll.	Minor. enroll.	Underrep. minor.[a]	Racial/ethnic category				
					Black	Hispanic	Amer. Indian	Asian	Other
Public health	1992-93[f]	100.0	21.9	15.8	7.1	7.9	0.8	6.1	78.1[f]
Allied health	1991-92[g]	100.0	21.0	17.3	10.6	6.2	0.6	3.7	79.0
Chiropractic	1992-93[h]	100.0	9.3	4.7	1.7	2.6	0.3	4.6	78.9

Source: Bureau of Health Professions. Minorities and Women in the Health Fields, edited. (Rockville, MD: U.S. Department of Health and Human Services, Health Resources and Services Administration, Bureau of Health Professions, 1994.)
na = Data not available.
[a]Includes black Americans, Hispanic Americans, and American Indians.
[b]Includes nine individuals for whom race/ethnicity data were not available.
[c]Includes 121 students enrolled in Puerto Rico: nonminority, 3; black, 1; Hispanic, 117.
[d]Estimated numbers. Detail may not sum to total due to rounding. Data for all nursing categories are based on 1,484 reporting basic registered nursing programs. Excludes American Samoa, Guam, Puerto Rico, and the Virgin Islands.
[e]Excludes foreign nationals.
[f]Minority composition of total enrollment not available.
[g]Includes only programs accredited by the Committee on Allied Health Education and Accreditation (CAHEA) of the American Medical Association.
[h]Total enrollment includes data from eight reporting schools. Detail does not sum to total due to missing racial/ethnic data from one school.

TABLE 15.4. First Professional Degrees Conferred by Institutions of Higher Education, by Field of Study and Racial/Ethnic Category, Biennially, 1984 to 1991

Field of study and year	Total[a]	All minor.	Underrep. minor.[b]	Black	Hispanic	Amer. Indian	Asian	Other[c]	White
All health fields									
1984-85[d]	28,375	3,106	1,964	1,073	746	145	1,142	419	24,850
1986-87	29,043	3,739	2,320	1,292	889	139	1,419	468	24,836
1988-89	29,210	4,332	2,316	1,193	1,014	109	2,016	492	24,386
1990-91	27,821	5,035	2,514	1,308	1,095	111	2,521	499	22,287
Allopathic medicine									
1984-85[d]	14,972	1,881	1,298	730	479	89	583	176	12,915
1986-87	15,429	2,141	1,336	786	484	66	805	151	13,137
1988-89	15,460	2,567	1,423	793	569	61	1,144	113	12,780
1990-91	15,043	3,054	1,514	882	578	54	1,540	142	11,847
Osteopathic medicine									
1984-85[d]	1,489	86	55	29	18	8	31	3	1,400
1986-87	1,618	109	64	26	25	13	45	11	1,498
1988-89	1,635	158	105	40	56	9	53	7	1,470
1990-91	1,459	163	80	17	51	12	83	5	1,291

TABLE 15.4 *(continued)*

Field of study and year	Total[a]	All minor.	Underrep. minor.[b]	Black	Hispanic	Amer. Indian	Asian	Other[c]	White
Dentistry									
1984-85[d]	4,732	620	331	177	123	31	289	84	4,028
1986-87	4,739	763	444	262	169	13	319	120	3,856
1988-89	4,265	824	395	183	199	13	429	158	3,283
1990-91	3,699	900	454	205	235	14	446	142	2,657
Optometry									
1984-85[d]	1,114	121	44	14	28	2	77	14	979
1986-87	1,082	125	51	18	29	4	74	14	943
1988-89	1,093	140	61	30	27	4	79	17	936
1990-91	1,115	176	58	17	34	7	118	21	918
Pharmacy									
1984-85[d]	648	139	43	30	12	1	96	53	456
1986-87	861	270	160	112	42	6	110	60	531
1988-89	1,074	296	84	51	31	2	212	45	733
1990-91	1,244	335	125	61	58	6	210	39	870
Podiatric medicine									
1984-85[d]	582	62	47	35	10	2	15	3	517
1986-87	591	58	46	33	11	2	12	12	521

1988-89	636	75	57	40	15	2	18	20	541
1990-91	589	117	83	52	28	3	34	12	460
Veterinary medicine									
1984-85d	2,177	96	76	36	34	6	20	9	2,072
1986-87	2,230	174	150	29	90	31	24	4	2,052
1988-89	2,157	119	90	32	44	14	29	9	2,029
1990-91	2,032	142	110	44	56	10	32	13	1,877
Chiropractic									
1984-85d	2,661	101	70	22	42	6	31	77	2,483
1986-87	2,493	99	69	26	39	4	30	96	2,298
1988-89	2,890	153	101	24	73	4	52	123	2,614
1990-91	2,640	148	90	30	55	5	58	125	2,367

Source: Bureau of Health Professions. *Minorities and Women in the Health Fields*, edited. (Rockville, MD: U.S. Department of Health and Human Services, Health Resources and Services Administration, Bureau of Health Professions, August 1994.)

aWithin the fifty states and the District of Columbia.
bIncludes black Americans, Hispanic Americans, and American Indians.
cIncludes nonresident aliens.
dData for 1984-1985 exclude awards to persons whose gender or race/ethnicity could not be imputed.

337

TABLE 15.5. Enrollment of Students in Health Professional Schools by Race/ Nationality, 1999-2000

Field	Number	Percent
Dentistry		
White	11,106	64.4
Black	808	4.7
Hispanic	912	5.3
American Indian	99	0.6
Asian	4,317	25.0
Total	17,242	100.0
Medicine (Allopathic)		
White	42,589	65.0
Black	5,051	7.7
Hispanic	4,322	6.6
American Indian	574	0.9
Asian	12,950	19.8
Total	65,486	100.0
Medicine (Osteopathic)		
White	8,019	77.2
Black	399	3.8
Hispanic	370	3.6
American Indian	65	0.6
Asian	1,535	14.8
Total	10,388	100.0
Nursing		
White	193,061	81.0
Black	23,611	9.9
Hispanic	9,227	3.9
American Indian	1,816	0.8
Asian	10,529	4.4
Total	238,244	100.0
Optometry		
White	3,619	68.1
Black	108	2.0
Hispanic	269	5.1
American Indian	30	0.6
Asian	1,287	24.2
Total	5,313	100.0
Pharmacy		
White	22,184	68.2

Field	Number	Percent
Black	2,697	8.3
Hispanic	1,086	3.3
American Indian	156	0.5
Asian	6,414	19.7
Total	32,537	100.0
Podiatry		
White	1,576	69.8
Black	192	8.5
Hispanic	122	5.4
American Indian	10	0.4
Asian	358	15.9
Total	2,258	100.0

Source: Center for Latin American, Caribbean, and Latino Studies, Latino Population of the U.S. Data Bases. Enrollment of Students in Health Professional Schools by Race/Nationality, 1999-2000 (n.d.). Available online at <http://web.gc.cuny.edu/laststudies/Latinodatabases.htm>.

and 1.3 percent to Hispanics. None were awarded to American Indians, while 7.8 percent were awarded to Asian Americans.[5]

Almost ten years later, in 2002, a total of 7,573 professional degrees (baccalaureate and PharmD) were awarded to all pharmacy graduates. Out of that total, 4,648 (61.4 percent) were awarded to whites; 1,625 (21.5 percent) to Asians, Native Hawaiians, or Pacific Islanders; 575 (7.6 percent) were awarded to blacks; 303 (4.0 percent) to Hispanics; 47 (0.6 percent) American Indians or Alaska Natives; 177 (2.3 percent) to foreign students; and 198 (2.6 percent) to other/unknown racial or ethnic identity. In 2002 (compared to ten years ago) the number of first professional degrees in pharmacy awarded to minorities increased slightly, the Asians had the largest increase while the Hispanics had the smallest increase. Although Hispanics are probably the largest racial minority group in the general population, representing 12.5 percent, they are poorly represented in the pharmacy profession. Only 4 percent of the pharmacy professional degrees in pharmacy in 2002 were awarded to Hispanics, compared to 21.5 percent of the degrees awarded to Asians, who represent only about 3.6 percent of the general population.[6] African Americans represent about 12.3 percent of the population and they received 7.6 percent of the first professional degrees in pharmacy awarded in 2002.

The representation of minorities in graduate degrees in pharmacy awarded is worse when compared to first professional degrees. in 2002 a total of 443 master of science degrees in pharmaceutical sciences were awarded. Of that

TABLE 15.6. Total Enrollment of Minorities in Schools for Selected Health Occupations, According to Detailed Race and Hispanic Origin: United States, Academic Years 1970-1971, 1980-1981, 1990-1991, and 1999-2000

Occupation, detailed race, and Hispanic origin	Number of students				Percent distribution of students			
	1970-1971[a]	1980-1981	1990-1991	1999-2000[b]	1970-1971[a]	1980-1981	1990-1991	1999-2000[b]
Dentistry[c]								
All races	19,187	22,842	15,951	17,242	100.0	100.0	100.0	100.0
White, non-Hispanic[c]	17,531	20,208	11,185	11,106	91.4	88.5	70.1	64.4
Black, non-Hispanic	872	1,022	940	808	4.5	4.5	5.9	4.7
Hispanic	185	519	1,254	912	1.0	2.3	7.9	5.3
American Indian	28	53	53	99	0.1	0.2	0.3	0.6
Asian	490	1,040	2,519	4,317	2.6	4.6	15.8	25.0
Medicine (Allopathic)								
All races[d]	40,238	65,189	65,163	66,444	100.0	100.0	100.0	100.0
White, non-Hispanic	37,944	55,434	47,893	42,589	94.3	85.0	73.5	64.1
Black, non-Hispanic	1,509	3,708	4,241	5,051	3.8	5.7	6.5	7.6
Hispanic	196	2,761	3,538	4,322	0.5	4.2	5.4	6.5
Mexican	–	951	1,109	1,746	–	1.5	1.7	2.6
Mainland Puerto Rican	–	329	457	482	–	0.5	0.7	0.7
Other Hispanic[e]	–	1,481	1,972	2,094	–	2.3	3.0	3.2
American Indian	18	221	277	574	0.0	0.3	0.4	0.9
Asian	571	1,924	8,436	12,950	1.4	3.0	12.9	19.5
Medicine (Osteopathic)								
All races	2,304	4,940	6,792	10,388	100.0	100.0	100.0	100.0
White, non-Hispanic[d]	2,241	4,688	5,680	8,019	97.3	94.9	83.6	77.2
Black, non-Hispanic	27	94	217	399	1.2	1.9	3.2	3.8
Hispanic	19	52	277	370	0.8	1.1	4.1	3.6

Category	Number				Percent distribution			
American Indian	6	19	36	65	0.3	0.4	0.5	0.6
Asian	11	87	582	1,535	0.5	1.8	8.6	14.8
Nursing, registered c,e								
All races	211,239	230,966	221,170	238,244	100.0	100.0	100.0	100.0
White, non-Hispanic d	—	—	183,102	193,061	—	—	82.8	81.0
Black, non-Hispanic	—	—	23,094	23,611	—	—	10.4	9.9
Hispanic	—	—	6,580	9,227	—	—	3.0	3.9
American Indian	—	—	1,803	1,816	—	—	0.8	0.8
Asian	—	—	6,591	10,529	—	—	3.0	4.4
Optometry c,e								
All races	3,094	4,540	4,650	5,313	100.0	100.0	100.0	100.0
White, non-Hispanic d	2,913	4,148	3,706	3,619	94.1	91.4	79.7	68.1
Black, non-Hispanic	32	57	134	108	1.0	1.3	2.9	2.0
Hispanic	30	80	186	269	1.0	1.8	4.0	5.1
American Indian	2	12	21	30	0.1	0.3	0.5	0.6
Asian	117	243	603	1,287	3.8	5.4	13.0	24.2
Pharmacy g								
All races	17,909	21,628	22,764	32,537	100.0	100.0	100.0	100.0
White, non-Hispanic d	16,222	19,153	18,325	22,184	90.6	88.6	80.5	68.2
Black, non-Hispanic	659	945	1,301	2,697	3.7	4.4	5.7	8.3
Hispanic	254	459	945	1,086	1.4	2.1	4.2	3.3
American Indian	29	36	63	156	0.2	0.2	0.3	0.5
Asian	672	1,035	2,130	6,414	3.8	4.8	9.4	19.7
Podiatry								
All races	1,268	2,577	2,226	2,258	100.0	100.0	100.0	100.0
White, non-Hispanic d	1,228	2,353	1,671	1,576	96.8	91.3	75.1	69.8
Black, non-Hispanic	27	110	237	192	2.1	4.3	10.6	8.5

TABLE 15.6 (continued)

Occupation, detailed race, and Hispanic origin	Number of students				Percent distribution of students			
	1970-1971[a]	1980-1981	1990-1991	1999-2000[b]	1970-1971[a]	1980-1981	1990-1991	1999-2000[b]
Hispanic	5	39	148	122	0.4	1.5	6.6	5.4
American Indian	1	6	7	10	0.1	0.2	0.3	0.4
Asian	7	69	163	358	0.6	2.7	7.3	15.9

Source: Centers for Disease Control and Prevention, National Center for Health Statistics. Total Enrollment of Minorities in Schools for Selected Health Occupations, According to Detailed Race and Hispanic Origin: United States, Academic Years 1970-71, 1980-81, 1990-91, and 1999-2000 (2003). Available online at <http://www.cdc.gov/nchs/data/hus/tables/2003/03hus104.pdf>.

Notes: Total enrollment data are collected at the beginning of the academic year. Data for chiropractic students and occupational, physical, and speech therapy students were not available for this table. Data are based on reporting by health professions associations.

– = Data not available.

[a] Data for osteopathic medicine, podiatry, and optometry are for 1971-1972. Data for pharmacy and registered nurses are for 1972-1973.

[b] Data for podiatry exclude New York College of Podiatric Medicine. Data for registered nurses are for 1996-1997, optometry are for 1998-1999, and dentistry are for 1999-2000.

[c] Excludes Puerto Rican schools.

[d] Includes race and ethnicity unspecified.

[e] Includes Puerto Rican Commonwealth students.

[f] In 1990 the National League for Nursing developed a new system for analyzing minority data. In evaluating the former system, much underreporting was noted. Therefore, race-specific data before 1990 would not be comparable and are not shown. Additional changes in the minority data question were introduced for academic years 1992-1993 and 1993-1994 resulting in a discontinuity in the trend.

[g] Prior to 1992-1993 pharmacy total enrollment data are for students in the final 3 years of pharmacy education. Beginning in 1992-1993 pharmacy data are for all students.

total 181 (40.9 percent) were awarded to whites, 43 (9.7 percent) to Asians, 17 (3.8 percent) to African Americans, 16 (3.6 percent) to Hispanics, none to American Indians, 15 (3.4 percent) to other/unknown race, and 171 (38.6 percent) to foreigners. Foreigners received more master of science degrees in pharmacy than all the minority racial groups combined.

Most of the doctor of philosophy degrees in pharmaceutical sciences (PharmD) in 2002 were awarded to foreigners. In 2002, a total of 376 doctor of philosophy degrees in pharmaceutical sciences were awarded. A total of 151 (40.2 percent) were awarded to whites, 27 (7.2 percent) to Asians, 8 (2.1 percent) to African Americans, 5 (1.3 percent) to Hispanics, 2 (0.5 percent) to American Indians, 7 (1.9 percent) to other/unknown racial groups, and 176 (46.8 percent) to foreigners.

There are several reasons why it is important to increase the number of minorities in the health professions and adapt to diversity.

1. It reduces internal conflict in the work environment, which in turn improves patient care.
2. It creates a work environment that is conducive to improved communication skills and encourages individual professional growth and creativity, which will result in enhanced patient care.
3. It is good business. Patients tend to be more responsive to providers they can relate to and who can communicate with them in their own native language. The success of some pharmacists has been attributed to the ability of these pharmacists to tailor their services to meet the needs of the cultural and ethnic groups in their service area. [7-9]
4. It reduces ethnic, racial, sexual, and other forms of discrimination lawsuits.
5. Diversity in the health professions can play an important role in eliminating possible discrepancies in the pattern of care among different racial groups, even after controlling for socioeconomic status.
6. Social good is served by having more equitable representation and diversity in all facets of society, especially in a critical area such as health care.
7. Minority health professionals can serve as role models for minority youth. These professionals therefore serve the unique role of being positive images to be emulated and sought after by our young people.
8. Minority health professionals are more likely to provide care in inner cities and less attractive neighborhoods, from which they may have come, because of greater commitment to these communities. Some minority health professionals have experienced the negative

effect of not having adequate health services in such neighborhoods and are more determined to bring about positive changes by serving in them.

9. Greater diversity of the health professions may improve patient-provider relationships and result in better follow-up, better patient care, and ultimately better patient outcomes and a healthier population.

10. Minority health professionals serve as a voice for minority health issues, research, and concerns. Minorities are more likely to be more concerned, involved, and take an active role in health issues concerning them.

11. Diversity cultivates better understanding and racial harmony in our ever more diverse society.

CULTURE, RACE, ETHNICITY, AND HEALTH CARE

Culturally diverse immigrants bring to the United States diverse cultures, attitudes, and beliefs on illness and health care. Several factors, including culture, affect a patient's response to health care services. The pharmacist is an integral member of the health care team in providing primary care and, to some extent, secondary and tertiary care to patients. The pharmacist as a health care provider needs to understand the importance of culture in providing health care services. Epidemiology and ethnic variations, cultural sensitivity, and treatment outcome variations are important issues in providing effective pharmaceutical care to a culturally diverse patient population.

CULTURAL SENSITIVITY

Cultural sensitivity is essential in understanding a patient's cultural value and how it influences his or her decision to comply with recommended treatment. A patient is not likely to accept a treatment modality that is contrary to his or her cultural values and beliefs.

Developing culturally sensitive health care requires being open to issues surrounding patient cultural health beliefs and the traditional medical system, which may be interwoven with spiritual belief. Some cultures, such as that of the Native Americans, have a deep spiritual foundation and family ties. Unlike the majority of white American culture, family means *all* relatives. These relatives may also be influential in the patient's health care decision making. Making the U.S. health care system culturally inclusive can be challenging, but it is necessary in light of our diversity.

During patient counseling, it is important to understand that in some cultures direct eye contact may be a sign of aggression and disrespect to one's superior. With this understanding, the pharmacist will not misinterpret a patient's lack of eye contact during counseling and will not attempt to force eye contact. It cannot be overemphasized that the patient's belief in the treatment provided by the health care professional is one of the most important elements responsible for producing a successful patient outcome.

EPIDEMIOLOGY AND ETHNIC VARIATIONS

Certain health problems and illnesses appear to be more prevalent among different population groups. Differences in mortality rates and prevalence of disease such as sickle-cell anemia exist among different ethnic groups. Therefore, understanding the basic culture-related epidemiology of any population will lead to improving the quality of pharmaceutical care and other health services provided to that population.

Some diseases affect different ethnic groups disproportionately.[10-13] African-American patients are overrepresented among sickle-cell anemia, hypertension, and prostate cancer patients. Since hypertension is the primary cause of heart and kidney disease, it is not surprising that African Americans have greater incidences of strokes, kidney failures, and heart failure related to high blood pressure when compared to whites. Hispanic patients have a high incidence of diabetes, and Hispanic men have a higher incidence of Hodgkin's disease. Chinese Americans have high rates of liver cancer. Native American women have a higher incidence of cervical cancer than white women. Native Americans appear to have the highest rate of diabetes. There are also ethnic and cultural differences in patient response to medicine and health care.

ETHNIC AND RACIAL DIFFERENCE IN TREATMENT OUTCOME VARIATIONS

It is also important that we pay close attention to treatment efficacy among different racial and ethnic groups. For several years, the typical model used during medical training in health professional schools and studying medication efficiency was a white male or female. To better serve all patients, this model needs to be expanded to include minorities. Providing better health care includes recognizing that responses to specific treatments may vary from one ethnic subpopulation to another. We must then realize that what may be effective treatment for a typical white male or female may not be equally effective for a typical African American, Hispanic, Indian, or Asian male or female. Genetic factors play a crucial role in drug metabolism and response to medications.[14] There are significant differences among racial and ethnic groups in drug metabolism. Genetic polymorphisms (enzymes) may influence a drug's actions, altering its pharmacokinetics and/or pharmacodynamic properties and necessitating dosage adjustments for some individuals.[15-17]

African Americans with hypertension treated with one agent respond better to diuretics than beta-blockers or angiotensin-converting enzyme (ACE) inhibitors.[18-20] Chinese are more sensitive to the effects of propranolol on heart rate and blood pressure compared to whites.[21] Substitution of one beta-blocker with another may be especially problematic for African Americans because of clinical differences in their response to propranolol when compared to labetalol.[22] For several psychotropic drugs such as lithium, antidepressants, and neuroleptics, Asians require lower doses and are more likely to have side effects at lower doses compared to whites.[23] Asians are also more sensitive to the adverse effects of alcohol such as tachycardia, palpitations, and facial flushing. American Indians metabolize alcohol at a faster rate when compared to whites.[24] These studies show the serious clinical implications in treating patients from diverse ethnic groups without regard to their ethnic differences. Ethnic and racial considerations must be taken into account in developing restrictive drug formularies and prescribing decisions to avoid putting minority subpopulations at great risk. Ethnic variations in diet may also significantly affect drug metabolism.

CULTURAL INFLUENCES
AND UTILIZATION OF PHARMACEUTICAL SERVICES

It is well known that culture influences health behavior, illness response, and attitude toward health care. It is no secret that patients engage in folk healing without informing their health care providers. Folk or alternative medical care can have a significant affect on treatment. It can complement, interfere, or complicate drug therapy.

Cultural explanation of an individual's illness is also important. This is because it affects the patient's decision whether to seek care or not. To provide better health services to patients, the health care provider should pay attention to the patient's cultural explanation of his or her health problem. This will often provide helpful insight into the patient's perception of the disease process, ethnology, illness experience, and health belief. The ways an individual will evaluate, respond, or treat a symptom and comply with recommended treatment is deeply embedded in the patient's culture. By considering a patient's culture when providing health services, health care providers can begin to see patients as heterogeneous and avoid generalizing treatment across all patients, which is central to effective clinical care.

Social and cultural values greatly influence individual decisions to seek care even in the absence of pathological processes or to delay health care for a serious health condition.[25-29] The decision to seek care is often affected by the social and cultural values, regardless of type or severity of the illness. A patient's culture influences what a patient may perceive as a health problem and what is ignored.

Reports in the pharmacy literature have found that diversity in the workplace is instrumental in improving patient outcomes, saving lives, and having successful community pharmacy practice.[30] Pharmacists in various professional settings are recognizing the importance of having a diverse workplace and creating a bond by having a pharmacist who can speak the patient's native language. Having a diverse workforce in pharmacy practice has resulted in serving patients better. Given the current trends, it may soon be necessary for health care professionals (especially those in culturally diverse communities) to have at least one individual in the workplace who can speak another language in addition to English, and who has an in-depth understanding of a specific culture. Health professionals who learn about cultural differences are more likely to build trust and loyalty with their patients. A pharmacist who speaks a patient's native language is better able to emphasize the importance of complying with medication orders and explain the role of alternative medical care, if any, than one who does not speak the patient's language. Remember that it is not unusual for foreign-born individuals to have less-than-adequate English communication skills. As a result, even simple instructions in English can easily be misunderstood by the patient, possibly leading to disastrous results.

Whether pharmacists practice in communities or institutional settings, their activities are interrelated with those of other medical care personnel. Of all the health care professionals, pharmacists are often the most easily accessible and may serve as the gateway to health care. As a result, the patient may first consult the pharmacist for a specific health problem because the pharmacist is found more conveniently in the community.

Pharmacists, therefore, play a significant role in patient self-medication. It is estimated that for more than 70 percent of health care problems consumers use over-the-counter (OTC) medication.[31] It also has been documented that pharmacists are a very important factor in influencing consumers to buy an OTC medication for the first time.[32] People who use the pharmacy for OTC products as the first line of defense against a health problem are likely to have more confidence in someone who understands their culture and can communicate with them. Understanding how some cultural and ethnic groups view health care and medication is important in counseling and improving patient outcomes. Some racial and ethnic groups, such as the Chinese, believe in healing the whole body. Some ethnic groups are more inclined to take herbal remedies or Eastern remedies in combination with their OTC and/or prescription drugs. Such combinations have a greater potential for side effects.

Pharmacists, by their education, are knowledgeable about drugs and drug therapy. However, effective and efficient drug therapy is better achieved if the patient's ethnic, racial, and cultural background are understood and taken into consideration during patient-pharmacist interaction in the pharmacy. The importance of one's culture in health and illness behavior cannot be overemphasized. From the onset of symptoms to the time a patient arrives at a pharmacy to the time the patient leaves the health care system, he or she makes several decisions and responses that are under cultural influence.

The patient utilizing the services of a pharmacy or pharmacist goes through several stages in the decision-making process. These stages can be viewed as a process occurring over time, in which both the patient and the pharmacist interact, each playing an important role—the patient at one time and the pharmacist at another. However, the key decision to continue or terminate the health utilization process is made by the patient. These stages include the following:

1. Perception of a need for a pharmacist's advice regarding a health problem.
2. Decision and selection of a pharmacy or pharmacist to go to for consultation.
3. Actual consultation with the particular pharmacist or any pharmacist at the pharmacy of a patient's choice.
4. If the patient complies with a pharmacist's recommendation and is satisfied with the outcome, the process is terminated. If, however, the patient chooses not to comply or is dissatisfied with the consultation and if the health problem persists, the patient may either end the process or seek another consultation, thus reinitiating the process (see Figure 15.1).

How long it takes a patient to go through the stages will vary from patient to patient.

To initiate the use of pharmacy services, the patient must first be able to perceive a need. During this stage, the patient may seek advice from friends or relatives, a process that often has been called the lay-referral network.[33]

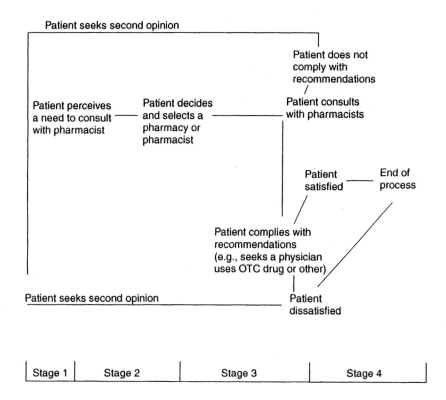

FIGURE 15.1. Stages in the Use of Pharmacy (Pharmacist) Services

A patient is more likely to seek advice from those within the same racial and ethnic group than from those outside the group. Any consultation with friends or relatives is often crucial to the patient's opinion about his or her own health problems and the subsequent decision to seek advice from a pharmacist or health care professional.

The choice of a pharmacy is often a function of the lay-referral system. A layperson often makes the recommendations regarding where to seek health care, which is sometimes based on that person's experiences with a similar health problem or with a particular pharmacy or pharmacist. Also influencing the selection of a pharmacy is the type of service offered and the pharmacist's ability to communicate in the patient's language.[34] Consumers do take advantage of professional services from a pharmacy if they are made aware of them.[35,36] Various studies have indicated that location, convenience, and low cost are among the most important considerations in selecting a specific type of pharmacy.[37,38] It is possible to distinguish among pharmacy patrons on the basis of their involvement and expertise in their choice of pharmacy. Patient involvement with a pharmacy and expertise in pharmacy selection are related to demographic characteristics and patient experience.[39] As more of the patient population belongs to a health care organization, such as health maintenance organizations (HMOs) or managed care, these organizations will continue to play a significant role in determining where patients receive their pharmacy services. Patients who are members of health plans and who do not wish to pay out of pocket for services or medications can use only those pharmacies selected by their health plan to receive benefits such as partial or full reimbursement for pharmacy services. However, where a consumer can culturally relate to a pharmacist or pharmacy, there is a greater likelihood of increased use of that pharmacist's or pharmacy's services. As competition in community pharmacy practice increases, diversity in the pharmacy creates an added differential advantage to help the pharmacy to remain financially viable. Once a pharmacy is identified in the community as being very effective in meeting the needs of an ethnic group, especially those of foreign origin who speak little or no English, the lay-referral system will further promote the services provided by that pharmacy. Thus the pharmacy may get into a health plan to provide pharmaceutical care to health plan enrollees when patients learn to use outcome data to select pharmacy services.

The next stage in the decision process involves actual consultation with the chosen pharmacist or pharmacy. The patient evaluates the pharmacist before and during the consultation. After consultation, and possibly during the consultation based on the patient's perception on how he or she was treated and the patient's confidence in the pharmacist, the patient decides whether to comply with the pharmacist's recommendation(s). The recommendation could be to see a physician, use an OTC drug, or some other recommendation. Decisions at this stage also can be influenced by the lay-referral network. If the pharmacist meets the expectations of the patient, the patient often will comply, as long as compliance does not make an undue demand on the patient's social functioning or involve a behavioral change contrary to the patient's belief and culture. Where the recommendation is in conflict with the patient's expectations or culture, noncompliance becomes inevitable. A successful outcome after the interaction between the pharmacist and the patient is beneficial in effective treatment of a health problem.

It is only by understanding the patient's cultural background that the pharmacist may be better able to effectively serve the needs of that patient. Once a pharmacist recognizes that a patient has perceived a major health problem to be a minor one because of cultural background and belief, then the pharmacist can more effectively communicate with the patient about the importance of consulting a physician rather than using an OTC product.

As already indicated, regardless of what recommendations a health care professional makes to a patient, these recommendations will be influenced by a host of sociocultural and psychological factors. If the patient decides not to comply, for whatever reason, either the process is terminated or the patient may decide to seek a second opinion from another health care provider, sometimes utilizing the lay-referral system again. If the recommendations result in a desirable outcome, the patient may continue to consult with that pharmacist as a community health care provider.

CULTURE AND TREATMENT COMPLIANCE

The importance of culture, race, and ethnic background in the lay-referral system must be emphasized. Each racial and ethnic group respects and accepts certain values, attitudes, and beliefs within its culture. The value system of an ethnic group is deeply seeded, bringing strong adherence to a set of beliefs. Different cultures use varying standards for judging normality and abnormality, so that what is regarded as illness or disease in one cultural setting may not be so in another. The range of normality and abnormality in different cultures therefore does not always coincide. Mechanic provided a good example with a skin disorder called dyschronmatic spirochestosis; it was so prevalent in a South American tribe that tribal members who did not have the disease were regarded as abnormal.[40] In this instance, having the disease was perceived by tribal members as normal rather than a disease process. Recommendation for a treatment in such a situation is likely to fail because it is in conflict with the patient's belief.

Cultural perspectives of illness and disease operate at different periods in the illness determination process. The experience of illness and the decision to seek help and to comply with a prescribed regimen are as much a function of the ability to cope and adapt to one's culture as they are a biological phenomenon. Where the lines between health and illness are not clear to the average person, cultural factors typically intervene before a perception of illness and a need for health care are realized. When the need for health care is not realized, then the patient will not comply with even the recommendation to seek care.

A patient's social group structure, which includes ethnic exclusivity and family tradition (that is, the importance placed on custom and traditions), is one of Suchman's measures of illness behavior. Suchman found that ethnic exclusivity was associated with a high degree of skepticism toward medical care, thus making effective communication with patients crucial.[41] Because of variations in patient response to illness and in the tendency to seek health care, several other researchers have suggested various health belief models to summarize and explain these differences.[42-45] Stoeckle's definition of the factors that cause patients to seek health care in response to symptoms included the following:

- Patient's perception, belief, and attitude about the health problem
- Patient's attitude and expectation of the health care system
- Patient's definition of health and sickness, including when health care becomes necessary[46]

A close look at these health belief models explaining patient response to illness shows that they appear to have one basic and essential element in common—the patient's culture. Although culture is not emphasized in these models, they do recognize that culture clearly influences how one handles sickness, including the decision to comply with recommended treatment.

Another good example of how cultural differences affect the way people react to symptoms was provided by Zborowski in his description of the response to pain by members of ethnocultural groups, specifically Jews, Italians, Irish, and "Old Americans" in New York City hospitals.[47] In this study, he reported substantial ethnic variations in the respondents' reaction to pain. Thus, symptom sensitivity seems to have a cultural correlation that affects the use of health care services and, consequently, compliance with recommendations.

Unsuccessful consultation with the pharmacist obviously has several negative ramifications for the patient, including loss of confidence in the pharmacist as a health care professional, increased health care expenses, wasted time, and perhaps increased morbidity and mortality. For a successful outcome, it is usually necessary for the patient to comply with health care recommendations. The health care professional must understand the patient in order to improve patient compliance.

The literature is rich in information and various reasons why patients may not comply with a prescribed regimen. These reasons include side effects, taste, cost, and attitude toward health care providers and illness. A patient's attitude is often influenced by the culture. Therefore, the health care professional should pay more attention to the patient's cultural background. Culture not only influences the patient's decision to seek care but also the decision to comply or not comply with recommended therapeutic regimens.

It has been documented that conflicting cultural beliefs across ethnic groups may affect medication compliance and drug and placebo responses, as well as responses to standardized clinical psychiatric and psychological tests.[48-50]

Where culture and compliance are in conflict, the importance of an effective pharmacist-patient relationship and communication cannot be overemphasized. Reassuring the patient that the recommendation is essential for effective treatment of the health problem will help improve compliance, patient care, and outcomes.

CONCLUSION

The United States population is becoming more diversified than ever. Projections by the U.S. Bureau of the Census indicate that racial minority populations will continue to increase. Different ethnic and racial groups have different cultures with real implications for health care and services. Although racial minority enrollment and graduation from health professional schools appear to be increasing, they are very much underrepresented compared to their proportions in the population. Asians have made more significant progress in entering the health professions compared to other racial minorities. There are several advantages to having a racially diverse workforce in the provision of health services.

Certain diseases and health problems appear to be more prevalent among certain ethnic and racial groups. Racial minorities also show different responses to different classes of drugs when compared to Caucasians. Genetic factors play an important role in drug metabolism, which may explain the difference in drug responses by different ethnic and racial groups.

Ethnic and racial minorities can be subjected to greater health risks if they receive the usual or standard doses of some drugs because they cannot tolerate the standard dosage of these drugs. Racial minorities should be included in all clinical drug trials and metabolic studies for better determination of therapeutic efficacy, effectiveness, and side effects among minority populations. Health care professionals should individualize treatment and take racial and ethnic origin into consideration. The extent and nature of cross-racial variability in metabolism and response to all classes of drugs are not known. Health care providers should watch for atypical responses or unexpected side effects in therapeutic management of racial and ethnic minorities.

Ethnic, racial, and cultural background play a significant role in patient responses to therapy, illness, disease, and health care services.[51] Different cultures use differing standards in judging ill health. The patient's culture not only influences the patient's decision to seek care but also whether to comply with recommended therapy. Pharmacists must consider a patient's ethnic, racial, and cultural background to provide optimal drug therapy, especially to racial minorities.

NOTES

1. Laabs, J. Interest in diversity training continuing to grow. *Personnel Journal* 1993; October: 18.

2. U.S. Bureau of Census, Current Population, series P-25, Nos. 917, 952, 995, 1095. *U.S. Bureau of Census Population Estimates by Age, Sex, Race, and Hispanic Origin: 1990 to September 1993.*

3. U.S. Bureau of Census. *United States Census 2000.* (U.S. Department of Commerce, Economic, and Statistics Administration, July 2002.)

4. American Association of Colleges of Pharmacy. AACP Institutional Research Report Series: *Profile of Pharmacy Students 1995* (Alexandria, VA: American Association of Colleges of Pharmacy, 1995).

5. Ibid.

6. American Association of Colleges of Pharmacy. AACP Institutional Research Report Series: *Profile of Pharmacy Students 2003* (Alexandria, VA: American Association of Colleges of Pharmacy, 2003).

7. Anonymous. Community commitment. *NARD Journal* 1995; 39 (August).

8. Anonymous. Investing in diversity. *American Druggist* 1995; 22 (September).

9. Gorey, K.M. and Vena, J.E. Cancer differentials among U.S. blacks and whites: Quantitative estimates of socioeconomic-related risks. *Journal of the National Medical Association* 1994; 86(3): 209.

10. Ibid.

11. U.S. Department of Health and Human Services. *Health status of the disadvantaged: Chart Book 1990* (U.S. Department of Health and Human Services, Public Health Resources and Services Administration, 1990).

12. National Institutes of Health. *Cancer among blacks and other minorities: Statistical profiles* (U.S. Department of Health and Human Services, National Institutes of Health, 1991).

13. Jones, A.L. (ed.), *Minorities and cancer* (New York: Springer-Verlag, 1992).

14. Meyer, U.A. Drugs in special patient groups: Clinical importance of genetics in drug effects. In Morreli, H.F., Hoffman, B.B., and Nierenberg, D.W. (eds.), *Melmon and Morrelli's clinical pharmacology: Basic principles in the therapeutics,* Third edition (New York: McGraw-Hill, 1992), pp. 875-894.

15. Eichelbaum, M. and Cross, A.S. The genetic polymorphism of debrisoquine/sparteine metabolism—Clinical aspects. *Pharmacology and Therapeutics* 1990; 46: 377-394.

16. Wood, A.J.J. and Ahou, H.H. Ethnic differences in drug disposition and responsiveness. *Clinical Pharmacokinetics* 1991; 20: 350-373.

17. Dayer, P., Merrier, G., Perrenoud, J., Marmy, A., and Leeman, T. Interindividual pharmacokinetics and pharmacodynamic variability of different beta-blockers. *Journal of Cardiovascular Pharmacology* 1986; 6(Suppl.): 20-24.

18. Hall, D. Pathophysiology of hypertension in blacks. *American Journal of Hypertension* 1990; 3: 366S-371S.

19. Veterans Administration Cooperative Study Groups on Antihypertensive Agents. Comparison of propranolol and hydrochlothiazide for initial treatment of hypertension: Results of short-term titration with emphasis on racial differences in response. *Journal of the American Medical Association* 1982; 248: 1996-2003.

20. Freis, E.D. Antihypertensive agents. In Kalow W., Goedde, H.W., and Agarwal, D.P. (eds.), *Ethnic differences in reactions to drugs and zenobiotics* (New York: Alan R. Liss, Inc., 1986), pp. 313-322.

21. Zhou, H.H., Adeloyin, A., and Wilkinson, G.R. Difference in plasma binding of drugs between Caucasians and Chinese subjects. *Clinical Pharmacokinetics and Therapeutics* 1990; 48: 10-17.

22. Frishman, W.H. Clinical difference between beta-adrenergic blocking agents: Implications for therapeutic substitution. *American Heart Journal* 1987; 113: 1190-1198.

23. Binder, R.I. and Levy, R. Extrapyramidal reactions in Asians. *American Journal of Psychiatry* 1981; 138: 1243-1244.

24. Kalow, W. Ethnic difference in drug metabolism. *Clinical Pharmacokinetics* 1982; 7: 374-400.

25. Zola, I.K. Culture and symptoms: An analysis of patients presenting complaints. *American Sociological Review* (1966) 31: 615-630.

26. Stocker, J.D. and Barsky, A.J. Attributions: Uses of social sciences knowledge in the "doctoring" of primary care. In Eisenburg, L. and Kleinma, A. (eds.), *The relevance of social science for medicine* (Hingma, MA: D. Reidel Publishing Co., 1980), pp. 223-240.

27. Ludwig, E.G., and Gibson, G. Self-perception of sickness and the seeking of medical care. *Journal of Health and Social Behavior* 1969; 10: 125-133.

28. Battistella, R.M. Factors associated with delay in initiation of physicians' care among late adulthood persons. *American Journal of Public Health* 1971; 61: 1348-1961.

29. Zborowski, M. Cultural components in response to pain. *Journal of Social Issues* 1952; 84: 16-30.

30. Anonymous, Community commitment; Anonymous, Investing in diversity.

31. Knapp, D.A. and Knapp, D.E. Decision making and self-medication: Preliminary findings. *American Journal of Hospital Pharmacy* 1972; 29: 1044-1012.

32. Knapp, D.A., Oeltjen, P.D., and Knapp, D.E. OTC decision making using nonprescription drug for the first time. *Medical Marketing Media* 1975; 10: 26-29.

33. Freidson, E. *Patients' views of medical practice* (New York: Russell Sage Foundation, 1961).

34. Anonymous, Community commitment; Anonymous, Investing in diversity.

35. Angevine, E. The consumer's consumer. *Journal of the American Pharmaceutical Association* 1972; 12(NS): 356.

36. The Dichter Institute of Motivation Research, Inc. *Communicating the value of comprehensive pharmaceutical services to the consumer: Final report* (Washington, DC: American Pharmaceutical Association, 1973).

37. Kabat, H.F. Choice of pharmaceutical service. *Journal of the American Pharmaceutical Association* 1969; (NSG): 73.

38. Hammel, R.W. and Mayers, M.J. Patterns of prescription patronage. *The Wisconsin Pharmacist* 1965; 34: 224.

39. Lipowski, E.E. How consumers choose a pharmacy. *American Pharmacy* 1933; NS 33(12): S14-S17.

40. Mechanic, D. *Medical sociology* (New York: Free Press, 1968).

41. Suchman, E.A. Social patterns of illness and medical care. *Journal of Health and Human Behavior* 1956; 6.

42. Stoeckle, J.D., Zola, I.K., and Davidson, G.E. On going to see the doctor: The contributions of the patient to the decision to seek medical aid. *Journal of Chronic Disease* 1963; 6: 975-989.

43. Rosenstock, I. Why people use health services. *Milbank Memorial Fund Quarterly* 1966; 44: 94-127.

44. Zola, I. Illness behavior of the working class. In Shostak, A. and Gomberg, W. (eds.), *Blue collar world: Studies of the American worker* (Englewood Cliffs, NJ: Prentice-Hall, 1964).

45. Anderson, R. *A behavioral model of families' use of health services: Center for Health Administration Studies.* Research Series 25 (Chicago, IL: University of Chicago Press, 1968).

46. Stoeckle et al., On going to see the doctor.

47. Zborowski, Cultural components in response to pain.

48. Smith, M., Lin, K.M., and Mendoza, R. Nonbiological issues affecting psychopharmocotherapy: Cultural considerations. In Lin, K.M., Poland, R.E., and Nakaski, G. (eds.), *Psychopharmacology and psychobiology of ethnicity* (Washington, DC: American Psychiatry Press, 1992).

49. Lin, K.M., Poland, R.E., and Lesser, I.M. Ethnicity and psychopharmocology. *Cultural Medicine and Psychiatry* 1986; 10: 151-165.

50. Lawson, W.B. Racial and ethnic factors in psychiatric research. *Hospital and Community Psychiatry* 1986; 37: 50-54.

51. Harwood, A. (ed.), *Ethnicity and medical care: A commonwealth fund book* (Cambridge, MA: Harvard University Press, 1981).

Chapter 16

New Technologies:
Understanding the Basics of Biotechnology

Nicholas Bartone
Robert J. Amend
Richard S. Hurd
Sandip Singh

We wish to suggest a structure for the salt of deoxyribose nucleic acid (D.N.A.). This structure has novel features which are of considerable biological interest.

> James Watson and Francis Crick,
> in a brief letter to the journal *Nature,*
> April 2, 1953

Over fifty years ago Watson and Crick successfully identified the structure of deoxyribonucleic acid (DNA) and, perhaps unknowingly, opened the eyes of the world to the promise of biotechnology. Their discovery has been the platform for unrelenting efforts that have only recently culminated in the successful characterization of a complete human genome sequence. Along the way, modern biotechnology was born through advancements in genetic manipulation, allowing for the control of selective gene expression and the determination of resultant protein products. Once harnessed, this technology allowed for the development of novel products such as recombinant human insulin for diabetes and monoclonal antibodies used to treat autoimmune disorders, thus revolutionizing pharmacotherapy.

In order to achieve a greater understanding of biotechnology, it is essential to first gain a basic understanding of the underlying science that drives its innovation. It is equally important to understand the implications of this "new" industry in terms of its affect on current economic, regulatory, and ethical environments. This chapter attempts to guide the reader from an understanding of the basic components that are currently shaping biotechnology to how biotechnology is quickly influencing our world today.

ESSENTIALS OF BIOTECHNOLOGY

Within each cell are strands of genetic code called DNA, the basic blueprint of life. This DNA is composed of a series of base pairs that match nucleosides such as adenosine to thymidine and cytidine to guanidine. An organism's physical traits are determined by the order of these bases, which, when taken together, comprise its genome, or complete set of DNA for an organism. In order to study the effects of each pairing and derive medical advances from this strand of bases, researchers must use the tools at their disposal to dismantle and scrutinize genomes. The following sections will provide a brief background into some of the most common avenues of biotechnology that aid in accomplishing this rather daunting task.

Molecular Cloning

Molecular cloning is, perhaps, the most important and widely utilized component of biotechnology. Different from animal cloning, molecular cloning is a technique that allows researchers to create multiple copies of genes in a relatively short period of time, taking entire genomes and deconstructing them into smaller, more useful portions. Molecular cloning aids in the quest to identify the structure and function of individual genes (a sequence of DNA nucleotides that comprise physical or metabolic traits) and their products.

The first step of this process is to isolate specific DNA sequences (i.e., targeted genes) from a heterogeneous mixture of DNA fragments.[1] Once isolated, the next step of the process is to amplify the separated DNA by extensively duplicating it to allow for further study.[2] The amplification process involves inserting the isolated target gene into a loop of DNA called a plasmid, forming recombinant DNA. This plasmid is then introduced into a host cell, such as a bacterial cell, where it can be replicated unharmed by degrading enzymes. This technology can be applied to entire genomes by taking a specific organism's cumbersome DNA and dividing it up into manageable portions that can be cloned. This allows researchers to concentrate on smaller portions of the genetic material, and when completed, these cloned bits of DNA can be connected to create the genome of the organism.[3]

Genomics

Once a DNA strand has been isolated and amplified through cloning, genomics is the first step in unraveling its code. Broken down, genomics is a combination of two natural roots. The first word, *genome,* is a hybrid of two Greek words: *gene* and *chromosome,* while the suffix "-ics" means, aptly, "the study of." [4,5] This study of genes is further broadened to encompass the two very similarly minded objectives of mapping and sequencing. The goals of mapping and sequencing, and thus of genomics, are to analyze the structure, organization, and function of genes. [6] They differ, however, in that sequencing takes the information gathered by the mapping of DNA and connects it in such a manner as to discern a final picture of an organism at a genetic level. This picture is called the "genome." Genomics is the study and comparison of various genomes that sheds light on the way different organisms act, react, and develop in the context of diversity.

The human genome contains between 25,000 and 35,000 genes, and sequencing initiatives such as the Human Genome Project are excellent examples of genomics. [7,8] This veritable sea of untapped information has caused the field of genomics to differentiate into specialties. These offshoots of genomics focus on specific parts of the gene itself, and the products that they may produce. The following sections will take you through some of the subordinate research tools that fall under the umbrella of genomics.

Structural Genomics

This portion of genomics relies heavily on genome sequencing and mapping and focuses on the architecture of the gene itself. Structural genomics has further evolved to include assignment of three-dimensional structures to the protein products of genes. [9,10]

Proteins are responsible for many cellular processes, and a protein's function is directly related to its shape and orientation. Each protein has an idiosyncratic, three-dimensional structure determined by the interactions of the amino acids that comprise it and cause it to fold. Structural genomics thrives on generating the structures of selected proteins from which most others can be predicted with reasonable accuracy. [11]

Once a protein's structure has been delineated, analysis of the structure can begin. Some of the information that can be gathered from the structure might include identification of surface structure and shape, as well as identification of structures buried within the protein. [12] These data can lead researchers to determine if a given protein is available for pharmacologic modification.

Functional Genomics

Although genomic research is responsible for identifying the pattern of a genome, it is important to realize that sequence alone cannot identify a gene's function. This is where the field of functional genomics steps forward as an application of structural genomics. Functional genomics allows researchers to translate gene classification and DNA sequence information, discerned from structural genomics, into a biological function. [13]

In order for the leap from sequence to function to be made, researchers must first identify what genes affect what traits. In its infancy, functional genomics strictly studied traits or characteristics expressed in the presence of genes, altered genes, or the absence of various genes altogether.[14] The problem with this rudimentary method is that idiosyncratic traits are the products of interactions among numerous genes, not just one. Through progressive research efforts, functional genomics has the potential to take a trait and tease out every gene that contributes to its expression, putting into perspective the nature and timing of each gene's involvement.[15]

As stated earlier, structural genomics, in and of itself, will not lead directly to the next blockbuster drug. Taking the information learned from structural genomics, however, and building upon it with functional genomics can lead to the identification of potential new drug targets. For example, throughout the life cycle of a cell, certain genes switch on and off in response to various stimuli, especially disease. By monitoring normal cells as they mutate and grow cancerous, researchers can selectively identify genes responsible for tumor origin, division, and growth. If researchers know the genes responsible for these actions, we will gain a greater understanding of the life cycle of cancer, which may lead us one step closer to the development of novel cancer therapies.[16]

Comparative Genomics

Comparative genomics is the culmination of recent research that realizes that sequencing all genomes is not necessarily feasible. This is due to the vast number of species that exist and the immense amount of time necessary to model genomes, even those of small organisms. Since most organisms share a good portion of their genetic code, examination of smaller model organisms allows for the comparison and ultimate translation of larger genomes. In humans, for instance, comparative genomics uses model organisms such as chimpanzees, mice, flies, and even worms to reveal the functions of our genes.[17-22]

Early comparative genomic studies focused on gene content and the order of chromosomes, hoping to identify what caused intra- and transspecies differentiation.[23] As this research progressed, researchers began to evaluate entire genomes, rather than just the sequence of chromosomes, and attempted to discern differences in the nucleotide sequencing. By comparing genomes at this level, it is possible to identify single points at which genomes might differ and ultimately lead to diversity within a population. The specific genetic deviations in a nucleotide sequence that constitute these differences are termed single nucleotide polymorphisms, or SNPs.[24] It is estimated that these SNPs occur once every 1,000 to 5,000 bases of the human sequence, which, when totaled, yields roughly a million potential points of differentiation from one human being to another.[25]

One such application of this technology lies in the modulation of human disease. In the case of mice, for example, resistance to such infections as *Mycobacterium bovis* and *Salmonella typhimurium* is controlled by one gene in the mouse genome and, depending upon the expression of that gene, the mouse is either resistant or susceptible to these organisms.[26,27] Through comparative genomics, this very same gene was found in humans; however, in humans it is responsible for susceptibility to such pathogens as tuberculosis and leprosy.[28,29] In this case, genetic dissection of the mouse genome in response to *M. bovis* infection has led researchers to the identification of similar mechanisms that determine the human response to leprosy and tuberculosis. Further applications of genomics will be discussed in the following section.

Pharmacogenomics versus Pharmacogenetics

Pharmaco*genetics* is often used interchangeably with pharmaco*genomics*. Although the line does seem to blur between the two, there is a distinct difference that separates one from the other. Although both disciplines focus on the variability of a drug response in the context of genetic diversity, the difference lies in the level at which it is addressed. Pharmaco*genetics* examines the sequence variations within single genes that have been isolated and linked to a specific action or response to a pharmacologic agent.[30] Pharmaco*genomics*, however, is the much broader science that examines the entire genome and takes into consideration that various genes are responsible for different ethnic, racial, or geographic variations in response to medication.[31]

The practical application of both these technologies form the gateway to making drug therapy personalized to an individual's genetic constitution. Take, for instance, the enzyme arylamine N-acetyltransferase, which is responsible for metabolizing such drugs as isoniazid, caffeine, and procainamide.[32] Phenotypically, there are two basic types of abnormalities in individuals with this enzyme, either they are fast or slow acetylators. Normally, there is no way to differentiate between individuals, until an agent that is metabolized by this enzyme is administered. If it is known ahead of time through pharmacogenetic testing that the patient in question is a slow acetylator the prescriber may lower the administered dose, since it will not be cleared as quickly, thereby avoiding any potential toxicity. In the case of a fast acetylator, a subtherapeutic response can be avoided. In addition to this, pharmacogenetics has the potential to be applied to the cytochrome-P450 enzymes, catechol O-methyl transferase, and possibly to many other enzyme families as well.

Pharmacogenomics pieces together pharmacogenetic information and seeks to explain how all of the variations within the genome taken together affect an individual's response to drugs.[33] This type of analysis also has the potential to identify disease-susceptible genes and target them for future drug therapy.[34] Combining these two concepts together, pharmacogenomics is the realization that one day medication will be tailored to an individual's genetic framework.[35,36]

Proteomics

Strictly speaking, a proteome is a complete set of proteins that are encoded by a specific gene. In common use, however, the term *proteome,* first coined in 1995, has been defined as the "total protein complement of a genome."[37] Similar to genes, not all encoded proteins are produced or "expressed" at the same time. Certain proteins are expressed only in times of cellular distress, such as disease or growth, while others are expressed only during periods of equilibrium, or for maintenance purposes. The difference, however, is that genomics studies the static gene sequence while proteomics studies the dynamic nature of the protein products of genes.[38] The systematic analysis of the properties of these proteins within and between cells and in the context of disease or pharmacological influence has been labeled proteomics.[39,40]

Essentially, proteomics strives to understand the interactions of proteins on physiologic states. This research is essential in understanding the disease process at the level of protein interaction. To accomplish this task, proteomic studies are carried out on a grand scale so as to completely understand a disease at the molecular level. This research can provide critical information about the life cycle of an invading organism and, based on proteomic studies, weaknesses can be found and treatments may be identified.[41]

Antisense

Antisense allows for the selective inhibition of cellular translation, or the transfer of the information contained in the double-stranded DNA into a single-stranded RNA, and ultimately the ability to block the production of a specific protein. Consequently, antisense is the name given to the technology that utilizes small bits of DNA or its reciprocate, RNA, to prevent gene expression and ultimately the production of a protein.[42]

Taking a step back, when a cell requires a specific protein, the process begins by unzipping the DNA in the nucleus and creating an inverse replication known as mRNA. This single-stranded product, also referred to as the "sense" strand, is released from the nucleus, after which it travels to the protein production centers of the cell. Here, ribosomes read the instructions on this "sense" strand and create the protein in demand.[43] Sometimes the process will produce proteins that can inhibit normal cellular functions, regulate viral replication, or disturb the pharmacologic actions of drugs. To illustrate this process, consider the cytomegalovirus (CMV), which has been linked in causing retinitis in acquired immunodeficiency syndrome (AIDS) patients. This infection is propagated by the overactive production of proteins that govern the creation of the virus. In this specific type of infection, it is necessary to inhibit the production of these proteins, which can be achieved through antisense technology. The process of this inhibition begins with an injected "antisense" oligonucleotide, which is reciprocal to the base sequence of the cell's "sense" mRNA strand. Once the antisense strand makes its way into the cell, it binds to the mRNA to prevent the production of the proteins that support the replication of CMV. An example of a product that operates by this mechanism is fomivirsen sodium (Vitravene, Isis Pharmaceuticals, Inc.). As you might imagine, this product overcomes significant delivery obstacles. Not only does the injected vector need to be targeted to access the tissue in question but it must also penetrate both the cell wall and nucleus and then integrate with the proper mRNA strand.

Of course, this technology has been applied to other therapeutic arenas. Currently, researchers are using antisense to combat viral diseases and infections, fight cancer, inhibit the inflammatory process, and treat asthma.[44] Theoretically, any disease that is either caused or mediated by protein function can be influenced by antisense technology.

Signal Transduction

In its most basic element, signal transduction refers to the transfer of a signal from the outside of a cell to the inside, where the signal is converted into a specific response such as gene expression or cell division.[45] These signals, which can be produced by hormones, neurotransmitters, growth factors, and other substances, can either pass through the cell wall via passive or active diffusion, or can bind to an external ligand.* Once inside, the signal can instigate a cascade of events that ultimately results in changing the activity of one or more proteins.[46]

APPLICATIONS OF BIOTECHNOLOGY IN HEALTH CARE

With the aid of genomic technologies, researchers have a clearer understanding of the genetic components of such conditions as breast cancer, Alzheimer's disease, colorectal cancer, and Parkinson's disease.[47-52] Genomics also contributes to the understanding of such important infectious diseases as AIDS and tuberculosis.[53] These diseases can be classified as multifactorial because their manifestations are dependent not only on environmental factors but also the interactions of multiple genes.[54] Human genetic variation may have a protective or pathologic role in the expression of disease, and these variations ultimately become the targets of drug development.[55] One example of this is the development of gene therapy, or the use of genes to treat disease. Researchers have attempted to use this technology to treat a number of different diseases. Clinical trials have utilized gene therapy to successfully treat patients with severe combined immunodeficiency (SCID), or "bubble-boy disease." Although this treatment is not free of complications, it has allowed some afflicted individuals to lead almost normal lives.[56]

Vaccines offer another route by which this technology may flex its muscle. Other arenas for biotechnology include stem-cell-based therapies, diagnostic testing, as well as other agricultural and social applications such as the development of alternative energy sources and cleaning up of toxic waste.[57,58] Some of these topics will be discussed later in this chapter.

Since the human genome has been outlined we have come much closer to making disease management more preventive than therapeutic.[59] The previous sections have presented a brief overview of the most common components of biotechnology. Included in those sections were examples of how each one individually might be applied to the health care sector. Used synergistically, these technologies may prove to be a principal foundation for the future of medicine.

Monoclonal Antibodies

Before the term *monoclonal antibody*, or mAb, is defined, it is crucial to grasp the physiology of the antibody itself. Cells in the immune system,

---

*A molecular group that binds to another entity to form a larger structure

more specifically B-lymphocytes, produce proteins called antibodies in an effort to ward off and defend the body against foreign invaders. Each B-lymphocyte is responsible for producing a distinct antibody that binds specifically to a single antigen, or target site, on the surface of an invader. Although there are a variety of shapes, the most commonly associated form of an antibody is the "Y" orientation, which is particularly important to its function. The two prongs of the "Y" are used to bind antigens, while the remaining stem portion is used primarily for interacting with other proteins or immune cells. When an antigen instigates an immune response, antibodies are produced that bind specifically to certain parts, or epitopes, of these invading substances. These antibodies are referred to as "monoclonal" because they are produced by a single type of B-cell and are specific to a single epitope.[60] Each invading toxin carries with it many epitopes, and thus many different antibodies can bind to it, resulting in a polyclonal antibody response. Monoclonal antibodies can be synthesized and have a great deal of use as both diagnostic and therapeutic agents.

Production of Monoclonal Antibodies

In order to produce monoclonal antibodies, first the specific antigen to which a humoral, or antibody, response is desired must be determined. Next, the designated source of antibody production, commonly a mouse, must be immunized by receiving enough antigen to elicit a humoral response. Subsequently, the B cells that produce the desired antibody must be selected and then fused with a myeloma cell line. This fusion produces "hybridoma" cells, or the fusion of specific antibody-producing plasma B cells with immortal myeloma cells. The hybridoma cell is then able to produce monoclonal antibodies indefinitely.[61]

The usefulness of murine, or mouse-derived mAbs, is limited by their high antigenicity, or ability to stimulate antibody production.[62] One way to rectify this is to make a combination product of both murine and human antibodies, which is termed "chimeric." Another way to reduce this antigenicity is to alter the protein sequences on the murine mAbs through recombinant DNA technology to resemble the human antibody more closely. The resulting murine antibody is considered "humanized" and offers a much lower degree of antigenicity. This humanizing technique has now been taken to the next level, where researchers have begun to genetically alter mice to produce the already humanized form of the antibodies. A newer method of mAb production uses bacteriophages* to deliver target genes—

---

*A virus that infects bacteria

coding for specific human antibody regions—into bacterial hosts. These genes are then integrated with the host cell's DNA, expressed, and the resulting antibodies are incorporated onto the surface of the bacteriophage, where they are subsequently harvested.[63]

Nomenclature of mAbs

Monoclonal antibodies, like most pharmaceutical agents, have a highly specialized nomenclature. Each name is broken into four fragments, as represented below:

Prefix – Target – Source – Suffix

Starting in reverse order, which is to say going from general to specific, all mAbs share the same suffix, -mab, identifying the product as a monoclonal antibody, but this is where the similarities begin to diverge. The source will fall into one of four categories and precede the suffix. The four sources are as follows: -u- for human, -o- for murine, -xi- for chimeric (a mix of both mouse and human), and –zu- for humanized.[64]

From this, the next stage is to isolate the antibodies' intended target. Although there are quite a few targets, the most commonly used are those that point to viral targets (-vir-), immune targets (-lim-), infectious lesions (-les-), bacterial targets (-bac-), cardiovascular targets (-cir-), and miscellaneous tumors (-tum-). There are a variety of specific tumor targets as well, but for the sake of brevity they will not be mentioned here. As a general note, the prefix has no specialized meaning and the target and source are often blended together for aesthetics. Both the prefix and the target/source blend are necessary to make each mAb's identity unique.

Take for instance, *Infliximab:*

Prefix	Target	Source	Suffix
Inf-	-li(m)-	-xi-	-mab

Antibody Applications

Monoclonal antibodies are highly specific for a single epitope and, as such, it should be no surprise that these agents have earned the nickname "magic bullets."[65] Using the extremely precise nature of mAbs, pharmacologic agents, such as chemotherapy drugs, can be attached to the mAb to produce a product referred to as a "conjugated monoclonal antibody." In the case of treating cancer, these conjugated proteins have the distinct ability to guide the medication to the site of action on the tumor. Radioactive chemicals have also been attached to mAbs and are currently used as highly specific cancer diagnostic agents by directing the agent to the site of the tumor and emitting radiation.

These specific antibodies have also found a niche in the treatment of certain autoimmune disorders, such as graft versus host disease (GVHD), rheumatoid arthritis, and Crohn's disease.[66-73] Other useful applications of monoclonal antibodies include the inhibition of IgE for the treatment of asthma and inhibition of α_4 integrin in the treatment of relapsing multiple sclerosis.[74-76] Monoclonal antibodies have demonstrated mixed results in the treatment of septicemia and in the therapy of substance abuse.[77-79]

Cytokines

When an immune system is activated by, for example, an invading pathogen or a healing wound, the way that immune cells communicate with each other is through a tightly knit, complex network of cytokines. These agents are endogenous proteins that are secreted by specific cell types in response to stimuli, and they act on target cells to precipitate growth, proliferation, differentiation, and activity. Cytokines regulate the production of one another, as well as hematopoiesis, wound healing, and a variety of other biological functions. They work via circuits of positive and negative feedback and have offered many clinical applications. Cytokines that may be familiar to the health care practitioner include interferons, interleukins, tumor necrosis factor, and a variety of growth factors, including erythropoietin. Therapeutically, these agents fall into broad and poorly defined categories, although many of them share similar purposes. To make classification even more arduous, many of these agents are considered pleiotropic, or acting on multiple cell types. One classification system, however, offers a simplistic way to view these cytokines and divides them based upon their empirical action: immunomodulatory, proinflammatory, or those that regulate cell proliferation and differentiation.[80] It should be noted that not all cytokines are currently used therapeutically, and for the purposes served here only a few will be discussed.

Immunomodulatory Cytokines

The immunomodulatory cytokines are released by and act on lymphocytes to influence growth, differentiation, and proliferation of the immune response. Examples of specific cytokines that can be grouped under this heading include the interleukin (IL) numbers 2, 4, and 10; transforming growth factor-β; and the interferons, but only the interferons and IL-2 will be explored here.

Interleukin-2 (IL-2). Released by T-lymphocytes, IL-2 is a lymphokine, or soluble cytokine released in response to a lymphocyte's contact with an antigen, which is involved with amplifying immune responses to specific antigens by increasing the proliferation of their parent T-cells. IL-2 also serves to regulate itself. Although short-term exposure to the cytokine will induce the T-cells to produce more IL-2, extended contact can actually inhibit its future release. Through negative feedback this inhibitory mechanism ultimately limits the intensity and extent of some immune responses. IL-2 is available on the market as a product called aldesleukin (Proleukin, Chiron) and is produced via recombinant DNA technology. As a therapeutic agent, IL-2 can be used as immunotherapy in many cancer types, including metastatic renal-cell carcinomas, melanoma, and possibly non-Hodgkin's lymphoma.[81-84] There has also been some supporting evidence that IL-2 could play a therapeutic role in the treatment of HIV/AIDS by stimulating the body's innate production of natural killer cells, a type of lymphocyte.[85,86] The use of this agent, however, is limited by its rather toxic side-effect profile. Among the most serious side effects, IL-2 has been known to cause vascular leak syndrome, cardiovascular disorders, and, unfortunately, has even proven fatal to a few patients.[87]

Interferons (INF). Interferons are another type of immunomodulatory cytokine. They are soluble proteins that interfere with the replication, proliferation, and immunomodulation of viral invaders in addition to regulating other cytokines. Although they do share some overlapping properties, each type of interferon is biologically and structurally distinct. The interferon family is a broad category of cytokines that can be divided into one of two subcategories, type I and type II, based on their intrinsic activity.

The type I interferons are highly antiviral in nature and most commonly include INF α and INF β, but also INF ω. These "interfere"-ons do not actually possess any antiviral activity themselves but, rather, prevent the virus from replicating by making the environment inside the host cell hostile to the virus.[88] They are synthesized and secreted in response to infection by viruses, bacteria, or upon exposure to specific cytokines. In addition to their antiviral nature, type I interferons have been found to modulate cell growth, differentiation, and proliferation. Type I interferons can be derived from lymphoblasts or leukocytes, or manufactured through the use of recombinant DNA technology. INF α is most commonly used to treat Hepatitis B and C infections and INF β has demonstrated efficacy in multiple sclerosis.[89-92] These two interferons have also demonstrated efficacy in the treatment of HIV as well as inflammatory bowel disease.[93-96] Used as a single agent or in combination with chemotherapy, INF α has been shown to be effective in treating hairy cell leukemia, chronic lymphocytic leukemia, as well as non-Hodgkin's lymphoma.[97-99] INF ω has been effective in treating hepatitis, especially in cases that have shown resistance to other interferons, but is still in clinical trials.[100]

Like the type I interferons, INF γ, the only Type II interferon, also possesses antiviral properties, but to a much lesser extent. The core biologic activity of INF γ is to regulate most phases of both the immune and inflammatory responses. It promotes T-cell and macrophage activation, operation, and differentiation, and as a result is most commonly used to stimulate the body's immune system. INF γ is manufactured through the use of recombinant DNA technology using bacteria and is clinically used to treat severe malignant osteopetrosis and chronic granulomatous disease.[101,102]

Proinflammatory Cytokines

The proinflammatory cytokines, such as interleukin-1 (IL-1) and tumor necrosis factor (TNF), are aptly named due to their ability to induce and propagate the processes of inflammation. This, however, is not necessarily a negative response, as inflammation is directly related to the isolation and repair of injury and is necessary for the preservation of health. It is only when the inflammatory process carries on for an extended period of time or is of a particular intensity that it becomes deleterious. In the endogenous setting, these effects can cause permanent damage, as is often seen in rheumatoid arthritis.[103] Realizing the dual nature of these particular cytokines, it stands to reason that they may serve multiple roles in the progression and, ultimately, the treatment of certain diseases. Consequently, these cytokines may be used in different capacities, either through their expression or inhibition, to alter various physiological functions or to treat different disorders.

TNF and IL-2 have multiple biologic roles within the context of inflammation and immunity. They are both responsible for activating T-lymphocytes, which in turn produce interleukin-2 and interferon γ, factors that increase the proliferation of B cells, colony-stimulating factors, and lymphotoxin, which is another type of TNF.[104] In addition, these cytokines also interact with B-lymphocytes to regulate the production of antibodies and promote the further release of ancillary colony stimulating factors.

Agonism of proinflammatory cytokines. With names such as "tumor necrosis factor" one may be led to believe that this class of cytokines possess tremendous tumorcidal activity but, in truth, these promises have gone largely unfulfilled. Therapeutically, recombinant human TNF, rHuTNF, has been noted to be cytotoxic to a select number of tumor-cell lines, yet it is generally nontoxic to normal cells.[105] This fact might suggest that rHuTNF might have a high therapeutic index.[106] Unfortunately, the reality is that its use as a chemotherapeutic agent is precluded by its high side-effect profile. Among other side effects, TNF has been noted to cause cardiovascular, nephrotic, hepatic, neuro, and pulmonary toxicity.[107-109] Most of the data that support the use of rHuTNF as a chemotherapeutic have been the result of animal studies. These studies have determined that the cytokine lacks any direct antitumor activity but, rather, affects tumor growth by destroying its vasculature and indirectly through T-cell–mediated immunity (i.e, through TNF's activation of macrophages, natural killer and natural cytotoxic cells, neutrophils, and cytotoxic T-cells).[110-113]

Antagonism of proinflammatory cytokines. The inhibition of certain endogenous cytokines has shown efficacy in treating chronic inflammatory diseases such as rheumatoid arthritis and inflammatory bowel disease.[114] The therapeutic cytokines that block the actions of these endogenous cytokines via receptor antagonism are quickly becoming a mainstay in clinical practice.

Cytokine Downregulators

Just as recombinant proteins that mimic certain cytokines are used as therapeutic agents, other recombinant products act by downregulating cytokines. Different mechanisms of downregulation have been successfully employed.[115] Cytokine antagonists act by binding to cytokine receptors without transmitting a signal. Interleukin-1 receptor antagonists are examples of receptor antagonists that inhibit IL-1 from regulating the intensity of an inflammatory response.[116] Soluble cytokine receptors are made by enzymatically cleaving the extracellular portion of a cell-membrane-bound receptor.[117] These soluble receptors can bind free cytokine molecules before they reach the cell-membrane receptors, thus preventing them from eliciting their intended response. One example, etanercept, is a soluble TNF receptor involved in the inflammatory response.[118]

Colony-Stimulating Factors (CSFs)

Generally speaking, each of the CSFs is structurally distinct, yet they do have overlapping therapeutic activity. Each acts on pluripotent stem cells, but they stimulate the development of different cell lines, with the exception of interleukin-3, which has been implicated in cultivating all cell lines.[119]

These genetically produced agents are administered to reverse deficiencies in specific cell lines and, contrary to other cytokines, yield surprisingly few harmful side effects. As for applications of these agents, take, for instance, a patient who is undergoing chemotherapy or radiation therapy. Patients such as these may develop any one of a number of deficiencies, including granulocytopenia, which, if untreated, can be life threatening. This particular deficit has responded to treatment with granulocyte colony-stimulating factor, or G-CSF (filgrastim—Neupogen, Amgen), as well as to granulocyte-macrophage colony-stimulating factor, or GM-CSF (sargramostim—Leukine, Berlex). In addition, both GM-CSF and G-CSF can be used to treat chronic neutropenia, even in the face of aplastic anemia.[120-123]

Another class of CSFs increases the growth and maturation of red blood cells from pluripotent stem cells. More commonly referred to as erythropoietin or EPO (Procrit, Ortho Biotech Products, L.P.), this CSF is used clinically to increase the production of erythrocytes to reverse anemia associated with chemotherapy, HIV treatment, chronic kidney disease, and within the critical care setting.[124,125] Another agent that falls into this category is darbepoetin (Aranesp, Amgen) a version of endogenous erythropoietin modified to extend half-life.[126]

Another class of hematopoietic cell stimulators includes those that increase the production of platelets as well as escalate the proliferation and maturation of megakaryocytes. Cytokines that function in this capacity are interleukin-11, or oprelvekin (Neumega, Wyeth), and thrombopoietin, or TPO.[127,128] Both have been used to treat chemotherapy-induced thrombocytopenia.[129,130]

Clotting Disorders

Clotting disorders such as hemophilia were previously treated with blood transfusions, which exposed patients to severe potential complications. Such diseases can now be treated using recombinant versions of the clotting factors that these patients lack, such as Factors VIII and IX.[131]

Vaccines

One of the most important advances in medicine over the past decade has been the development of new vaccines through the use of biotechnology.[132] Recombinant technology has allowed researchers to design specific triggers of immunity by isolating the antigen that directly elicits a response and recombinantly producing that moiety, while avoiding the virulent, or disease causing, organism. Since this next generation of vaccines will consist of only the antigen, not the actual microbe, the recipient of the vaccine will be protected from ever contracting the associated illness.[133] Thus, the recombinant vaccine can elicit a targeted, safer, and more effective response than traditional vaccines.[134] In addition, these vaccines can often be developed much faster and are cheaper than their traditional counterparts.[135]

Another generation of vaccines that are currently in development are those that fight cancer. These vaccines differ from traditional vaccines in that they are administered *after* the person develops the disease. Their job is, therefore, not to prevent the cancer, but to locate and terminate the tumor by amplifying the body's natural immune response.[136]

The majority of recombinant vaccines currently in use are for animal diseases, which are used to protect livestock and poultry in order to avoid transmitting diseases to humans who consume them.[137] In addition to protecting against bacterial and viral diseases, recombinant technology is now being used to produce vaccines against parasitic infections.[138] At present, Hepatitis B vaccine is the only human recombinant vaccine in clinical use.[139]

Gene Therapy

Some common diseases, such as diabetes and chronic kidney disease, are associated with defective or damaged genes that do not produce enough of a certain protein. With the advent of recombinant technology, these diseases have been treated in part by giving injections of the missing proteins such as human insulin (Humulin, Eli Lilly and Company) or epoetin alfa (Procrit, Ortho Biotech Products, L.P.). In the future, gene therapy may be used to supply defective cells with functional genes, thereby allowing for the in vivo production of these vital substances.

Gene therapy is a process that attempts to either modify the expression of genes or correct aberrant genes in order to fight disease.[140] Generally, a gene cannot be directly inserted into a cell; instead it must be delivered using a carrier known as a "vector."[141]

Gene therapy can be divided into three procedural categories. During ex vivo gene transfer, certain cells, usually blood cells, are removed from the body, incubated with a vector containing a gene in order to allow transduction, the incorporation of desired gene into DNA. Then, the genetically modified cells are returned to the body.[142] The injection of a gene-containing vector directly into the blood stream is termed in vivo gene therapy and, although a challenging task, holds the most promise for tolerable and convenient gene therapeutics in the future.[143] In situ gene therapy avoids issues of target location by placing the vector containing a therapeutic gene directly into a specific tissue of the body (i.e., a tumor injected with a gene coding for a cytokine or a toxin).[144]

The most important factor in any gene-transfer process, apart from production of the actual gene that is being transferred (transgene), is the choice of vector used to deliver the gene to the target site. The type of vector chosen can decide whether the gene therapy is a success or a failure. Unfortunately, a universally ideal vector does not currently exist, as all have advantages and disadvantages. For example, one vector may be able to reach the target cells but, once there, may cause an immune response that results in cell death. Many factors must be considered when choosing a vector to deliver a gene product, the most important of which include: the length of time that the transgene needs to be expressed, the dividing state of the target cells, the type of target cell, the size of the transgene, and the potential for an immune response against the vector. Other factors to consider in vector selection include the ability to administer the vector more than once, the ease of producing the vector, the facilities available, and any safety and regulatory implications.[145]

Vectors that have been developed to deliver transgenes to cells are generally viral or nonviral. Viruses, by their nature, are able to transfer genetic material into target cells. Advantages of viral vectors include specific cell-binding and entry properties, efficient targeting of the transgene to the nucleus of the cell, and the ability to avoid degradation once within the cell.[146] Prior to use, viral vectors are rendered innocuous by removing specific genes responsible for the virus' infectious capability (i.e., viral replication).[147] Next, a transgene to be delivered by the virus must be inserted into the viral genome, usually into the space created by gene removal, therefore limiting the size of transgene that can be used.[148] Last, the recombinant virus must be grown to high titer levels and can then be used to transduce cells or tissues in vivo or ex vivo.[149] Viral-type vectors include retroviral vectors (i.e., Moloney murine leukemia virus and lentivirus), adenoviruses, adeno-associated viruses, herpes simplex virus type 1, and vaccinia virus.[150]

Often in the viral vector development process, nonessential genes are removed to make room for the incorporation of transgene material.[151] In the extreme example, only a viral shell may remain, designed for a high level of gene expression for a controlled amount of time.[152] Research efforts to achieve this same result have led to the development of nonviral vectors such as liposomes, DNA-ligand conjugates, and naked DNA.[153] Advantages of these systems include their virtually infinite capacity, lack of infectious or mutagenic capability, and potential for large-scale production.[154] However, delivery using these methods may not be as efficient or cell specific when compared with viral vectors.

To date, the most successful method of gene therapy delivery has been achieved using a vector derived from the Moloney murine leukemia virus. By inserting a gene coding for the adenosine deaminase (ADA) enzyme, children suffering from ADA deficiency and the resulting severe immunodeficiency, have been able to live normal lives.[155] However, the use of this vector has resulted in the development of two cases of leukemia in patients participating in a single gene therapy trial.[156] Initial research into these events has found points of insertional mutagenesis, possibly responsible for the lymphoproliferation. Future investigations will attempt to determine whether these serious adverse events were a direct result of the retroviral gene therapy treatment and, if so, what steps can be taken to increase the safety of this seemingly efficacious and very important therapy.

Stem Cells

A stem cell is a cell that has a unique capacity to reproduce itself and give rise to specialized cell types.[157] Most cells in the body, such as heart cells or skin cells, are committed to a specific function, while a stem cell remains uncommitted until it receives a signal to differentiate.[158] Stem cells have the potential to provide information about human cellular development, specifically the factors involved in cellular differentiation.[159] Human stem-cell lines serve as test models, allowing researchers to infer the safety and efficacy of drugs prior to their use on animals or humans.[160] More specific to medical practice, stem cells may be used in the future to treat diseases and disorders that destroy or impair certain cells and tissues, such as Parkinson's and Alzheimer's diseases, heart disease, and diabetes.[161] Sources of stem cells include embryos, fetal tissue, umbilical cord blood, and certain adult tissues. All sources are accompanied by variable differentiation potentials, and some by a certain degree of ethical controversy, as discussed later in this chapter.

DRUG DELIVERY OF PROTEIN PRODUCTS

The delivery of therapeutic proteins in a convenient, safe, and efficient way has always been a goal of biotech manufacturers. Advancing the delivery of protein products (including currently marketed products such as insulin and interferon, as well as those still in development) beyond the basic subcutaneous (SC), intramuscular (IM), and intravenous (IV) methods, may be the key to commercial success in upcoming years. This success will likely be based on more convenient drug delivery, which may increase patient compliance and willingness to undergo therapy. Ultimately, this will allow for greater response to therapy and reduced prevalence of disease and disease complications.[162]

When new options are considered for the delivery of proteins, variations of parenteral administration are usually the most convenient.[163] These methods avoid enzymes found in the gut that promise efficient protein destruction and also provide a natural progression from the injectable methods employed by most animal and early clinical research.[164]

Traditionally, drugs requiring daily injections have been delivered via a small-diameter needle and a low-volume syringe. This process can be relatively complicated for the layperson, and fairly traumatic for any patient. To improve convenience and compliance, external pumps, prefilled syringes, auto injectors, pen devices containing cartridges loaded with the protein, and needleless injectors have been used.[165]

Depot delivery systems provide an alternative to pumps and repeated injections by enabling the protein to be continuously delivered from an implanted reservoir or injected slow-release solution.[166]

"Next generation" parenterally administered proteins such as peginterferon alfa-2b (PEG-Intron, Schering-Plough) and darbepoetin alfa (Aranesp, Amgen) have incorporated pegylation and increased glycosylation, respectively, in order to extend drug half-life. Although still associated with the trauma and complexity of injection, these formulations offer patients the option of less-frequent dosing.

In the future, proteins may be delivered via the lungs, a physiologically sensible route due to the large surface area and rapid absorption rate across alveolar membranes and into circulation.[167] Limitations of pulmonary delivery include the potentially toxic effects of certain compounds such as growth factors and cytokines, mass limitations for proteins requiring higher doses for therapeutic effect, and the lack of ability to titrate dose.[168] Overall, taking current limitations into consideration, the pulmonary delivery of proteins may be limited to agents that necessitate moderate to low doses and are unaffected by high peak levels.[169] Novel devices are in development to improve pulmonary delivery by offering metered dosing, minimal protein holdup, particles with greater lung penetration, and improved aerosol characteristics.[170] The reliability of insulin delivery via the lungs has been questionable in the past; however, multiple companies have progressed to phase III clinical trials evaluating the long-term safety and efficacy of pulmonary insulin delivery utilizing their respective novel devices.[171,172] A pulmonary device for the systemic delivery of interferon alfa, a recombinant protein to treat hepatitis B and C, as well as some cancers, is also currently in clinical trials.[173]

The nasal route of delivery for therapeutic proteins is often plagued by poor or variable bioavailability and nasal irritation. Calcitonin-salmon (Miacalcin, Novartis) is an example of a polypeptide successfully delivered via this route, and one that displays the aforementioned limitations.[174]

Extensive research has also focused on the delivery of proteins via transdermal and oral routes. However, development has been unsuccessful thus far, and future efforts will be needed to find ways to penetrate the respective barriers of these methods, namely the stratum corneum and the gut mucosa.[175]

BIOTECHNOLOGY MANUFACTURING PRACTICES

Synthesis of biologics, specifically recombinant proteins, is often a painstaking process requiring considerable time, precision, and technological resources. As newer techniques become available, the production processes are refined to address previous limitations. Once the production of a small quantity of product is perfected, the great challenge becomes how to optimally and efficiently produce the drug in mass quantities.

Recombinant Proteins

After a desired gene has been isolated and cloned (see Molecular Cloning in the Essentials of Biotechnology section of this chapter) it must be expressed in an appropriate host cell. First, a decision must be made as to what host cell to use for protein expression. Whereas microbial hosts (i.e., *E. coli* bacteria) have a very quick doubling time, the protein is more difficult to harvest because of the cell's intracellular storage of protein product. Conversely, mammalian host cells (i.e., Chinese hamster ovary (CHO) cells) have a slower doubling time, but protein product is relatively easy to harvest because of the cell's ability to excrete protein extracellularly.[176,177] Another type of cell host, the yeast cell, appears to have some of the combined benefit of high yield, as seen with bacterial cells, as well as many of the protein modification systems found in mammalian cells.[178] Often, the final decision affecting which host-cell type to choose is dependent upon the degree of protein complexity and posttranslational modification (i.e., glycosylation) required, for which a higher degree favors mammalian host cells, although yeast cells may prove adequate as well.[179] Examples of proteins produced in microbial-cell hosts include insulin, filgrastim, and interferons.[180] Mammalian host-cell-produced proteins include tissue plasminogen activator (tPA, alteplase), EPO (erythropoietin, epoetin alfa), and clotting factors.[181]

Newer protein production mechanisms, such as baculovirus expression systems, are gaining popularity. These systems produce recombinant viruses containing a desired gene. The viruses are then transfected into insect cells, where the resultant proteins are expressed. Baculovirus expression systems offer the advantages of supporting growth of proteins requiring a high degree of posttranslational modification as well as allowing for simultaneous expression of multiple genes.[182]

After an appropriate host cell is selected, the foreign gene must be introduced into the cell. This can be accomplished by first inserting the desired gene into a vector. The most common vectors are plasmids, which are circular rings of DNA found in bacteria that can replicate autonomously when introduced into a host cell. Next, the vector must be inserted into the host DNA.[183] Recombination occurs by using enzymes (restriction endonucleases) to cut open plasmids at compatible sites for introduction of the foreign gene. After inserting the gene, another enzyme (DNA ligase) recombines the foreign gene with the plasmid. Next, the recombined plasmid is transferred into the host cell. As the plasmid DNA replicate, the host cell expresses the gene that was inserted into the plasmid. In this manner, the desired protein is produced.

Large-Scale Manufacturing

Determination of the best method for commercial production of a biotechnology product is influenced by the unit value of the agent and the volume of the agent required.[184] In cases of high-potency products with a relatively small volume, production in multiple small-unit systems will suffice. However, with vaccines and therapies requiring greater quantities (i.e., mAbs), production can only be cost-effectively achieved through the use of large-scale bioreactors. Each product and its application determine at what scale a break-even point is reached.[185]

Multiple-unit production (i.e., using multiple flasks or roller bottles), which is generally not very economical unless demand is low, is easy to handle and allows for direct transfer from the laboratory to production without requiring a scale-up procedure. However, this process type is heterogenous, generally involves considerable time and cost, and frequently results in contamination. An example of a product that uses roller-bottle production is recombinant human erythropoietin, for which yearly demand is satisfied with only a few kilograms of product.[186]

Large-batch reactors have the advantages of being homogenous, easy to scale up and partially controllable. Disadvantages include depletion of nutrients and accumulation of toxic metabolites, with subsequent decreased viability during a run.[187] To address these issues, fed-batch reactors allow for replacement of essential nutrients during a run in order to prolong viability. Perfusion reactors allow for ongoing removal of toxic metabolites during production, thus requiring a smaller scale of batch cultures than usual to obtain a desired amount of product. The major drawbacks to perfusion reactors are the long and complicated validation procedure required and decreased flexibility due to design specifications for individual products.[188]

The major rate-limiting factor for large-scale production of biologic products is the purification process, which can account for 50 to 90 percent of production costs.[189] There is an unmet need for more efficient, effective and economic large-scale bioseparation techniques that can be used to achieve high purity and high recovery while maintaining a molecule's biological activity.[190] The previously mentioned problem of toxic waste-product buildup can add to the difficulty in the purification process. By increasing the use of serum-free media and perfusion reactor systems, the buildup of these waste products can be decreased.[191] Furthermore, in order to address these issues on a broad scale, there is an increasing trend in the use of "production platforms" or, specifically, common sets of cell lines, for which processes can be duplicated and streamlined across products.[192]

Transgenic animals have also become an efficient method of large-scale production of biologics.[193] This concept is based on the fact that some proteins require posttranslational modification, such as glycosylation, that cannot occur in bacterial hosts. A large farm animal, such as a pig, sheep, goat, or cow, however, can be used as a mammalian host for complex protein production, as has been done for clotting factors VIII and IX.[194] The gene coding for the desired human protein can be inserted into an animal's regulatory sequences that cause expression in its mammary tissue. Thus, following transformation of an embryo with the desired gene and introduction of that embryo into a foster mother, the genetically engineered offspring that produce the desired protein in their mammary tissue can be selected.[195] These animals will then secrete the desired protein in their breast milk, which can subsequently be isolated and purified for use. It is possible, for example, with certain clotting factors, to meet the national demand of recombinant protein with the use of only a few animals.[196]

Government Regulation of Biologics

In 1902, the Center for Biologics Evaluation and Research (CBER) was created by the passage of the Biologics Control Act.[197] This act was in response to nearly two-dozen deaths that occurred in 1901 after children re-

ceived contaminated vaccines. Over 100 years later, CBER continues to regulate biologics in the United States. The mission of CBER is to protect and enhance the public health through this regulatory process.[198]
In recent years, general CBER responsibilities have included

- the safety of the nation's blood supply and the products derived from it;
- the production and approval of safe and effective childhood vaccines;
- the proper oversight of human tissue for transplantation;
- an adequate and safe supply of allergenic materials and antitoxins;
- the safety and efficacy of biological therapeutics, defined as those products derived from living sources rather than chemical synthesis.

Rather than a new drug application (NDA) that is required for new molecular entities, biologics require the submission of a biologic license application (BLA) to gain approval.[199] In 2002, nine new biologic therapeutics and vaccines were approved for use in the United States, including adalimumab (Humira, Abbott Laboratories) and pegfilgrastim (Neulasta, Amgen).

In contrast to the role held by CBER, the Center for Drug Evaluation and Research (CDER) has been responsible for the review of all nonbiologic pharmaceuticals. However, in September 2002 the Food and Drug Administration (FDA) introduced an initiative to shift the review of some biological therapeutics from CBER to CDER, a move expected to produce a more efficient, effective, and consistent review program for human drugs and biologics.[200,201] A reorganization template lists three classes of therapeutics that will be transferred to CDER, including

- monoclonal antibodies intended for therapeutic use;
- cytokines, growth factors, enzymes, and interferons (including recombinant versions); and
- proteins intended for therapeutic use that are extracted from animals or microorganisms.[202]

CBER will continue to regulate

- monoclonal antibodies, cytokines, growth factors, or other proteins when used solely as an ex vivo constituent in a manufacturing process or when solely used as a reagent in the production of a product that is under the jurisdiction of CBER;
- viral-vectored gene insertions;
- products composed of human or animal cells or from physical parts of those cells;

- blood, blood components and fractions, and recombinant versions of typical blood component or fraction transfusion products;
- plasma expanders;
- allergen patch tests;
- allergenics;
- antitoxins, antivenins, and venoms;
- in vitro diagnostics;
- vaccines, including therapeutic vaccines; and
- toxoids and toxins intended for immunization.[203]

With this regulatory shift, many of the categories of biologics that have revolutionized modern medicine (i.e., monoclonal antibodies and interferons) will now be under the jurisdiction of CDER. Although left with decreased responsibilities, CBER will continue to regulate the development of many biologics, including gene therapy, a field of exceptional regulatory complexity.

In addition to the reorganization of regulatory divisions, approval of biologic generics is another challenge currently facing the FDA. No approval process is established at this time. This can be attributed to the inherent structural complexity and extensive, complicated manufacturing processes of biologics, which can make establishing and maintaining bioequivalence extremely difficult. However, FDA Commissioner Mark McClellan appears to offer some hope to proponents of a generic path for biologics, saying that the "feasibility of interchangeable or generic biologics should be assessed further."[204] The Generic Pharmaceutical Association continues to pressure the FDA to create such a path, with representatives citing the excessive cost of the NDA-approval route as their primary reason.[205]

IMPACT OF BIOTECHNOLOGY ON HEALTH CARE COSTS

Currently, over 130 biotechnology drugs and vaccines are approved by the FDA, of which over 70 percent have been approved within the past six years.[206] In addition, over 350 new products are currently in clinical trials.[207] This change in the landscape of health care will affect all facets of the health care system from payers such as the government to managed care insurers and employers; providers, such as hospitals and physicians; and end users, the patients and consumers. The pharmacy profession is currently in a position to greatly influence all parties involved, whether it be as consultants to managed care organizations, as clinical associates at institutions, or as dispensing pharmacists with end-user interface.

With the quickly increasing number of biotech products becoming available, the U.S. health care system is faced with the daunting task of delivering cutting-edge care while managing the high costs often accompanying such innovations. Pharmacoeconomic analysis will be required to determine the true value associated with these technologies.

Audiences Affected by Biotechnology Products

Government

As principal payers for the elderly, the government is being greatly affected by the rapid growth of the population that is becoming Medicare eligible. Senior citizens currently use over a third of all medications prescribed while they make up only 12 percent of the U.S. population.[208] With many biotech products targeting chronic conditions that largely affect the elderly, the cost of these medications is often falling on the government. Medicare enrollees currently have coverage for injectable products that are administered in a health care provider's office. Thus, products such as recombinant growth factors and monoclonal antibody agents are paid for by Medicare as long as a provider administers them, rather than the patient.

The cost of caring for an older person has increased significantly over the past several years, in terms of both medical and pharmaceutical intervention. As Uwe Reinhardt, respected Princeton University health care economist put it,

> 10-15 years ago the ratio of health-care spending for 55-year-olds to 25-year-olds used to be about 2.3 to 1. Now it's closer to 3.5 or 4 to 1. An older person now costs more. It's the new technology.[209]

Through its state-run Medicaid program, the government is also responsible for providing medical and prescription benefits to the indigent. Several states are now implementing preferred drug lists and organizing multistate purchasing groups as a bargaining tool to obtain discounted prescription products or value-added services such as disease management programs.[210]

Furthermore, there are over 40 million uninsured Americans, many of whom are lower-middle-class people not considered indigent and therefore are ineligible for government programs such as Medicaid.[211] The government is already trying to address this gap problem, which is further complicated by the high cost of biotech treatments.

The government is also charged with regulating the biopharmaceutical industry in terms of enforcing patents and simultaneously allowing introduction of generic competition to lessen the burden of prescription drug costs. However, to date, the introduction of generic biotech products has been prohibited due to strong safety concerns by the FDA.[212] Adding to this concern are safety issues resulting from the discovery of antibody production against some biologic compounds, underscoring the extremely painstaking process required to manufacture biotech/biologic products.[213]

Private Payers

As new and expensive biotech products are introduced into the health care system, managed care insurers, such as the government, must look for ways to control their increasing expenditures on prescription medications. The Academy of Managed Care Pharmacy (AMCP) in 1998 estimated that payers should expect to spend $5 to $8 billion annually on biotech products; as an estimated 7 to 12 percent of total drug expenditures, this makes them the fastest-growing component of this rapidly growing element of health care costs.[214]

In order to cope with these increasing costs, managed care organizations increase premiums paid by employers for their employees' health benefits, often forcing small employers who cannot absorb the incremental costs to cut these benefits. Other employers are forced to manage these higher costs by making changes to their employee coverage plans by either stiffening eligibility requirements (reducing categories of people eligible), reducing what types of plan options are available (substituting HMO for indemnity insurance), or making their employees pay higher premiums for less-restrictive plans.[215] There is currently movement by managed care companies to offer a wider array of plan options for employers from very low-cost, restrictive plans to high-cost, wider-access plans, so that employees can choose the model that best fits their needs.[216]

Providers

Hospitals and physicians are facing lower reimbursement rates due to changes in payment formulas used by Medicare and, subsequently, many private payers. This has made providers more cost conscious, specifically about ensuring that they do not lose money on high-cost products or procedures. The net result is that providers are forced to consider the short-term economics of medicine in addition to, and sometimes in place of, long-term benefits to patients to ensure that their practices are consistently viable.[217]

Whereas payers are feeling a great pinch from the introduction of high-cost prescription medications such as biotech products, providers are often finding monetary benefits in their use. Specifically, physicians and hospitals are finding the margins between product acquisition costs and reimbursement rates for certain biotech products to be a lucrative source of income to offset the diminishing payment received for other services that they provide.

Patients/Consumers

When employers are faced with increasing premiums from insurers, they often pass the additional costs directly to their employees. The employees, in turn, can be affected in a number of different ways. They may choose to pay a higher premium to stay in their current plan or be forced into a more restrictive plan, if unwilling to pay the additional cost. Employers may also opt to take the additional premium out of the employees' compensation by reducing employee salaries or slowing the rate of salary increases. Again, employees who work for small employers may be left without employee health benefits. Ultimately, patients/consumers may seek the benefit of new biotechnology products but may be unwilling to pay the high costs associated with these agents.

Manufacturers

Manufacturers justify the high prices of newer biotechnology products by pointing to the tremendous improvements these products can bring to human health. In addition, recent estimates for the cost of launching a new product exceed $800 million, in large part the result of costs associated with more stringent clinical trials.[218] Manufacturers are thus faced with added pressure to recoup their tremendous investments. This involves premium pricing and a great deal of work with the government, private insurance companies, and patient advocacy groups to ensure that their products will be covered for insured patients who will benefit from them. An additional responsibility of the manufacturers of biotech products is improving access to medications for the more than 40 million uninsured Americans who would not be able to otherwise afford these expensive medications. This improved access often comes in the form of manufacturer-sponsored discount prescription drug cards and patient assistance programs.

The Great Debate

The debate continues as to whether these newer, high-tech products will benefit the health care system by either reducing overall costs or, alternatively, by bringing greater benefit at an increased cost. In some cases, a biotechnology product is replacing what was once only treatable by a medical procedure, such as hemophilia. However, in other cases a new product is treating a previously inadequately treated or untreatable condition, such as transplant rejection or certain tumors, thereby increasing costs to the health care system that are accompanied by improvements in care. There is also a growing trend for biotech products to focus on enhancing quality of care and life and improving performance for sufferers of chronic conditions such as rheumatoid arthritis and chronic kidney disease.[219,220] These less tangible quality-of-life benefits further challenge our ability to demonstrate value through appropriate pharmacoeconomic analysis.

It is argued that improved technology in medicine increases health care demand as well as the proportion of the Gross Domestic Product (GDP) dedicated to health care. The counterpoint is that an increase in the percentage of GDP spending on health care may not be a negative outcome if it fuels the growth of other economic sectors, which is what extensive, detailed analysis of the biotechnology industry is predicting.[221,222]

Addressing the Problem

With nearly everyone in the health care system affected by biotechnology products, it is imperative that the issue of biotechnology's impact be properly assessed and managed. The pharmacy profession holds an increasingly important role in this environment.

With growing emphasis on cost justification of newer products, insurers are increasingly making coverage decisions based on economic considerations. Outcomes data is an essential component in making these important decisions.[223] As data on outcomes are compiled, insurers and managed care pharmacists are better able to make accurate assessments when comparing either one drug versus another, drug therapy versus no therapy, or drug therapy versus medical intervention. A commonly asked question in this regard is, what traditional health care costs will be saved by using new technologies and techniques?[224] However, in order to conduct appropriate pharmacoeconomic analysis of this question, which should account for indirect and secondary costs, a proper understanding of the therapeutic and regulatory environment is required.[225]

In late 2000 and early 2001, the Academy of Managed Care Pharmacy created a standardized tool for supporting formulary and drug policy decision making. The establishment of a uniform criteria to evaluate products on the basis of their costs and benefits when undergoing formulary review represents a significant step toward instituting "outcomes-based access," where a drug's proven "value" determines whether or not payers will provide coverage for the product.[226]

The current dilemma still facing the science and practice of pharmacoeconomics is the ability to appropriately quantify the value of extended survival or, perhaps more difficult yet, the value of enhanced survival. A secondary issue is the stark reality, from a business standpoint, of the disincentive for insurance companies to act on prospects of long-term cost-savings in the absence of near-term savings, when health plan switching is frequent among employees and employers. For example, the plan that makes the greatest investment in a person's care may not see the cost savings expected in return due to a patient changing his or her insurance plan.

Although several steps must be taken in order to be better prepared to assess and address the increasing effect of biotechnology products on health care, much of the thinking is still quite abstract and will require long-term solutions. For the present, and in the interest of those who are responsible for the daily viability of their practices, organizations, or institutions, several options can be explored, many of which rely on the premise of Specialty Pharmacy.[227]

Specialty Pharmacy provides the health care system (i.e., payers, providers, and patients) a means of increasing cost-effectiveness through improved operational efficiency with biotech products by realizing the considerable savings achieved by buying products in bulk, educating both patients and professionals on appropriate use, and facilitating the distribution process by eliminating middlemen and markups.[228] This rapidly growing specialty area of pharmacy is booming at a time when managed care is trying to catch up to the biotechnology boom that began several years before.

ETHICAL ISSUES CREATED BY BIOTECHNOLOGY

In 1973, soon after the first successful attempt to recombine DNA from one organism to another, a group of scientists called for a self-imposed moratorium on scientific research involving recombinant DNA technology.[229] The following year, the National Institutes of Health (NIH) formed the Recombinant DNA Advisory Committee (RAC) to oversee laboratory research using recombinant DNA.[230] Over the next few years, as recombinant DNA technology was proven safe, guidelines of this committee were revised accordingly.[231] During this same period, societal debate regarding the religious and ethical aspects of recombinant DNA nearly lead to a ban on such research.[232]

It is difficult to imagine practicing medicine today without the benefits of recombinant DNA products such as insulin, erythropoietin, granulocyte colony-stimulating factor, and interferons. They have become mainstays in medical practice, contributing to the health of millions.

However, accompanying these advancements, society and health care professions are faced with new ethical and moral dilemmas. Stem-cell research and cloning are at the forefront of political, medical, and religious debate. The use of gene therapy to alter human phenotypes remains controversial. Genetic discrimination and the patenting of genes continue to cause conflict. Difficulty lies in determining right and wrong regarding these topics but, at the very least, future medical practitioners are required to decide their own stance on such issues and how this stance will influence the patient care that they will provide.

Stem cells, as discussed earlier in this chapter, have a number of potential applications. However, the focus of the stem-cell debate involves the source of these cells. Stem cells can be derived from embryos, fetal tissue, umbilical cord blood, and certain adult tissues.[233]

Embryonic stem cells can come from excess embryos developed in fertility clinics for in vitro fertilization (IVF), from embryos created specifically for research purposes, or from embryos created via somatic cell nuclear transfer (SCNT).[234] The first two embryonic sources are self-explanatory; SCNT entails the removal of the nucleus from a donated egg, followed by the replacement of that nucleus with the nucleus from a somatic cell (a body cell that is neither an egg nor a sperm).[235] The process is concluded with division induction, after which stem cells are separated from the rest, and a cell line that is genetically identical to the somatic cell from which the nucleus was taken is created.[236]

IVF embryos from fertility clinics are seen by some as potential life, with their use in research being equated with mutilating and killing a child.[237] However, IVF clinics store excess embryos, commonly harvested in greater numbers than needed to lend ease to the IVF process, only for a limited time before their destruction.[238] The opposing argument, therefore, is that research involving embryos has potential medical benefits, while preventing the use of these embryos for research will simply support their frequent and calculated disposal.[239]

Policies limiting research on embryos are often based on the preservation of human life, with the premise that an embryo is a person or a potential person.[240] The debate that surrounds this viewpoint involves the questioning of when personhood begins. Some believe human life starts at conception, while others are of the opinion that one becomes a person at birth.[241] Still others have concluded that life begins with the development of the neurological tissue, which occurs after the stage most sought for research, the blastocyst stage.[242]

The use of stem cells from aborted or miscarried fetuses generates another set of concerns.[243] Antiabortion activists worry that the use of fetal tissue will encourage women who are against abortion or are unsure to pursue abortion. They insist women will reference the positive use of the fetus to justify an "immoral act."[244] Others argue it is unlikely that this slight moral comfort would swing a woman's opinion from childbearing to abortion.[245] Obtaining cells from spontaneously aborted fetuses, with parental permission, is viewed by some as equivalent to cadaveric organ donation.[246] This concept remains controversial, however, because the ability to obtain uncoerced informed consent from parents in such an emotional setting has been questioned.[247]

The issue of creating embryos through SCNT has produced the most conflict as of late. Although researchers claim to have no intention of reimplanting these embryos in the uterus and allowing them to grow, which would be defined as human cloning, some insist that cloning embryos for stem-cell research brings us one step closer to cloning humans, as recombinant DNA brought us one step closer to stem-cell research. Some governments have expressly prohibited human cloning and have allowed SCNT embryo use. Other countries, including the United States, however, seem to take the stance that cloning embryos through SCNT should not be allowed until the benefits of stem-cell research have been proven.

Stem cells from other sources, for instance, bone-marrow stem cells retrievable from adults, or stem cells from the blood of the umbilical cord, are associated with relatively few ethical concerns.[248] However, the full potential of these cells with regard to differentiation capability and therapeutic use has yet to be determined and, consequently, may create significant research limitations if used alone.[249]

On July 10, 2002, the Council on Bioethics appointed by President George W. Bush drew a distinction between two types of "cloning." They agreed unanimously to permanently ban cloning in order to produce children, which "is unethical, ought not to be attempted, and should be indefinitely banned by federal law."[250] However, they were divided on the "far more vexing" issue of cloning for research purposes, with seven of the eighteen members favoring the progression of this research under a strict set of guidelines and ten requesting a four-year moratorium to be applied to all researchers.[251] During the proposed moratorium, a federal review of current and planned human embryo research would take place, and the time would allow for public debate, policy formation, and a public consensus.[252] Almost thirty years after the moratorium inspired by the development of recombinant DNA technology, scientific research in the United States is heading toward another moratorium, this time inspired by stem-cell research and cloning. Similar to the development of recombinant DNA technology, it is likely that the true potential of stem-cell research will not be realized for many years, possibly limited in the United States to the stem-cell lines available today.

Gene therapy for the treatment of serious disease, like that used in those afflicted with SCID, is now generally accepted as ethically appropriate.[253] However, genetic engineering applications in the near future may not be disease-related but, instead, aimed at "functional enhancement" or "cosmetic" purposes.[254] The possibilities are vast and include obtaining size from growth-hormone gene alteration or introducing hair-stimulating genes into follicles to treat alopecia.[255] Advancements such as these, if successful, will need to be evaluated carefully by the medical community, as their long-term effects are unknown. In addition, in utero gene therapy of the fetus may become commonly performed in upcoming years and, if limited to the prevention of serious disease, will likely be considered ethical.[256] Again, caution will need to be exercised to prevent the development of fetal gene therapy targeting outcomes other than disease.[257] For example, technology progression may allow for the selection of human traits such as eye and hair color, and even gender, during the developmental stages of the fetus.[258]

Genetic screening has created additional ethical issues. With the progression of genetic research, certain genes have been isolated which have been associated with increased risk of developing specific diseases (i.e., sickle-cell disease and breast cancer). Conflict arises when genetic screening, particularly the examination of the genetic makeup of employees or job applicants by an employer, is used to eliminate those who may be predisposed to a certain disease.[259] Employers may use this information to eliminate workers or applicants with genes coding for conditions that could cause them to be less productive and more costly for health insurance purposes.[260] Cases of this type of discrimination appeared in the 1970s when laws dictating mandatory sickle-cell screening were passed in at least twenty states, resulting in work discrimination, rising insurance premiums, denial of employment, and employment termination.[261] The AMA advises that information gained through all types of medical testing should be kept confidential, available only to the employee and appropriate human resource and medical officers of the organization.[262] The AMA also states that employees and job applicants subjected to testing should be fully informed of test purposes and results. In addition, any employee who is able to perform job tasks and is not endangered by performing them should be free to apply for and retain such positions as long as performance standards are met.[263]

Research advances currently being attempted contribute an additional aspect to genetic screening. Some researchers are trying to locate specific genes or groups of genes that are predictive of certain behavioral traits.[264] Known as behavioral genetics, this field has the potential to discover genes that code for particular behavioral traits, including attention deficit disorder, depression, and susceptibility to aggression.[265] Even if these tests could not yield predictions of definite outcomes, as many would argue is impossible, they may be able to indicate increased susceptibility to certain conditions and could create future discriminatory practices.[266]

The patenting of genes has raised questions regarding both property rights and the accessibility of data and materials. Many wonder who "owns" the pieces of DNA that make up the human genome and if it is right to allow for the patenting of these entities. Furthermore, some believe that the patenting of these sequences will limit their accessibility and, as a result, their development into useful products.

CONCLUSION

Today, pegylated interferon will be dispensed to a patient attempting to cure their life-threatening hepatitis C, and a renal patient will be maintained on epoetin alfa therapy, replacing what chronic kidney disease has taken away. Tomorrow, a diabetic patient will avoid the discomfort of injections with the use of an insulin inhaler, and an HIV patient will halt the progression of his or her disease through the administration of gene therapy.

The products of biotechnology have changed the practice of medicine forever, and many more innovations are on the horizon. A comprehensive understanding of the field of biotechnology, however, encompasses far more than the end products it produces, delving into the science behind these agents and the awe-inspiring methods used to synthesize them. Furthermore, the field has managed to influence every segment of healthcare it touches, raising complex pharmacoeconomic questions for payers and patients, leading to regulatory debate and reorganization, and presenting society with intriguing ethical questions. In this chapter, we attempted to provide you with a brief glimpse into the vast and quickly changing world of biotechnology, and we hope that the information shared has advanced your understanding of this exciting field that promises to expand the practice of pharmacy in the future.

NOTES

1. Greene, J.J. and Rao, V.B. (Eds.). *Recombinant DNA Principles and Methodologies* (New York: Marcel Dekker, 1998).
2. Ibid.
3. Biotechnology Industry Organization. *The Technologies and Their Applications.* 2003. Available online at <http://www.bio.org/er/applications.asp>.
4. Rapoport, A. *Semantics* [Reprint of *Invitation to Semantics*, 1911] (New York: Crowell, 1975).
5. Rieger, R., Michaelis, A., and Green, M.M. *Glossary of Genetics and Cytogenetics* (Fourth Edition) (New York: Springer-Verlag, 1976).
6. McKusick, V.A. and Ruddle, F.H. A New Discipline, a New Name, a New Journal. *Genomics* 1987; 1: 1-2.
7. Ewing, B. and Green, P. Analysis of Expressed Sequence Tags Indicates 35,000 Human Genes. *Nature Genetics* 2000; 25: 232-234.
8. Roest-Crollius, H., Jailon, O., Bernot, A. et al. Estimate of Human Gene Number Provided by Genome-Wide Analysis Using *Tetraodon nigroviridis* DNA Sequence. *Nature Genetics* 2000; 25: 235-238.
9. Blundell, T.L. and Mizuguchi, K. Structural Genomics: An Overview. *Progress in Biophysics and Molecular Biology* 2000; 73: 289-295.
10. Teichmann, S.A., Chothia, C., and Gerstein, M. Advances in Structural Genomics. *Current Opinion in Structural Biology* 1999; 9: 390-399.
11. National Institutes of Health, National Institute of General Medical Sciences. Structural Genomics: The Cutting Edge. 2001. Available online at <http://www.nigms.nih.gov/funding/psi/catalyst.html>.
12. Thornton, J.M., Todd, A.E., Milburn, D., Borkakoti, N., and Orengo, C.A. From Structure to Function: Approaches and Limitations. *Nature Structural Biology* 2000; 7(11): 991-994.
13. Biotechnology Industry Organization, *The Technologies and Their Applications.*
14. Ibid.
15. Ibid.
16. Ibid.
17. Olson M.V. and Varki, A. Sequencing the Chimpanzee Genome: Insights into Human Evolution and Disease. *Nature Reviews Genetics* 2003; 4(1): 20-28.
18. Ansari-Lari, M.A., Oeltjen, J.C., and Schwartz, S. et al. Comparative Sequence Analysis of a Gene-Rich Cluster at Human Chromosome 12p13 and Its Syntenic Region in Mouse Chromosome 6. *Genome Research* 1998; 8: 29-40.
19. Hardison, R.C., Oeltjen, J., and Miller, W. Long Human-Mouse Sequence Alignments Reveal Novel Regulatory Elements: A Reason to Sequence the Mouse Genome. *Genome Research* 1997; 7: 966.
20. Bouck, J.B., Metzker, M.L., and Gibbs, R.A. Shotgun Sample Sequence Comparisons Between Mouse and Human Genomes. *Nature Genetics* 2000; 25(1): 31-33.
21. Celniker, S.E. The *Drosophila* Genome. *Current Opinion in Genetics and Development* 2000; 10(6): 612-616.

22. Rubin, G.M., Yandell, M.D., Wortman, J.R., et al. Comparative Genomics of the Eukaryotes. *Science* 2000; 5461 (March): 2204-2215.

23. UC Davis Genome Center. What Is Genomics?: The Emergence of Genomics As a Discipline. n.d. Available online at <http://www.genomecenter.ucdavis.edu/plan/proposed.pdf>.

24. Leeder, J.S. Pharmacogenetics and Pharmacogenomics. *Pediatric Clinics of North America* 2001; 48(3): 765-781.

25. UC Davis Genome Center. What Is Genomics?

26. Plant, J.E. and Glynn, A. Genetics of Resistance to Infection with *Salmonella ty, 959phimurium* in mice. *Journal of Infectious Disease* 1976; 133: 72-78.

27. Gros, P., Skamene, E., and Forget, A. Genetic Control of Natural Resistance to *Mycobacterium bovis* (BCG) in Mice. *Journal of Immunology* 1981; 127: 2417-2421.

28. Comstock, G.W. Tuberculosis in Twins: A Re-Analysis of the Prophit Survey. *American Reviews of Respiratory Disease* 1978; 117: 621-624.

29. Abel, L., Vu, V.D., Oberti, J., et al. Complex Segregation Analysis of Leprosy in Vietnam. *Genetic Epidemiology* 1995; 12: 63-82.

30. Cooper, D. What Is Pharmacogenetics? Paper presented at the Pharmacogenetics in Patient Care Conference of the American Association Clinical Chemistry. November 6, 1998, Chicago. Available online at <http://www.aacc.org/pharmacogenetics/>.

31. Mancinelli, L., Cronon, M., and Sadee, W. Pharmacogenomics: The Promise of Personalized Medicine. *AAPS PharmSci* 2000; 2(1): Article 4. Available online at <http://www.aapspharmsci.org/default.asp>.

32. Grant, D.M., Goodfellow, G.H., Sugamori, K.S., and Durette, K. Pharmacogenetics of the Human Arylamine N-Acetyltransferases. *Pharmacology* 2000; 61: 204-211.

33. Cooper, What Is Pharmacogenetics?

34. Mancinelli, Cronon, and Sadee, Pharmacogenomics: The Promise of Personalized Medicine.

35. Cooper, What Is Pharmacogenetics?

36. Persidis, A. The Business of Pharmacogenomics. *Nature Biotechnology* 1998; 16: 209-210.

37. Wasinger, V.C., Cordwell, S.J., Cerpa-Poljak, A., et al. Progress with Gene-Product Mapping of the Mollicutes: *Mycoplasma genitalium. Electrophoresis* 1995; 16(7): 1090-1094.

38. Persidis, A. Proteomics. *Nature Biotechnology* 1998; 16(4): 393-394.

39. Biotechnology Industry Organization, *The Technologies and Their Applications.*

40. Anderson, N.L. and Anderson, N.G. Proteome and Proteomics: New Technologies, New Concepts, and New Words. *Electrophoresis* 1998; 19: 1853-1864.

41. Persidis, Proteomics.

42. Biotechnology Industry Organization, *The Technologies and Their Applications.*

43. Robbins-Roth, C. Introduction to Antisense Technology. In C.L. Brakel (Ed.), *Advances in Applied Biotechnology Series.* Volume 2: *Discoveries in Antisense Nucleic Acids* (Houston: Gulf Publishing Company, 1989).

44. Biotechnology Industry Organization, *The Technologies and Their Applications*.

45. Persidis, A. Signal Transduction As a Drug-Discovery Platform. *Nature Biotechnology* 1998; 16(11): 1082-1083.

46. Biosource. n.d. Available online at <www.biosource.org>.

47. Armstrong, K., Eisen, A., and Weber, B. Assessing the Risk of Breast Cancer. *New England Journal of Medicine* 2000; 342: 564-571.

48. St. George-Hyslop, P.H. Molecular Genetics of Alzheimer's Disease. *Seminars in Neurology* 1999; 19: 371-383.

49. Lynch, H.T. Hereditary Nonpolyposis Colorectal Cancer (HNPCC). *Cytogenetics and Cell Genetics* 1999; 86: 130-135.

50. Mouradian, M.M. Recent Advances in the Genetics and Pathogenesis of Parkinson's Disease. *Neurology* 2002; 58: 179-185.

51. Michael, N.L. Host Genetic Influences on HIV-1 Pathogenesis. *Current Opinions in Immunology* 1999; 11: 466-474.

52. Small, P.M. and Fujiwara, P.I. (2001). Management of Tuberculosis in the United States. *New England Journal of Medicine* 2001; 345: 189-200.

53. Michael, Host Genetic Influences on HIV-1 Pathogenesis; Small and Fujiwara, Management of Tuberculosis in the United States.

54. Guttmacher, A.E. and Collins, F.S. Genomic Medicine—A Primer. *New England Journal of Medicine* 2002; 19(347): 1512-1520.

55. Ibid.

56. Biotechnology Industry Organization, *The Technologies and Their Applications*.

57. Ibid.

58. Human Genome Program, U.S. Department of Energy. Genomics and Its Impact on Science and Society: A 2003 Primer. March 2003. Available online at <http://www.ornl.gov/hgmis/publicat/primer2001/>.

59. Venter, J.C., Adams, M.D., Myers, E.W., et al. The Sequence of the Human Genome. *Science* 2001; 291: 1304-1351.

60. Nelson, P.N., Reynolds, G.M., Waldron, E.E., et al. Demystified . . . Monoclonal Antibodies. *Journal of Clinical Pathology: Molecular Pathology* 2000; 53: 111-117.

61. Ibid.

62. Berger, M., Shankar, V., and Vafai, A. Therapeutic Applications of Monoclonal Antibodies. *American Journal of Medical Science* 2002; 324(1): 14-30.

63. Medical Research Council. *Monoclonal antibodies*. Research in Focus Series. n.d. Available online at <http://www.mrc.ac.uk/pdf_mon_antibodies.pdf>.

64. Van Laan, S. Nomenclature for Biological Products: Monoclonal Antibodies. American Medical Association. 2003. Available online at <http://www.ama-assn.org/ama/pub/article/4781-4661.html>.

65. Panosian, C. Magic Bullets Fly Again. *Scientific American.com*. October 2001. Available online at <http://www.sciam.com/article.cfm?articleID=00007F6F-D588-1C6E-84A9809EC588EF21&pageNumber=1&catID=2>.

66. Wise, M. and Zelenika, D. Monoclonal Antibody Therapy in Organ Transplantation. In P. Sheppard and C. Dean (Eds.), *Monoclonal Antibodies: A Practical Approach* (New York: Oxford University Press, 2000), pp. 431-447.

67. Bachier, C.R. and LeMaistre, C.F. Immunotoxin Therapy of Graft-versus-Host Disease. In M.L. Grossbard (Ed.), *Monoclonal Antibody-Based Therapy of Cancer* (New York: Marcel Dekker, 1998), pp. 211-229.

68. Hengster, P., Pescovitz, M.D., Hyatt, D., et al. Cytomegalovirus Infections After Treatment with Daclizumab, an Anti-IL-2 Receptor Antibody, for Prevention of Renal Allograft Rejection. *Transplantation* 1999; 68: 310-313.

69. Mani, R.N., Breedveld, F.C., Kalden, J.R., et al. Therapeutic Efficacy of Multiple Intravenous Infusions of Anti-Tumor Necrosis Factor Alpha Monoclonal Antibody Combined with Low Dose Methotrexate in Rheumatoid Arthritis. *Arthritis and Rheumatism* 1998; 41: 1552-1563.

70. Choy, E.H.S., Kingsley, G.H., and Panayi, G.S. Monoclonal Antibody Therapy in Rheumatoid Arthritis. In P. Shepherd and C. Dean (Eds.), *Monoclonal Antibodies: A Practical Approach* (New York: Oxford University Press, 2000), pp. 449-461.

71. Pisetsky, D.S. Tumor Necrosis Factor Blockers in Rheumatoid Arthritis. *New England Journal of Medicine* 2000; 16: 810-811.

72. Present, D.H., Rutgeerts, P., Targan, S., et al. Infliximab for the Treatment of Fistulas in Patients with Crohn's Disease. *New England Journal of Medicine* 1999; 340: 1398-1405.

73. Bell, S. and Kamm, M.A. Antibodies to Tumor Necrosis Factor Alpha As Treatment for Crohn's Disease. *Lancet* 2000; 355: 858-860.

74. Milgrom, H., Fick, R.B., Su, J.Q., et al. Treatment of Allergic Asthma with Monoclonal Anti-IgE Antibody. Rhu Mab-E25 Study Group. *New England Journal of Medicine* 1999; 34: 966-973.

75. Salvi, S.S. and Babu, K.S. Treatment of Allergic Asthma with Monoclonal Anti-IgE Antibody. *New England Journal of Medicine* 2000; 342: 1292-1293.

76. Miller, D.H., Kahn, O.A.K., Sheremata, W.A., et al. A Controlled Trial of Natalizumab for Relapsing Multiple Sclerosis. *New England Journal of Medicine* 2003; 348: 15-23.

77. Hinds, C.J. Monoclonal Antibodies in Sepsis and Septic Shock. *British Medical Journal* 1992; 304: 132-133.

78. Abraham, E., Anzueto, A., Gutierrez, G., et al. Double-Blind Randomized Controlled Trial of Monoclonal Antibody to Human Tumor Necrosis Factor in Treatment of Septic Shock: NORASEPT II Study Group. *Lancet* 1998; 351: 929-933.

79. Wu, C. Antibodies May Treat Overdoses, Addiction. *Science News* 1999; 56: 134.

80. Harrison's Online. Cytokines. In *Introduction to the Immune System* (Chapter 305). August 13, 2002. Available online at <http://harrisons.accessmedicine.com/server-java/Arknoid/amed/harrisons/co_chapters/ch305/ch305_p07.html>.

81. Motzer, R.J., Bander, N.H., Nanus, D.M. Renal-Cell Carcinoma. *New England Journal of Medicine* 1996; 335: 865-875.

82. Noble, S. and Goa, K. Aldesleukin (Recombinant Interleukin-2): A Review of Its Pharmacological Properties, Clinical Efficacy and Tolerability in Patients with Metastatic Melanoma. *BioDrugs* 1997; 7: 394-422.

83. Kirkwood, J.M., Ibrahim, J.G., Sondak, V.K. et al. High- and Low-Dose Interferon Alfa-2b in High-Risk Melanoma: First Analysis of Intergroup Trial E1690/S911/C9190. *Journal of Clinical Oncology* 2000; 18: 2444-2458.

84. Dutcher, J.P. and Wiernik, P.H. Novel Biologic Approaches to Hematologic Malignancies. *Cancer Treatment & Research* 1999; 99: 275-306.

85. Kovacs, J.A., Vogel, S., Albert, J.M., et al. Controlled Trial of Interleukin-2 Infusions in Patients Infected with the Human Immunodeficiency Virus. *New England Journal of Medicine* 1996; 335(18): 1350-1356.

86. Piscitelli, S.C., Bhat, N., Pau, A. A Risk-Benefit Assessment of Interleukin-2 As an Adjunct to Antiviral Therapy in HIV Infection. *Drug Safety* 2000; 22: 19-31.

87. Sundin, D.J. and Wolin, M.J. Toxicity Management in Patients Receiving Low-Dose Aldesleukin Therapy. *Annals of Pharmacotherapy* 1998; 32: 344-352.

88. Baron, S., Tyring, S.K., Fleischmann, W.R. The Interferons: Mechanisms of Action and Clinical Applications. *Journal of the American Medical Association* 1991; 266: 1375-1383.

89. Niederau, C., Heintges, T., Lange, S., et al. Long-Term Follow-Up of HBeAg-Positive Patients Treated with Interferon Alfa for Chronic Hepatitis B. *New England Journal of Medicine* 1996; 334: 1422-1427.

90. Jaeckel, E., Cornberg, M., Wedemeyer, H., et al. Treatment of Acute Hepatitis C with Interferon Alfa-2b. *New England Journal of Medicine* 2001; 345(20): 1452-1457.

91. Andersson, P.B., Waubant, E., and Goodkin, D.E. How Should We Proceed with Disease-Modifying Treatments for Multiple Sclerosis? *Lancet* 1997; 349: 586-587.

92. Rudick, R.A., Sibley, W., and Durelli, L. Treatment of Multiple Sclerosis with Type 1 Interferons. In D.E. Goodkin and R.A. Rudick (Eds.), *Multiple Sclerosis: Advances in Clinical Trial Design, Treatment and Future Perspectives* (London: Springer-Verglag, 1996), pp. 223-250.

93. Brook, M.G., Gor, D., Forster, S. et al. Anti-HIV Effects of Alpha-Interferon. *Lancet* 1989; 1: 42.

94. Lane, H.C., Davey, V., Kovacs, J.A. et al. Interferon-Alpha in Patients with Asymptomatic Human Immunodeficiency Virus (HIV) Infection: A Randomized Placebo-Controlled Trial. *Annals of Internal Medicine* 1990; 112: 805-811.

95. Sumer, N. and Palabiyikoglu, M. Induction of Remission by Interferon-Alpha in Patients with Chronic Active Ulcerative Colitis. *European Journal of Gastroenterology and Hepatology* 1995; 7: 597-602.

96. Davidsen, B., Munkolm, P., Schlichting, P., et al. Tolerability of Interferon Alpha-2b, a Possible New Treatment of Active Crohn's Disease. *Alimentary Pharmacology & Therapeutics* 1995; 9: 75-79.

97. Jonasch, E. and Haluska, F.G. Interferon in Oncological Practice: Review of Interferon Biology, Clinical Applications, and Toxicities. *Oncologist* 2001; 6(1): 34-55.

98. Schrek, R. Intractable Chronic Lymphocytic Leukemia and Interferon. *Medical Hypotheses* 1991; 35(3): 182-183.

99. Fischer, A., Segal, A.W., Seger, R., and Weening, R.S. The Management of Chronic Granulomatous Disease. *European Journal of Pediatrics* 1993; 152(11): 896-899.

100. Bayes, M., Rabasseda, X., and Prous, J.R. Gateways to clinical trials. *Methods and Findings in Experimental and Clinical Pharmacology* 2002; 24(5): 291-327.

101. Key, L.L. Jr., Rodriguiz, R.M., Willi, S.M., et al. Long-Term Treatment of Osteopetrosis with Recombinant Human Interferon Gamma. *New England Journal of Medicine* 1995; 332(24): 1594-1599.

102. Fischer et al., The Management of Chronic Granulomatous Disease.

103. Old, L.J. Tumor Necrosis Factor. *Scientific American* 1988; 258: 59-60.

104. Ibid.

105. Old, L.J. Tumor Necrosis Factor. *Science* 1985; 230: 630-632.

106. Spriggs, D.R., Sherman, M.L., Frei, E., and Kufe, D.W. Clinical Studies with Tumor Necrosis Factor. In G. Bock (Ed.), *Tumor Necrosis Factor and Related Cytokines—Ciba Foundation Symposium 131* (Chichester, UK: Wiley, 1987), pp. 206-227.

107. Sherman, M.L., Spriggs, D.R., Arthur, K.A., et al. Recombinant Human Tumor Necrosis Factor Administered As a Five-Day Continuous Infusion in Cancer Patients: Phase I Toxicity and Effects on Lipid Metabolism. *Journal of Clinical Oncology* 1988; 6: 344-350.

108. Moritz, T., Niederle, N., Baumann, J., et al. Phase I Study of Recombinant Human Tumor Necrosis Factor Alpha in Advanced Malignant Disease. *Cancer Immunology, Immunotherapy* 1989; 29: 144-150.

109. Morice, R.C., Blick, M.B., Ali, M.K., and Gutterman, J.U. Pulmonary Toxicity of Recombinant Tumor Necrosis Factor. *Proceedings of the American Society of Clinical Oncology* 1987; 6: 29.

110. Urban, J.L., Shepard, H.M., Rothstein, J.L., Sugarman, B.J., and Schreiber, H. Tumor Necrosis Factor: A Potent Effector Molecule for Tumor Cell Killing by Activated Macrophages. *Proceedings of the National Academy of Sciences USA* 1986; 83: 5233-5237.

111. Degliantoni, G., Murphy, M., Koyabashi, M., et al. Natural Killer (NK) Cell Derived Haemopoetic Colony Inhibiting Activity and NK Cytotoxic Factor. *Journal of Experimental Medicine* 1985; 162: 1512-1530.

112. Shau, H. Characterization and Mechanism of Neutrophil-Mediated Cytostasis Induced by Tumor Necrosis Factor. *Journal of Immunology* 1988; 141: 234-238.

113. Nakano, K., Okugawa, K., Furuichi, H., et al. Augmentation of the Generation of Cytotoxic T Lymphocytes Against Synergistic Tumor Cells by Recombinant Human Tumor Necrosis Factor. *Cellular Immunology* 1989; 120: 154-164.

114. Bresnihan, B. Treatment of Rheumatoid Arthritis with Recombinant Human Interleukin-1 Receptor Antagonist. *Arthritis and Rheumatism* 1998; 41: 2196.

115. Izaguirre, A.G. Chemokine Receptor Family. 1997. Available online at <http://www.umdnj.edu/pathweb/genpath/lec_1/Chemokine_Receptor_Family/chemokine_receptor_family.htm>.

116. Ibid.

117. Ibid.

118. Amgen, Inc. *Enbrel* [Prescribing Information]. October 2002.

119. Eder, M., Geisler, G., Ganser, A. IL-3 in the Clinic. *Stem Cells* 1997; 15: 327.

120. Frampton, J.E., Lee, C.R., Faulds, D. Filgrastim: A Review of Its Pharmacological Properties and Therapeutic Efficacy in Neutropenia. *Drugs* 1994; 48: 731-760.

121. Nemunaitis, J. A Comparative Review of Colony-Stimulating Factors. *Drugs* 1997; 54: 709-729.

122. Young, N.S. Aplastic Anaemia. *Lancet* 1995; 346: 228-232.

123. Champlin, R.E., Nimer, S.D., Ireland, P., et al. Treatment of Refractory Aplastic Anemia with Recombinant Human Granulocyte-Macrophage-Colony-Stimulating Factor. *Blood* 1989; 73: 694-699.

124. Ortho Biotech Products, L.P. *Procrit* [Prescribing Information]. December 2000.

125. Evans, R.W., Rader, B., Manninen, D.L. The Quality of Life of Hemodialysis Recipients Treated with Recombinant Human Erythropoietin. *Journal of the American Medical Association* 1990; 263: 825-830.

126. Amgen, Inc. *Aranesp* [Prescribing Information]. July 2002.

127. Tepler, I., Elias, C., Smith, J.W., et al. A Randomized Placebo-Controlled Trial of Recombinant Human Interleukin-11 in Cancer Patients with Severe Thrombocytopenia Due to Chemotherapy. *Blood* 1996; 87: 3607-3614.

128. Kaushansky, K. Thrombopoietin. *New England Journal of Medicine* 1998; 339: 746-754.

129. Vadhan-Raj, S., Kavanagh, J.J., Freedman, R.S., et al. Safety and Efficacy of Transfusions of Autologous Cryopreserved Platelets Derived from Recombinant Human Thrombopoietin to Support Chemotherapy-Associated Severe Thrombocytopenia: A Randomized Cross-Over Study. *Lancet* 2002; 359(9324): 2145-2152.

130. Tepler et al., A Randomized Placebo-Controlled Trial of Recombinant Human Interleukin-11.

131. Boedeker, B.G.D. Production Processes of Licensed Recombinant Factor VIII Preparations. *Seminars in Thrombosis and Hemostasis* 2001; 27(4): 385-394.

132. Biotechnology Industry Organization. Top 10 Biotechnologies for Improving Health in Developing Countries. October 2002. Available online at <http://www.bio.org/globalhealth/topbiotech.asp>.

133. Biotechnology Industry Organization, *The Technologies and Their Applications.*

134. Biotechnology Industry Organization, Top 10 Biotechnologies for Improving Health in Developing Countries.

135. Ibid.

136. Biotechnology Industry Organization, *The Technologies and Their Applications.*

137. Access Excellence @ The National Health Museum. Animal Health Care— An Overview. 1992. Available online at <http://www.accessexcellence.org/RCAB/BA/ Animal_Health_Overview.html>.

138. Ibid.

139. Hardie, D. Anti-Viral Chemotherapy and Vaccines. Available online at <http://web.uct.ac.za/depts/mmi/jmoodie/vacc2.html>.

140. American Society of Gene Therapy. What Is Gene Therapy? 2002. Available online at <http://www.asgt.org/press_releases/basics.html>.

141. National Cancer Institute. *Questions and Answers About Gene Therapy.* June 7, 2000. Available online at <http://cis.nci.nih.gov/fact/7_18.htm>.

142. Anderson, W.F. Human Gene Therapy. *Nature* 1998; 392(30): 25-30.

143. Ibid.

144. Ibid.

145. Fry, J.W. and Wood, K.J. Gene Therapy: Potential Applications in Clinical Transplantation [Electronic version]. 1999. *Expert Reviews in Molecular Medicine.* Available online at <http://www.ermm.cbcu.ac.uk/99000691h.htm>.

146. Ibid.

147. Ibid.

148. Ibid.

149. Ibid.

150. Ibid.

151. Ibid.

152. Ibid.

153. Peel, D. *Virus Vectors & Gene Therapy: Problems, Promises & Prospects.* 1998. Available online at <http://www.micro.msb.le.ac.uk/335/peel/peel1.html>.

154. Ibid.

155. National Cancer Institute, *Questions and Answers About Gene Therapy.*

156. Novak, K. Gene Therapy Resumes. *Nature Reviews* 2002; 2(11): 813.

157. National Institutes of Health. *Stem Cells: Scientific Progress and Future Research Directions.* n.d. Available online at <http://www.nih.gov/news/stemcell/execsummary.pdf>.

158. Ibid.

159. Anonymous. A Comparative Look at the U.S. and British Approaches to Stem Cell Research. *Albany Law Review* 2002; 65(3): 831-855.

160. Ibid.

161. Ibid.

162. Cleland, J.L., Daugherty, A., and Mrsny, R. Emerging Protein Delivery Methods. *Current Opinions in Biotechnology* 2001; 12: 212-219.

163. Ibid.

164. Ibid.

165. Ibid.

166. Ibid.

167. Ibid.

168. Ibid.

169. Ibid.

170. Ibid.

171. Gene Therapy Weekly (Eds.). System to Administer Medications Has Several Applications. *Gene Therapy Weekly* 2002; November 21: 9.

172. Perera, A.D., Kapitza, C., Nosek, L., et al. Absorption and Metabolic Effect of Inhaled Insulin: Emerging Treatments and Technologies. *Diabetes Care* 2002; 25(12): 2276-2286.

173. Aradigm Corporation. Aradigm Presents Data from First Human Study of Interferon Administration via the AERx Technology Platform at International Controlled Release Society Meeting. 2002. Available online at <http://www.corporate-ir.net/ireye/ir_site.zhtml?ticker=ardm&script=410&layout=-6&item_id=318072>.

174. Novartis Pharmaceuticals Corp. *Miacalcin* [Prescribing Information]. November 2002.

175. Cleland, Daugherty, and Mrsny, Emerging Protein Delivery Methods.

176. Evens, R. and Witcher, M. Biotechnology: An Introduction to Recombinant DNA Technology and Product Availability. *Therapeutic Drug Monitoring* 1993; 15: 514-520.

177. Simonsen, C.C. and McGrogan, M. The Molecular Biology of Production Cell Lines. *Biologicals* 1994; 22(2): 85-94.

178. Carrol, J.M. and Trombetta, L.D. The Basic Principals of Recombinant DNA Technology. In S.W. Zito (Ed.), *Pharmaceutical Biotechnology: A Programmed Text* (Second Edition). (Lancaster, PA: Technomic Publishing Co., 1997), p. 20.

179. Evens and Witcher, Biotechnology: An Introduction to Recombinant DNA; Simonsen and McGrogan, The Molecular Biology of Production Cell Lines.

180. Kretzmer, G. Industrial Processes with Animal Cells. *Applied Microbiology and Biotechnology* 2002; 59: 135-142.

181. Evens and Witcher, Biotechnology: An Introduction to Recombinant DNA; Simonsen and McGrogan, The Molecular Biology of Production Cell Lines.

182. Pharmingin. Baculovirus Expression System: Applied Reagents for Heterologous Gene Expression. Available online at <http://www.pharmingen.com>.

183. Evens and Witcher, Biotechnology: An Introduction to Recombinant DNA.

184. Kretzmer, Industrial Processes with Animal Cells.

185. Ibid.

186. Ibid.

187. Ibid.

188. Ibid.

189. Cunha, T. and Aires-Barros, R. Large-Scale Extraction of Proteins. *Molecular Biotechnology* 20(1): 29-40.

190. Ibid.

191. Chu, L. and Robinson, D.K. Industrial Choices for Protein Production by Large-Scale Cell Culture. *Current Opinion in Biotechnology* 2001; 12: 180-187.

192. Ibid.

193. Kimball, J. Transgenic Animals. 2002. Available online at <http://users.rcn.com/jkimball.ma.ultranet/BiologyPages/T/TransgenicAnimals.html>.

194. Arizona State University, Genetic Engineering and Society. Transgenic Animals (Chapter 19). August 19, 2002. Available online at <http://photoscience.la.asu.edu/photosyn/courses/BIO_343/lecture/transan.html>.

195. Ibid; Kimball, Transgenic Animals.

196. Arizona State University, Genetic Engineering and Society, Transgenic Animals.

197. Center for Biologics Evaluation and Research. *CBER Vision Newsletter,* Special Commemorative Issue. July 2002. Available online at <http://www.fda.gov/cber/inside/centnews.htm>.

198. Center for Biologics Evaluation and Research. Commemorating 100 Years of Biologics Regulation. 2002. Available online at <http://www.fda.gov/cber/about.htm>.

199. Center for Drug Evaluation and Research. New Drug Application. 2002. Available online at <http://www.fda.gov/cder/handbook/ndabox.htm>.

200. F-D-C Reports, Inc. CBER/CDER Consolidation Working Group Unveils Product Transfer Plans. *The Pink Sheet* 2002; 64(44): 24-26.

201. U.S. Food and Drug Administration. *Phase Two of CBER/CDER Product Consolidation Concludes.* January 8, 2003. Available online at <http://www.fda.gov/bbs/topics/ANSWERS/2003/ANS01188.html>.

202. U.S. Food and Drug Administration, *Phase Two of CBER/CDER Product Consolidation Concludes;* F-D-C Reports, Inc., CBER/CDER Consolidation Working Group.

203. U.S. Food and Drug Administration, *Phase Two of CBER/CDER Product Consolidation Concludes;* F-D-C Reports, Inc., CBER/CDER Consolidation Working Group.

204. F-D-C Reports, Inc. FDA Generic Biologics Policy May Be One Change Under McClellan. *The Pink Sheet* 2002; 64(41): 7-8.

205. Ibid.

206. Biotechnology Industry Organization. Biotechnology Industry Statistics: Some Facts About Biotechnology. 2003. Available online at <http://www.bio.org/er/statistics.asp>.

207. Ibid.

208. Massachusetts Division of Healthcare and Finance Policy. Healthpoint: What's Driving Prescription Drug Costs? April 1999. Available online at <http://www.state.ma.us/dhcfp/pages/pdf/hp_13.pdf>.

209. Thottam, J., Altman, D., Reinhardt, U., and Shearer, G. Business, Heal Thyself: With Health-Care Costs Soaring, a TIME Round Table Takes a Look at the Causes—And Some Possible Cures. *Time.* October 6, 2002. Available online at <http://www.time.com/time/education/article/0,8599,361733-1,00.html>.

210. Tufts CSDD Institute for Professional Development. Outlook 2002. 2002. Available online at <http://csdd.tufts.edu/InfoServices/OutlookPDFs/Outlook2002.pdf>.

211. Reinhardt, U.E. The Predictable Managed Care Kvetch on the Rocky Road from Adolescence to Adulthood. *Journal of Health Politics, Policy & Law* 24(5): 897-910.

212. F-D-C Reports, Inc. Generic Biologics Cannot Use Waxman/Hatch As Model, Ex-FDAer Siegel. *The Pink Sheet* 2002; 64(44): 24-26.

213. F-D-C Reports, Inc. J&J Eprex "Dear Doctor" Letter in EU Recommends I.V. Administration, EU Labeling Changed. *The Pink Sheet* 2002; 64(29): 11-12.

214. Hargis, J.E. Biotechnology As a Pharmacy Specialty [Electronic version]. *Journal of Managed Care Pharmacy* 1998; 4(5).

215. Intelligent Healthcare, LLC. The New Economics of Health Care Inflation. August 2001. Available online at <http://www.intelhc.com>.

216. Kowalczyk, L. HMO Rates Climb Again for 2002: Increases Tied to Drug Costs, Fees for Care. *The Boston Globe* June 21, 2001.

217. Intelligent Healthcare, LLC, The New Economics of Health Care Inflation.

218. Tufts CSDD Institute for Professional Development, Outlook 2002.

219. Salvado, A.J. and Lawless, G. Biotechnology and Managed Care. *Journal of Managed Care Pharmacy* 2000; 6(4): 285-292.

220. Physicians for a National Health Program. The Center for Medicare and Medicaid Services, in New Projections Released Today in Health Affairs, Estimates That Health Spending Will More than Double to $2.8 Trillion by 2011 and Climb to More than 17 Percent of the GDP over the Next Decade, up from 13.2 Percent Currently. March 12, 2002. Available online at <www.pnhp.org/Press/2002/Quote_of_the_day/3.12.02.htm>.

221. Pardes, H., Manton, G., Lander, E., et al. Medicine: Effects of Medical Research on Health Care and the Economy. *Science* 1999; 283(5398): 36-37.

222. Biotechnology Industry Organization. Ernst & Young Economics Consulting and Quantitative Analysis, Economic Contributions of the Biotechnology Industry to the U.S. Economy: Prepared for the Biotechnology Industry Organization, May 2000. Available online at <http://www.bio.org/news/ernstyoung.pdf>.

223. Salvado and Lawless, Biotechnology and Managed Care.

224. Intelligent Healthcare, LLC, The New Economics of Health Care Inflation.

225. Salvado and Lawless, Biotechnology and Managed Care.

226. Balekdjian, D. and Russo, M. Outcomes Based Access: Raising the Bar. November 2002. *Pharmaceutical Executive.* Available online at <www.pharmexec.com/pharmexec/article/articledetail.JSP?id-36728>.

227. Hargis, Biotechnology As a Pharmacy Specialty.

228. Ibid.

229. Biotechnology Industry Organization. Guide to Biotechnology: Ethics. 2003. Available online at <http://www.bio.org/er/ethics.asp>.

230. Ibid.

231. Ibid.

232. Weissman, I.L. Stem Cells—Scientific, Medical and Political Issues. *The New England Journal of Medicine* 2002; 346(20): 1576-1579.

233. Anonymous. A Comparative Look at the U.S. and British Approaches to Stem Cell Research.

234. Ibid.

235. Biotechnology Industry Organization, Guide to Biotechnology: Ethics.

236. Anonymous, A Comparative Look at the U.S. and British Approaches to Stem Cell Research.

237. Ibid.

238. Ibid.

239. Ibid.

240. Ibid.

241. Ibid.

242. Ibid.

243. Ibid.

244. Ibid.

245. Ibid.

246. Balint, J.A. Ethical Issues in Stem Cell Research. *Albany Law Review* 2002; 65(3): 729-742.

247. Ibid.

248. Ibid.

249. Anonymous, A Comparative Look at the U.S. and British Approaches to Stem Cell Research; Balint, Ethical Issues in Stem Cell Research.

250. McLellan, F. U.S. Expert Panel Divided over Human Therapeutic Cloning. *Lancet* 2002; 360(9328): 231.

251. Ibid.

252. Ibid.

253. Anderson, Human Gene Therapy.

254. Ibid.

255. Ibid.

256. Ibid.

257. Ibid.

258. Ibid.
259. Pagnatarro, M.A. Genetic Discrimination and the Workplace: Employee's Right to Privacy v. Employer's Need to Know. *American Business Law Journal* 2001; 39(1): 139-145.
260. Ibid.
261. Ibid.
262. Ibid.
263. Ibid.
264. Nuffield Council on Bioethics. *Genetics and Human Behaviour.* 2002. Available online at <http://www.nuffieldbioethics.org/publications/geneticsandhb/rep0000001098.asp>.
265. Ibid.
266. Ibid.

Chapter 17

Unresolved Issues in Pharmacy

William A. Zellmer

"Why don't people's hearts tell them to continue to follow their dreams?" the boy asked the alchemist.
"Because that's what makes a heart suffer most, and hearts don't like to suffer."

Paulo Coelho
The Alchemist

INTRODUCTION

This chapter is based on a dream for the future of pharmacy. A dream that pharmacy will become a profession that is dedicated to helping people make the best use of medicines, and that this dedication will permeate the inner fiber of pharmacists and shape their interactions with patients and prescribers.

This dream has been nurtured by the following four beliefs:

• People need a readily accessible and knowledgeable professional advocate to help them make the best use of medicines.
• Pharmacists are better educated for this role than any other health worker.
• There is a profound gap between what pharmacists have been educated to do and how they typically behave in practice.
• It will be well worth the effort, from a broad societal perspective, to close this gap.

Two fundamental changes must be made for pharmacists to become a more meaningful force in the rational use of medicines:

- Pharmacists must adopt professionalism as the dominant guide to their behavior.
- Pharmacy must rationalize the development and deployment of its workforce.

Not everyone associated with the field of pharmacy will agree with this vision or with this prescription for achieving the vision. For example, the marketers of pharmaceuticals will continue to promulgate the myth that prescription medicines are safe and effective for widespread use and pose no unreasonable risks in their consumption; by implication, a patient-care role for pharmacists is unnecessary. Another example: The regulators of drug products will continue to pretend that the perfect rules can be written and enforced to ensure patient safety in the use of medicines. The bureaucratic system in which they function blinds them to the results that could be achieved if pharmacists were engaged more deeply in the medication-use process.

Pharmacists cannot look to the drug industry or government regulators to be their champions. They must be their own instruments of change. It is quite clear how that change *could* be achieved. It is not at all clear whether that change *will* be achieved. Pharmacists are well rewarded under the current method of practice, and there is ample reason to doubt that they will muster the desire and determination to transform their role in health care. Moreover, pharmacists are pegged with a well-entrenched stereotype that creates limited public expectations; it is easier to simply meet this low benchmark than create and fulfill a higher one.

THE PHARMACY PROFESSION

For purposes of this discourse, equated *pharmacy practice* is with the *pharmacy profession.* Pharmacy practice is conducted by individual pharmacists—individual *pharmacy practitioners*—not the corporate or institutional owners of pharmacy facilities (which have been called *pharmacy providers*):

> The pharmacy practitioner is the atom—the irreducible constituent—of the profession of pharmacy. If it were not for the personal health care service that individual pharmacists provide to individual clients, pharmacy would be merely an area of knowledge and an array of tech-

nical functions in the sequence of steps from drug discovery to drug consumption. It is pharmacy practitioners who have made personal commitments to attain and maintain the knowledge required to help people with their medication-related needs. It is pharmacy practitioners who have internalized the ethical standards of pharmacy. The core values of the profession, as well as the yearning for continued improvement of the profession, reside in the hearts of practitioners, not in the policies and procedures of providers.[1]

There is often confusion about what it means to be a pharmacy practitioner because individuals educated as pharmacists work in many sectors of society, inside and outside of health care. Such individuals are of great value to society, but, for purposes of this discussion, they are not included as practitioners or as components of the profession of pharmacy. Others may make different distinctions and it is their privilege to do so. This is not a question of right or wrong but simply a matter of communicating clearly.

PREVENTABLE PROBLEMS IN MEDICATION USE

The array of problems associated with medication use has been well documented and will be only briefly discussed here. When reviewing such information, it is important to look for details about the extent to which the problems documented were preventable and to think about how pharmacists could have helped prevent those problems.

Most medication use occurs among ambulatory patients, and significant medication-related morbidity and mortality occurs in this population. Based on a metaanalysis of various studies, it was estimated in 1994 that more than one million Americans were hospitalized because of adverse drug events (ADEs), which accounted for nearly 5 percent of hospital admissions.[2] One study showed that 17 percent of outpatients reported a problem with prescribed medications.[3] In a study of ambulatory Medicare patients, the rate of ADEs was 5 percent annually.[4]

Abundant evidence has shown that pharmacists who are appropriately engaged with ambulatory patients can help them improve the outcomes of their medication therapy.[5] Some medical researchers have become believers in the value of pharmacists in improving patient outcomes. Consider, for example, a study involving four medical practices in Boston in which 25 percent of patients who had one or more prescriptions experienced ADEs. Of these ADEs, 28 percent were ameliorable and 11 percent were preventable, suggesting that assertive community pharmacists could have made a significant difference in the well-being of many patients. In fact, the authors of this study stated, "Increasing patients' access to outpatient pharmacists (to discuss medications and side effects)" would be a good strategy to improve patient outcomes.[6]

There have been many studies of preventable ADEs in hospitals. Just to cite one example, the rate of ADEs was 6.5 per 100 nonobstetrical admissions at two tertiary care hospitals, with an extrapolated mean of approximately 1,900 ADEs per hospital. Twenty-eight percent of the ADEs were preventable.[7] Studies in intensive care units and in general medical units of hospitals demonstrated that pharmacists attending rounds reduced preventable ADEs by more than 70 percent.[8,9]

Based on the available evidence, the Institute of Medicine, in its report, *To Err Is Human,* listed the following two strategies among fourteen ideas for improving medication safety:

- Ensure the availability of pharmaceutical decision support (i.e., the availability of pharmacists to consult with prescribers).
- Include a pharmacist during rounds of patient care units.[10]

The National Quality Forum, which is developing and implementing a national strategy for health care quality measurement and reporting, has included the following point in its list of thirty "practices that have been demonstrated to be effective in reducing the occurrence of adverse health care events":

> Pharmacists should actively participate [in all acute care settings] in the medication-use process, including, at a minimum, being available for consultation with prescribers on medication ordering, interpretation and review of medication orders, preparation of medications, dispensing of medications, and administration and monitoring of medications.[11]

In summary, preventable ADEs are a serious public health problem, solid evidence has proven that pharmacists can significantly reduce the severity of this problem, and health care leaders are calling on practicing pharmacists to address this issue.

CURRENT DEPLOYMENT OF PHARMACISTS

Let's conduct a mind experiment. Think about all of the pharmacy practitioners in the various sectors of health care delivery in the United States. Now imagine a linear scale that could be used to differentiate among pharmacists based on their primary roles irrespective of practice site. At the left end of the scale is a classification for those who engage in only technical, impersonal functions related to order fulfillment in the dispensing process. At the right end is a classification for those who spend essentially all of their time interacting with patients, caregivers, and prescribers in giving advice or making decisions about appropriate medication use. Impersonal, technical services on the left; personal, high-judgment services on the right; mixed roles in between.

It is in the best interest of society for the profession of pharmacy to seek the optimal distribution of pharmacists along this scale. The need for services is certainly great at both ends of the scale, but where does society achieve the maximum benefit from its investment in developing the knowledge, skills, and abilities of the pharmacist?

Currently, the distribution of pharmacists is clustered around the left end of the scale. However, given the immense societal needs related to achieving the best use of medicines, pharmacy should encourage a mass migration of practitioners toward the right.

The majority of pharmacists practice in community pharmacies and most of them are extremely insular. They are preoccupied by the mechanics and rudiments of their work. They define their role in production-line terms: processing all the prescriptions that come in as quickly as possible without compromising accuracy. This is a valuable service; no consumer should expect anything less. However, the expertise of the pharmacist is misapplied in the performance of this service. Other valuable services that should be provided in tandem with transferring a powerful medicine from the pharmacy's shelves to the patient are not being performed because the pharmacist is immersed in the mechanics of dispensing.

For example, does the pharmacist concern herself or himself with whether the medication regimen is appropriate for the patient's condition and health-related behavior? Does the pharmacist care whether the patient understands how to use the medicine? Does the pharmacist want to know if the patient has any questions or concerns about the medicine? It is utterly astounding that in the vast majority of settings in which prescription medicines are dispensed, the answer to all these questions is no!

In institutional practice, too many pharmacy staffs restrict their sights to the activities within the confines of their departments. The expertise and oversight of the pharmacist are needed in the entire medication-use process, the major steps of which are prescribing, transcribing, dispensing, administering, and monitoring. Just as this process transcends professional and departmental boundaries, so must the pharmacist transcend her or his department and ensure that safe systems and appropriate expertise are applied to all steps in medication use.

WEAK PULSE OF PROFESSIONALISM

In too many practice settings, the pulse of pharmacist professionalism is weak or nonexistent. Resuscitation is urgently needed. Unless that revival occurs, there is no assurance that pharmacists will continue to be required in the prescription dispensing process.

A major characteristic of a profession is the compact that exists between the discipline and society. In exchange for an exclusive franchise to practice a profession, the individuals in the discipline promise to use their knowledge and expertise to help members of society and to put their clients' interests and welfare above their own. These ideas about professionalism have been captured in a code of ethics for pharmacists.[12] The code's principles convey some sense of what it means to be guided by professionalism as a pharmacist; the first five of these principles focus on responsibilities related to serving individual patients:

- A pharmacist respects the covenantal relationship between the patient and the pharmacist. (This is the exchange mentioned previously—in return for the gift of trust from society, the pharmacist promises to help people achieve the best use of medications.)
- A pharmacist promotes the good of every patient in a caring, compassionate, and confidential manner.
- A pharmacist respects the autonomy and dignity of each patient.
- A pharmacist acts with honesty and integrity in professional relationships.
- A pharmacist maintains professional competence.

Pharmacy educators have devoted significant attention to explaining the importance of professionalism and have recommended how to foster the behavioral attributes of professional health care workers among pharmacy students and new pharmacy practitioners.[13]

Why do so many pharmacists who are blessed with an outstanding professional education regress to technicians when they enter practice? Among the components of an answer to this complex question may be the following points: Most pharmacists do not control the policies and procedures of their practice setting. Current practice procedures are so firmly entrenched that many pharmacists with leadership skills self-select for roles in other sectors of pharmacy. Years of neglecting the obvious have conditioned everyone to expect no more.

This problem cannot be corrected overnight. However, it can be corrected over time, with sufficient forethought and will. Here are a few of the things that could be done:

- Encourage ambulatory patients to select a personal pharmacist. Not a pharmacy, but a pharmacist.
- Teach pharmacists how to recognize and resist corporate edicts, both blatant and subtle, that undermine their ability to care for patients.
- Recognize and honor pharmacists who have demonstrated an authentic professional commitment to patients. We need more heroes in the frontline ranks of pharmacy.
- Increase efforts to develop and enrich the work of frontline pharmacists in all practice settings. Let's remember that the true nature of pharmacy is defined in the everyday interface between pharmacists and patients.
- Limit entry to colleges of pharmacy to students who have already demonstrated their capacity for compassion and caring.[14]

The *field* of pharmacy (which includes the employers of pharmacists) is in the process of adjusting the need for pharmacists in the mechanics of dispensing; as evidenced, for example, by the growth of mail-service pharmacies and the immense investments hospitals are making in automated dispensing technology. However, no evidence has been found so far that these changes are resulting in any greater contact between patients and pharmacists. The *profession* of pharmacy needs to be more fully engaged in this process, and it must assertively ensure that the public's interests are protected as these changes occur.

OPTIMUM USE OF PHARMACISTS

Some sense of what the optimum distribution of pharmacists would look like may be gained by reviewing the work of an important conference conducted in 2001.[15] This program occurred at a time when there was a lot of worry and talk about the shortage of pharmacists. The solution-seeking discussions were generally based on the current roles of pharmacists. This led the conference organizers to ask what the projections of future need for pharmacists would look like if we assumed that pharmacists will be performing the roles for which they have been educated?

The conference participants examined the current use of pharmacists in four areas:

- outpatient prescription dispensing and inpatient drug-order fulfillment,
- patient care services in primary care settings,
- patient care services in secondary and tertiary care settings, and
- non–patient-care functions that require pharmacists.

The conference participants assumed that the public and the profession of pharmacy want the services of pharmacists to contribute to medication use that is safe, effective, patient centered, timely, efficient, and equitable. (These are attributes that the Institute of Medicine has said should characterize the entire health care system.[16]) Based on this assumption, the conference participants forecasted the need for pharmacists in the year 2020. The remarkable conclusions are summarized in Table 17.1.

These projections, of course, are very rough estimates based on a particular set of assumptions and should not be taken as the last word on pharmacist needs two decades from now. Nevertheless, several important points are revealed by the numbers. First, the need for pharmacists in patient care probably cannot be fully met by simply redeploying pharmacists from order fulfillment; if the profession is to meet the needs that patients, caregivers, and health professionals have relating to the best use of medicines, the output of new pharmacists over the next twenty years must accelerate significantly. Currently, it is estimated that 69 percent of practicing pharmacists are engaged in order fulfillment; the comparable figure in the 2020 projection is 38 percent (based on an estimated supply of 260,000 pharmacists). Given the legal requirements imposed on the order-fulfillment process, the demands in this area of practice may take precedence over the demands in patient care. Hence, if nothing is done to expand the output of pharmacists, only about 140,000 practitioners will be available for patient care services in 2020 (54 percent of pharmacists in practice, compared with 24 percent today). Based on conference projections, at least twice that many pharmacists will be needed in primary, secondary, and tertiary patient care. It may take far longer than twenty years for the profession to be able to completely satisfy the need for pharmacists in patient care.

TABLE 17.1. Estimates of Current Use and Projected Need for Pharmacists (Full-Time Equivalents)

Function	Use of pharmacists, 2001	Need for pharmacists, 2020
Order fulfillment	136,400	100,000
Primary care services	30,000	165,000
Secondary/tertiary care services	18,000	130,000
Indirect/other services	12,300	22,000
Total	196,700	417,000
Total estimated supply (based on currently known plans for school-of-pharmacy capacity)		260,000
Shortfall		157,000

Many questions are raised by the previous discussion. Will other health workers step in to fill the void in medication-related patient care? If traditional pharmacies (and the pharmacists they employ) continue to be perceived as conveying only a commodity, not a professional service, will the rate of evolution of alternate sources of that commodity accelerate? (An example is the use of technology to deliver the medicine for the initial course of therapy before the patient leaves the doctor's office, with the remaining supply delivered by mail.) Will PharmD-educated pharmacists migrate to patient care positions regardless of opposing salary incentives, leaving the pickings scarce for those who are hiring pharmacists for order fulfillment? Would such a migration, especially in the face of the retirement of BS-educated pharmacists, force the chain drug stores and state regulators to invent a new model for the safe dispensing of prescriptions to outpatients, empowering lower-trained personnel to assume most of the work? Can the nation's capacity for postgraduate pharmacy residency training be expanded sufficiently to prepare an adequate number of practitioners for patient care?

CREDENTIALING PATIENT CARE PHARMACISTS

Ambulatory patients who use medicines need pharmacists for two broad types of patient care services. The first type of service relates to oversight and communication at the time the prescription is dispensed. Many pharmacists have been well educated to provide this service. The second type of service relates to the management of a patient's drug therapy in collaboration with the prescriber. This type of advanced practice is especially valuable to patients taking multiple medicines or medicines that are particularly risky to use.

It is one thing to call for the profession to become more engaged in collaborative drug therapy management, but it is quite a different proposition for the public to understand and support such a shift. This issue often comes to the fore in the public policy arena when pharmacist organizations advocate for an expanded scope of pharmacist practice and for payment of pharmacists for services such as collaborative drug therapy management. The typical initial reaction to such advocacy from a legislator or government bureaucrat is, "What?! Tell me again what you want to be authorized to do and to be paid for? Isn't that what the doctor is supposed to do? Is the pharmacist I see behind the counter in my pharmacy even interested in doing what you say you want to be paid for?"

The profession should face up to its well-entrenched dispensing stereotype and public skepticism about an advanced role for pharmacists. The most powerful way to bust out of its monolithic image would be for the profession to create a specific category of licensed pharmacists who have demonstrated their qualifications for collaborative drug therapy management. Optometry has developed a system of licensure and certification that may be a model for pharmacy. Basic licensure of the optometrist empowers the practitioner for traditional roles related to eye examination and prescription of corrective lenses. In addition, the optometrist can become certified by the state board of optometry, through examination, for advanced practice that entails use of diagnostic and therapeutic pharmaceutical agents. [17]

Pharmacy should develop a similar system to distinguish between practitioners who are qualified only for traditional practice roles versus those who have demonstrated the knowledge, skills, and abilities for advanced practice such as collaborative drug therapy management. This system would assure the public that pharmacy has a mechanism to verify the competence of individual practitioners for advanced roles and provide a framework for compensation for such services.

CONTINUING THE DEVELOPMENT OF PHARMACY TECHNICIANS

The shortage of pharmacists and the escalation in pharmacist salaries has stimulated sharp growth in the employment of pharmacy technicians. This has been particularly notable in recent years among chain drug store corporations (hospitals have used pharmacy technicians for decades), many of which, since the late 1990s, have encouraged their technicians to become certified by the Pharmacy Technician Certification Board (PTCB). The creation of PTCB in 1995, and its certification of more than 140,000 technicians (as of 2003), have been important milestones in pharmacy's development of a technical corps of workers to perform routine tasks and free up the pharmacist for higher-order functions. In many states, pharmacists are allowed to delegate more tasks to technicians who are certified compared with noncertified assistants. However, this aspect of rationalizing the pharmacy workforce is not yet complete. Pharmacy should now assertively move to establish appropriate standards for the education and training of technicians.

Let's consider this issue from the layperson's perspective. Walk into almost any community pharmacy today and take a careful look at the personnel in the prescription department. A common model is for a sales clerk to be positioned for primary contact with the customer. Behind the sales clerk is typically a short wall of shelves filled with merchandise and bags of dispensed prescriptions. Behind that wall, sometimes on a raised platform, is the dispensing area, populated with a number of workers. There is rarely any distinction in garb between pharmacists and technicians, so consumers are unable to tell exactly what type of worker is in the dispensing area, although they may assume that everyone there is a pharmacist.

Now let's examine this picture from a public health perspective. The pharmacist is required to be licensed by the state. Nationwide, the minimum qualifications for pharmacist licensure include graduation from an accredited school of pharmacy. This is in line with general public expectations about governmental oversight of health professionals. However, what about the certified technician? There is no education and training requirement for certification. All that is necessary is high school graduation or equivalency and satisfactory completion of the PTCB exam. About half the states require some type of on-the-job training for technicians, but no uniform standards exist for such training. For the most part, the quality of the education and training of pharmacy technicians is left up to the employer.

Imagine what a muckraking television journalist could do with this situation:

When you take a prescription to your local pharmacy, you trust that you will be getting the right medicine and that it will be labeled correctly. Is your trust warranted? How much do you know about the people who are dispensing your medicine? Can you be assured that they have the necessary qualifications for interpreting your doctor's order correctly, choosing the right medication, and labeling it properly? The answer may surprise you.

Although pharmacists are required to have five or six years of college education and pass a nationally standardized licensure exam, there is no standard for the education and training of the nonpharmacists who assist them. Some of the assistants—called pharmacy technicians—may have passed a test of their knowledge to receive national certification, but there is no requirement that only certified individuals be hired. Further, the only educational requirement for certified technicians is high school graduation. As many as three technicians are allowed to work with each pharmacist. Individual pharmacies and drug store corporations have their own methods for training technicians, but no national standard has been established for the content and quality of that training. With a national shortage of pharmacists and with more new medications coming on the market every year, the number of prescriptions dispensed by the nation's pharmacies is mushrooming. With this growth come more opportunities for mistakes. A report in the *Boston Globe* in 1999 stated that in Massachusetts alone there are 2.4 million prescriptions filled improperly every year; 86 percent of these errors involved the consumer getting the wrong medicine or the wrong strength.

Why do pharmacies permit such a notable gap in the education and training of personnel who handle your prescription medicines? We have nationwide educational standards for most occupations in the health field; why is an exception made for pharmacy technicians? Will your health be put at risk the next time you have a prescription filled?

Uniform national standards for the education and training of pharmacy technicians should be developed and enforced because anything less poses a tremendous risk to public confidence in pharmacy. The current lack of standards for technician education and training inhibits the extent to which pharmacists are willing to delegate tasks to technicians. Identification of appropriate standards for the education and training of technicians can be done more effectively and efficiently nationwide by a body such as the Accreditation Council for Pharmacy Education (which performs a similar function for pharmacist education) than by the thousands of individual employers of technicians.

AN ALTERNATIVE SCENARIO

What if, the dreams of dreamers notwithstanding, it turns out to be impossible to professionalize frontline pharmacy dispensing practice? If such a hypothetical reality were to become widely accepted inside and outside of pharmacy, what type of rational system could be devised to ensure public safety when prescription medicines are dispensed? Among the action steps that could be contemplated to make this scenario acceptable are the following:

- Standardize the ambulatory-care prescription dispensing process in all pharmacies, such that a worker moving from Pharmacy A in Town X to Pharmacy B in Town Y would be stepping into the same process.
- Imbue the process with advanced, computer-driven quality assurance techniques with appropriate checks and balances to avoid essentially all dispensing error. Require ongoing documentation of the safety of the process that is available for inspection at any time by the state board of pharmacy.
- Based on an objective task analysis, outline the minimum knowledge, skills, and abilities that a worker in this system must have to ensure patient safety. Establish national standards for the education and training of workers in the minimum requirements. Test workers on the mastery of the minimum knowledge, skills, and abilities and certify those who pass. Require retesting based on updated requirements every few years.
- Train personnel thoroughly in the dispensing process. Verify competency in the process often.
- Require that the prescriber enter the prescription into an electronic system, which transmits the order automatically to the pharmacy, to avoid the problem of illegibility.

- Require that a licensed pharmacist be available at a central call center to consult with the on-site pharmacy workers regarding any unusual situations that arise and to broker any adjustments in therapy with the prescriber.

Under such a system, the vast majority of pharmacists would be available for patient care roles in medical offices, clinics, hospitals, nursing homes, other health care settings, and private clinical pharmacy practices. All hope and pretense of making community pharmacies anything other than retail outlets would be removed. (This may be what pharmacists in prescription departments, through their insularity and reticence, are signaling they want.)

Although this alternative scenario is not one the author favors, the marketplace, in fact, will decide whether pharmacy moves in this direction over the course of time. Among the forces at play in the marketplace are the vision and motivation of pharmacists, the decisions of retail chain drug store executives, and consumer beliefs about the safety and value of medicines. The first factor—the vision and motivation of pharmacists—is both a source of despair and a source of hope: Despair in the sense that so few contemporary pharmacy practice leaders are speaking and living the language of professionalism. Hope in the sense that if enough pharmacists are true to their hearts, an unstoppable force for change will be unleashed.

CONCLUSION

People need a readily accessible and knowledgeable professional activist to help them make the best use of medicines. Pharmacists have an opportunity to fulfill this vital public health role. However, profound changes in attitude and orientation of practitioners will be required for this to happen on a large scale, and it may take generations before those changes become instilled into pharmacy practice.

The profession should make its workforce development and deployment more rational. Pharmacists should migrate from routine technical functions in dispensing to patient care functions that produce better value for society's investment in the education of pharmacists. Two specific workforce changes needed are the development of a system of credentialing pharmacists who are qualified to collaborate with prescribers in managing drug therapy and the establishment of minimum standards for the education and training of pharmacy technicians.

These are the big unresolved issues in pharmacy, and although they are not new issues, it is not too late to face them head on.

NOTES

1. Zellmer, W.A. Distinguishing between pharmacy practitioners and providers [editorial]. *Am J Hosp Pharm* 1994; 51: 2314.

2. Lazarou, J., Pomeranz, B.H., and Corey, P.N. Incidence of adverse drug reactions in hospitalized patients: A meta-analysis of prospective studies. *JAMA* 1998; 279: 1200-1205.

3. Gandhi, T.K., Burstin, H.R., Cook, E.F., et al. Drug complications in outpatients. *J Gen Intern Med* 2000; 15: 149-154.

4. Gurwitz, J.H., Field, T.S., Harrold, L.R., et al. Incidence and preventability of adverse drug events among older persons in the ambulatory setting. *JAMA* 2003; 289: 1107-1116.

5. Posey, L.M. Proving that pharmaceutical care makes a difference in community pharmacy. *J Am Pharm Assoc* 2003; 43: 136-139.

6. Gandhi, T.K., Weingart, S.N., Borus, J., et al. Adverse drug events in ambulatory care. *N Engl J Med* 2003; 348: 1556-1564, p. 1561.

7. Bates, D.W., Cullen, D.J., Laird, N.M., et al. Incidence of adverse drug events and potential adverse drug events: Implications for prevention. *JAMA* 1995; 274: 29-34.

8. Leape, L.L., Cullen, D.J., Clapp, M.D., et al. Pharmacist participation on physician rounds and adverse drug events in the intensive care unit. *JAMA* 1999; 282: 267-270.

9. Kucukarslan, S.N., Peters, M., Mlynarek, M., et al. Pharmacists on rounding teams reduce preventable adverse drug events in hospital general medicine units. *Arch Intern Med* 2003; 163: 2014-2018.

10. Institute of Medicine Committee on Quality of Health Care in America. *To err is human—Building a safer health system* (Washington, DC: National Academy Press, 1999), p. 158.

11. National Quality Forum. Safe practices for better healthcare (Washington, DC: National Quality Forum, 2003), p. 7.

12. American Society of Health-System Pharmacists. Code of ethics for pharmacists. Available online at <www.ashp.org/bestpractices/ethics/Ethics_End_Code. pdf>.

13. Hammer, D.P., Berger, B.A., Beardsley, R.S., et al. Student professionalism. *Am J Pharm Educ* 2003; 67 (03): Article 96. Available online at <http://www. ajpe.org/view.asp?art=aj670396+pdf.yes>.

14. Zellmer, W.A. Searching for the soul of pharmacy. *Am J Health-Syst Pharm* 1996; 53: 1911-1916.

15. Knapp, D.A. Professionally determined need for pharmacy services in 2020—Report of a conference sponsored by the Pharmacy Manpower Project Inc. Available online at <http://www.aacp.org/site/page.asp?TRACKID-+VID-1+CID-1056+DID-6195>.

16. Institute of Medicine Committee on Quality of Health Care in America. *Crossing the quality chasm—A new health system for the 21st century* (Washington, DC: Institute of Medicine, 2001).

17. New York State Education Department. Optometry license requirements. Available online at <http://www.op.nysed.gov/optom.htm>.

Chapter 18

Pharmacy Looks to the Future

Jon C. Schommer
Richard R. Cline
Tom A. Larson
Donald L. Uden
Ronald S. Hadsall
Stephen W. Schondelmeyer

INTRODUCTION

When looking to the future, it is impossible to predict it with 100 percent accuracy and certainty. A story is told of an individual who developed an algorithm that correctly predicted 95 percent of the time whether a stock would go up or down in price the following day. Armed with such a seemingly accurate way to predict the future, some thought that they could apply this to their decision making about buying and selling stocks and make a fortune. Alas, those who used the algorithm lost money. Upon review, it was learned that the algorithm was quite good at predicting when a stock would go up the following day and when a stock would go down just slightly. However, it was not very good at predicting when a stock would plummet in price the following day. Those few days during which a stock price would plummet resulted in losses that more than wiped out any previous gains.

The goal of this chapter is *not* to predict the future of pharmacy. Even if one were to be 95 percent accurate, that would not be enough information to be successful in the future. As the stock market shows us, it takes only a brief moment to wipe out many years of gains. Our goal for this chapter is to present a discussion of what might be important components within the environmental, economic, and political landscape of pharmacy.[1] The purpose of this chapter is to first describe some trends and issues related to pharmacy practice. Next, we will highlight the process of the diffusion of new innovations and the "tipping point" principle, which helps understand why new innovations might be adopted slowly at first and then seem to "take off" and become adopted by whole populations. We will conclude the chapter with four possible pharmacy practice models of the future that we developed based on our discussions as faculty members who work at the same university. These discussions mostly were lunchtime musings and are presented as a point of discussion for others. We will make the argument that no one model is likely to dominate. Rather, the mix of these models over time might depend on how pharmacy develops in three areas: technicians, technology, and transitions in practice and the rate of diffusion of innovations in these areas.

TRENDS AND ISSUES

Pharmacists' place in American culture has been tied to the vision of the pharmacist as the proprietor of a drug store. The drugstore itself, a special combination of soda shop, prescription department, and general emporium, is something of a cultural icon.[2] By the early 1900s in the United States, physicians had agreed to dispense medicines only rarely and pharmacists reciprocated by limiting their diagnosing and prescribing to cases of minor ills and emergencies.

During the 1950s, the number of prescriptions dispensed by pharmacists increased by over 50 percent, transforming the prescription department into the economic engine of the drugstore.[3] Pharmacists gained respect from their connection with new, effective drugs coming on the market but were restricted to machinelike tasks in which they "counted and poured" these medications into bottles. The 1951 Durham-Humphrey Amendment to the Food, Drug, and Cosmetic Act removed much of the pharmacist's autonomy in practice, and the American Pharmaceutical Association Code of Ethics made the pharmacist's limited role quite clear.

> The pharmacist does not discuss the therapeutic effects or composition of a prescription with a patient. When such questions are asked, he suggests that the qualified practitioner [that is, a physician or dentist] is the proper person with whom such matters should be discussed.[4]

The era of clinical pharmacy (1965 to 1990) emerged in which pharmacists asserted themselves as "drug information experts." During this period of change, Brodie and Benson stated that "the ultimate goal of the services of pharmacy must be the safe use of drugs by the public. In this context, the mainstream function of pharmacy is clinical in nature, one that may be identified accurately as drug-use control."[5] Rooted in hospitals, clinical pharmacy came to encompass unit-dose distribution systems, the use of pharmacy technicians, the establishment of drug information centers, and the development of patient drug profiles. As clinical pharmacy demonstrated its utility, the number of pharmacists in institutional practice more than doubled to about 40,000, or nearly one-quarter of all practitioners, during the 1970s and 1980s.[6]

In the community pharmacy practice sector, the change to clinical pharmacy was more gradual, but the person who stood across the counter from the pharmacist was undergoing a transformation from "the customer" to "the patient." After 150 years of caring about the wants of customers, pharmacists were beginning to care about the needs of patients.[7] Such a paradigm shift prompted a revision of the American Pharmaceutical Association's Code of Ethics in 1969. The new code began, "A pharmacist should hold the health and safety of patients to be of first consideration; he should render to each patient the full measure of his ability as an essential health practitioner."[8]

The clinical pharmacy era is best characterized as a transitional period between the years of "count and pour" practice and the dawning era of "pharmaceutical care," which is considered the new period in pharmacy's history.[9] The pharmaceutical care concept grew out of Donald Brodie's drug-use control and has developed into a generally accepted definition. Pharmaceutical care is "the responsible provision of drug therapy for the purpose of achieving definite outcomes that improve a patient's quality of life."[10]

The Emergence of Pharmaceutical Care

Justification for the provision of pharmaceutical care is targeted at correcting the problem of "drug misadventuring," which covers the broad array of phenomena associated with negative drug experiences.[11,12] Drug misadventuring is a hazard or incident

1. which is an inherent risk when drug therapy is indicated,
2. which is created through either omission or commission by the administration of a drug or drugs during which a patient is harmed,
3. whose outcome may or may not be independent of the preexisting disease process,
4. which may be attributable to error, immunological response, or idiosyncratic response, and
5. which is unexpected and thus unacceptable to patient and prescriber.

According to Hepler and Strand, drug misadventuring can result from

1. inappropriate prescribing,
2. inappropriate delivery,
3. inappropriate behavior by the patient,
4. patient idiosyncrasy, and
5. inappropriate monitoring.[13]

Thus, drug misadventuring not only includes issues of harm (safety) but also issues of treatment failure (efficacy). For example, a patient who took tetracycline with an antacid, which inhibits the absorption of the drug, would have experienced a drug misadventure if the treated condition was not cured.

Reported research provides evidence of the seriousness of drug misadventuring. In a summary of reviewed literature, Schommer reported that noncompliance with drug regimens ranged between 4 and 77 percent, medication errors between 25 and 90 percent, and the incidence of adverse drug reactions between 2 and 51 percent of the subjects studied.[14] These wide ranges may be due to differences in study methods, but also may be due to the variety of medications, disease types, and populations investigated. Other estimates suggest that over half of the 2 billion medications prescribed each year may be taken incorrectly and result in one-sixth of all hospital admissions, over one-fourth of nursing home admissions, almost 2.5 million serious medical emergencies per year, and about 28 percent of all malpractice suits.[15-17] The abuse of prescription drugs results in more injuries and deaths to Americans than all illegal drugs combined.[18] Also, improper use may be related to over 50 percent of the failures of prescription medication therapy.[19] Overall, the estimated cost of drug-related morbidity and mortality for the ambulatory setting in the United States was $76.6 billion in 1995 and $177.4 billion in 2001.[20,21]

According to Hepler and Strand, pharmaceutical care can improve health care outcomes and decrease costs by preventing or detecting and resolving drug-related problems that can lead to drug misadventures, both by increasing the effectiveness of drug therapy and by avoiding adverse effects.[22] In 1998, Cipolle, Strand, and Morley proposed that pharmaceutical care is "a practice in which the practitioner takes responsibility for all of a patient's drug-related needs and held accountable for this commitment." Further, it is "a health care professional practice designed to meet the patient's drug-related needs by identifying, resolving, and preventing drug therapy problems."[23]

There is evidence to justify pharmacy's claim of a mandate to help the patient obtain the best possible drug therapy and especially to protect the patient from harm.[24-26] Literature reviews of the effects of "pharmaceutical care" based on over 400 studies showed that its provision to patients can increase appropriate use of medications; compliance; patient knowledge; understanding and recall of medication regimens; therapeutic outcomes (e.g., blood-pressure control); patient satisfaction; patient acceptance of medical care; and quality of life (e.g., increased school attendance).[27-29] Also, pharmaceutical care can decrease adverse drug reactions, number and cost of medications, emergency room visits, hospitalizations, length of stay in hospitals, and overall health care costs. Most of these studies were limited in scope, utilized different methods, and compared the provision of just a component of pharmaceutical care with doing nothing at all. However, the results of these diverse studies do support the assumption that pharmaceutical care can improve outcomes and reduce costs of health care.

The pharmacy profession is undergoing a transition in which the profession's goal is to adopt the practice philosophy of pharmaceutical care.[30-34] Such a practice requires the establishment of a therapeutic relationship with the patient, an assessment, a care plan, an evaluation, and continuous follow-up.[35] To make such a transition in practice, corresponding changes in pharmacist work activities are expected.[36] However, it is quite likely that pharmacists will experience heavy workloads, as they may need to continue to engage in traditional pharmacist activities as well as add the new activities that their evolving roles will require.

A number of trends have combined to increase pressure on pharmacists in their traditional medication-dispensing roles. The population of older adults (those age sixty-five and older) in the United States grew by 12.0 percent from 1990 to 2000 to approximately 35 million persons.[37] This group of Americans uses twice the number of prescription medications as any other demographic group.[38] In this same decade, the number of pharmacists per 100,000 U.S. residents increased only slightly, growing from 68 in 1991 to 71 in 2000.[39] Concurrently, the proportion of female pharmacists increased from 32 to 46 percent, a trend that is important because this group presently is more likely to work part-time than males.[40] Together, these trends contributed to an increase in the number of prescriptions dispensed per year per retail pharmacist from 16,500 in 1992 to 22,200 in 2000.[41]

Work activity research conducted in 1999 and 2000 supports the notion that pharmacists are experiencing workload pressure as pharmacy goes through a transition period.[42-50] For example, results of work activity research showed that U.S. pharmacists working full-time were on the job an estimated forty-four hours during a typical week. On a typical day, community pharmacists engaged in 141 interpersonal interactions, hospital inpatient pharmacists reported an average of 76 per day, and pharmacists working in other noncommunity settings reported 99 interactions per day. Community staff pharmacists, working in high-volume pharmacies reported the highest average number of interactions per day at 161. These interactions were comprised of sixty-seven face-to-face interactions (sixty-five of which were with patients), and ninety-four through another medium (thirty-two of which were with patients).

These findings reflect a heavy load of interpersonal interaction for community staff pharmacists working in high-volume pharmacies. For example, assuming a ten-hour workday with no breaks, this means that these pharmacists had over sixteen interactions per hour, or approximately one every four minutes. Assuming an eight-hour workday without breaks, the interaction rate is over twenty per hour, one every three minutes. Sixty-seven face-to-face interactions translate into more than eight face-to-face interactions per hour over the span of an eight-hour day without breaks, or one every 7.5 minutes. Ninety-four interactions through another medium translate into almost twelve of these types of interactions per hour, about one every five minutes.

Based on research conducted in 2000, 56 percent of U.S. community pharmacists' time was spent in medication-dispensing responsibilities, 19 percent was spent in consultation responsibilities, 16 percent was devoted to business management responsibilities and nine percent was spent in drug-use management responsibilities.[51] In comparison, these pharmacists would prefer to spend 38 percent of their time in medication-dispensing responsibilities, 34 percent in consultation responsibilities, only nine percent in business management responsibilities, and 21 percent in drug-use management responsibilities

Research suggests that, as of 2000, pharmacist workload still was focused on prescription-drug dispensing responsibilities. In addition, pharmacists had interpersonal interactions with others outside of their pharmacy practice once every three minutes in some practice settings, and may engage in face-to-face interaction with someone not working in their pharmacy at a rate of one every 7.5 minutes.[52] In light of pharmacists' workload and the effects that these workloads can have on pharmacy practice, the transition to the pharmaceutical care practice era has been slow. In the next section, we propose that understanding how new ideas might be adopted over time in pharmacy can be important for decision making as we move forward as a profession.

DIFFUSION OF INNOVATIONS
AND THE TIPPING POINT PRINCIPLE

Sociologists have developed the diffusion model, which is a way of looking at how an innovative idea or product is adopted by a population. A famous diffusion study was conducted by Ryan and Gross, in which they analyzed the adoption of hybrid seed corn in Greene County, Iowa, during the 1930s.[53] They found that the adoption was slow at first, during which time only a small number of innovative farmers tried the seed (Innovators). They were adventurous and willing to take a risk with the new seed. The opinion leaders (Early Adopters) in the community, the respected, thoughtful people who watched and analyzed what the Innovators were doing, followed suit after a few growing seasons had passed. Then came the big bulge of farmers, the Early Majority and the Late Majority, the deliberate and skeptical mass, who would never try anything until the most respected of farmers had tried it first. Finally, the Laggards, the most traditional of all, who see no urgent reason to change, started to adopt the new hybrid seed corn. A plot of the progression on a graph forms an S-shaped curve (see Figure 18.1). The "tipping point" occurs just as the Early Adopters started using the seed, with adoption rising sharply as the Majority catches on to the new product.[54]

Everett Rogers developed the "Diffusion of Innovations" model as a way to better understand this phenomenon that is often seen as new ideas or products are adopted.[55] In the pharmacy domain, examples of diffusion of innovations could include the adoption of

1. unit-of-use dosage forms,
2. third-party payment for prescription drugs,
3. patient profiles in community pharmacies, and
4. mail-order/Internet pharmacy.

For each example, one could plot the adoption curve and identify a tipping point. Recently, Shetty and Brooks developed and tested a statistical model for the diffusion of atypical antipsychotic drugs.[56] They found statistical evidence for the S-shaped adoption curve as posited by the diffusion of innovations theory and reported that the tipping point for adoption of atypical antipsychotic drugs in the Iowa Medicaid population started at fifty months after the drugs became available on the market.[57]

When a new innovation in health care is developed that has clear advantages, it is desirable from both a public policy perspective and from an individual patient perspective to have the new innovation adopted into patient

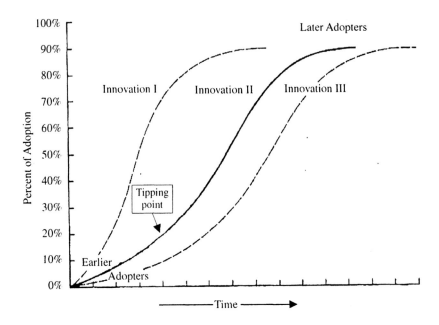

FIGURE 18.1. Diffusion of Innovation (*Source:* Adapted from Rogers, E. M. *Diffusion of Innovations,* Fourth Edition [New York: The Free Press, 1995].)

care as quickly as possible. According to the diffusion of innovations theory, the rate of adoption depends on a number of things. First, the perceived attributes of the innovation are important predictors for the rate of adoption. These include the product's relative advantage, compatibility with the user's goals, complexity of change, trialability of the product, and observability of the product's benefits. Second, the type of innovation decision affects the rate of adoption. For example, the more persons involved in making an innovation decision, the slower the rate of adoption. Third, communication channels (mass media or interpersonal) used to diffuse an innovation also may influence the innovation's rate of adoption. For complex innovations, interpersonal contact leads to quicker diffusion compared to mass media approaches. Fourth, the nature of the social system (norms, degree of network, interconnectedness) affects an innovation's rate of adoption. Adoption of a new pharmaceutical is expected to be quicker in a connected managed care network compared to a relatively unconnected fee-for- service healthcare network. Finally, the extent of change agents' promotion efforts affect the rate of adoption. This relationship is not linear, however. Greater payoff from a given amount of change-agent activity occurs at certain stages in an innovation's diffusion. The greatest response to change-agent effort (i.e., the tipping point) occurs when opinion leaders (Early Adopters) adopt the innovation, which usually occurs somewhere between 3 and 16 percent adoption in most systems.[58] In the Shetty and Brooks study, the tipping point occurred at fifty months in the cycle after there was a 7 percent adoption of the innovation (atypical antipsychotics).[59]

As one looks to the future of pharmacy, important questions must be asked so that relevant information can be collected and monitored over time to help make good decisions in the planning and implementation processes for pharmacy practice. Some of the questions are highlighted next.

What Will Be the Innovations?

An innovation is an idea, practice, or object that is perceived as new by an individual or other unit of adoption. It matters little whether or not an idea is new in terms of the lapse of time since its first use or discovery. The perceived newness of the idea for the individual determines his or her reaction to it. If the idea seems new to the individual, then it is an innovation.[60]

Innovations should not be viewed as independent from other innovations. Rather, one should remember that an adopter's experience with one innovation will influence that individual's perception of the next innovation. In reality, a set of innovations diffusing at about the same time in a system are interdependent. It is much simpler to try to study an innovation as an independent event, but such an approach would not be accurate.

An example of these principles might be the "concordance concept," which has been described as a new approach to the prescribing and taking of medicines (www.concordance.org). Concordance is an agreement reached after negotiation between a patient and a health care professional that respects the beliefs and wishes of the patient in determining whether, when, and how medicines are to be taken. Although reciprocal, this is an alliance in which health care professionals recognize the primacy of the patient's decisions about taking recommended medications. Concordance aims to help patients and prescribers to make as well-informed a choice as possible about diagnosis and treatment and benefit and risk, to collaborate fully in a balanced therapeutic alliance, and to optimize the potential benefits of medical care (www.concordance.org).

With the self-care movement and patients taking an active role in their health care, concordance could be useful for pharmacy practice. However, to understand the diffusion of this innovation into pharmacy practice and training, it would be helpful to collect and monitor information about other innovations that are taking place in the somewhat parallel areas of compliance, adherence, patient-centered care, pharmaceutical care, disease management, and other paradigms. Also, it would be useful to know that the concordance concept had its origins in the United Kingdom within medical school circles. Monitoring the parallel development and adoption of these various paradigms would be instructive for those who make decisions about the future of pharmacy.

Which Communication Channels Are Being Used?

Communication is the process by which individuals create and share information with one another in order to reach mutual understanding.[61] Diffusion of innovations is a type of communication in which the message content that is exchanged is concerned with a new idea. The essence of the diffusion process is the information exchange through which one individual communicates a new idea to others.

A communication channel is the means through which messages get from one individual to another. Mass media, marketing, interpersonal channels, conferences, meetings, trade journals, professional journals, and scientific journals are examples of how messages are delivered and exchanged in pharmacy practice.

One of the problems in the diffusion of innovations in health care is that the participants often are heterophilous. That is, the individuals who interact are different in certain attributes.[62] A change agent is often more technically competent than his or her clients or audience. This difference frequently leads to ineffective communication, as the participants do not speak the same language. Examples of this in pharmacy not only include the frustration pharmacists often experience as they try to convince patients to "buy into" new service offerings but also the frustration that opinion leaders in pharmacy have experienced in trying to convince practitioners to take on new roles and innovations.

However, when two individuals are identical regarding their technical grasp of an innovation (homophily), no diffusion can occur, as there is no new information to exchange. As innovations are developed and diffused, it is useful to monitor the extent to which communications are between individuals who are identical in their technical grasp of the innovation. Too often pharmacy seems to be "preaching to the choir" as it communicates about innovations in practice. By monitoring communication channels and the extent to which it is homophilous, innovations could be diffused more quickly and effectively in pharmacy.

In the future, new devices are likely to change the communication channels that individuals use. Some relatively new channels that already have emerged include the Internet, the World Wide Web, intranets, wireless communication, decision-support technologies (physician-order entry, bar coding, handheld personal digital assistants), electronic mail, telemedicine, and direct-to-consumer advertising for prescription drugs. Blumenthal proposed that these technologies are instruments of connectivity that allow information to be transferred among various parties in the health care system.[63] This new connectivity might change who is connected to whom, what kind of information flows between the parties, and the relative competencies of the interacting parties, since patients are likely to be much better informed participants in the health care system.[64]

New connections between parties might emerge as well. For example, patients might be more likely to exchange useful information with: (1) other patients, (2) health care organizations, or (3) organizations that pay for health care. There might also be new exchanges between health care organizations. From a diffusion-of-innovations point of view, the new connectivity that Blumenthal described might be able to not only link heterophilous individuals that have new information to share with each other but also decrease the unequal level of competence between a change agent and his or her clients or audience. The result of the new connectivity could be that health care innovations will diffuse at a faster rate than previously realized.

At What Time Will the Tipping Point Be Reached?

Time is an important element in the diffusion process. For example, how long will it take for individuals to pass from first knowledge of an innovation through its adoption or rejection? What will be the rate of adoption for innovations that ultimately are adopted? How long will individuals use the innovation before it is replaced with something else or no longer needed?

If the time period for adoption is too long, it might prohibit one from even embarking on trying to develop an innovation. If a new idea, product, or service is going to be rejected, it is best to "fail fast," so that a minimum amount of resources are wasted. Also, it is the goal to reach adoption as quickly as possible, so that the monetary rewards can be reaped as soon as possible.

Another time-related element to monitor in addition to the adoption or rejection of an innovation is the time to *discontinuance*. That is, decisions to adopt an innovation ultimately are reversed at a later point. Discontinuance may occur because an individual becomes dissatisfied with an innovation or because the innovation was replaced with an improved idea. It is also possible for an individual to adopt an innovation after a previous decision to reject it.

If one wishes to understand pharmacy's future, it would be prudent to monitor the adoption, rejection, and discontinuance of ideas in the practice domain. As changes are monitored over time, the tipping point principle provides some insight about how seemingly little or insignificant things can make a big difference in the diffusion process over time. Malcolm Gladwell provided an example of the tipping point principle with the case of Paul Revere's ride during the American Revolution.[65] At the same time that Revere began his ride north and west of Boston, a fellow revolutionary—William Dawes—set out on the same urgent errand, working his way to Lexington via the towns west of Boston. Both men carried the identical message, through the same number of towns, over just as many miles. However, Dawes' ride didn't set the countryside afire like Revere's did. The local militia leaders along Dawes' ride weren't alerted. The news was not spread through word-of-mouth like it was along Revere's ride.

Gladwell argued that this example shows that the success of any kind of social phenomenon is heavily dependent on the involvement of people with a particular and rare set of social gifts.[66] Revere's news "tipped" and Dawes' didn't because of the differences between the two men and the people who spread the news. Gladwell contends that for new ideas to be successfully diffused in a population, three types of individuals are needed: Connectors, Mavens, and Salesmen.

Connectors know lots of people and are the kinds of people who know everyone. Sprinkled among every walk of life are a handful of people with a truly extraordinary knack of making friends and acquaintances. They are connectors.[67] They have the desire and ability to create and enjoy what sociologists call the "weak tie," a friendly yet casual social connection.

When it comes to diffusion of innovations, connectors are important for more than simply the number of people they know. There importance is also a function of the *kinds* of people they know.[68] Connectors are people whom all of us can reach in only a few steps because, for one reason or another, they manage to occupy many different worlds and subcultures and niches. Paul Revere was a connector. He was intensely social. When he died, his funeral was widely attended. He had diverse interests such as fishing, hunting, card playing, theater, pubs, and business. Paul Revere was able to link the diverse group of revolutionaries. Revere became a kind of clearinghouse for the anti-British forces. He knew everyone and was the logical person to go to with information that needed to be spread quickly. William Dawes, on the other hand, was not noticed as he rode spreading the same message that Revere did. Dawes was not a connector. The word-of-mouth communication that Revere accomplished was not realized along Dawes' route.

Connectors are not the only people who matter for diffusion of new ideas and innovations. Usually, someone else is needed to tell the Connectors about the innovation. Whereas Connectors are people specialists, Mavens are information specialists. The word maven means one who accumulates knowledge. Marketplaces depend on information, and the people with the most information can be very important for the diffusion of new ideas. Mavens often take great pride in their expertise about a particular topic or new idea. However, researchers have reported that Mavens are not likely to be very good persuaders.[69] It is not until the information is conveyed to a Connector that the idea will start to spread to others.

The final piece of the puzzle is that the information must be persuasive to others before it will be adopted. This is the role of what Gladwell calls "Salesmen."[70] Mavens are experts and Connectors are social glue, but Salesmen have the skills to persuade us even when we are unconvinced of what we are hearing. Salesmen are as critical to the diffusion of innovations as the two other groups. These individuals tend to be outgoing, gregarious people. They love helping people. When Salesmen become convinced about the value of a new idea or innovation, they exhibit an evangelistic passion for persuading others. Studies show that persuasiveness is not just rooted in the information or the message. Rather, nonverbal cues, relationships, and subliminal messages sent through smiles and nods are very important in the persuasion process. Salesmen are gifted at the subtle, the unhidden, and the unspoken as they strive to help others with their message.

Gladwell concluded his argument by pointing out that if an innovation or new idea has value and meets a need (the stickiness factor); is introduced at the right time (power of context); and is spread through the use of Mavens, Connectors, and Salesmen, the tipping point can be reached and the innovation can become adopted. Through an understanding of this complex process and monitoring how innovations in health care are developing, one could make good predictions about the adoption of innovations in pharmacy. Once the tipping point is reached (usually when between 3 to 16 percent of a population adopts an innovation) a great deal production capacity is required. Just anticipating these tipping points in pharmacy practice would help make strategic planning decisions about pharmacy infrastructure, technology, workforce, education, and policy more accurate, certain, and adaptable.

Among Which Members of the Social System?

One other question to consider is which interrelated units will be engaged in joint decision making and joint problem solving to accomplish a common goal. Units of a social system may be individuals, informal groups, organizations, and/or subsystems.[71] The social system constitutes a boundary within which the innovation diffuses. It can affect norms of how diffusion takes place, the roles of opinion leaders and change agents, and even the consequences of innovations within that system. For pharmacy, diffusion of innovations might be different depending upon health care sectors, patient populations, or even countries that would be affected by the innovation.

Diffusion of innovations theory and the tipping point principle can be helpful for monitoring changes that are likely to take place in pharmacy over the next few years. What are the new practice models that might emerge? It is difficult to know, but based on our conversations we would like to propose four possible scenarios to monitor. In the next section, we provide a brief description of each and then provide our argument that the models that will emerge dominant will most likely depend on three main issues: technicians, technology, and transitions in pharmacy practice. We ask the reader to note that our descriptions of each model are extremes and are designed to serve as a basis for discussion.

PRACTICE MODELS OF THE FUTURE

"Patient As Unit of Analysis" Model

One possible model that may be used to project the roles and demand for pharmacists is the patient as unit of analysis (PUA). The PUA is based upon several assumptions. Briefly, the patient as unit of analysis attempts to foresee the impacts that current trends in pharmacy practice (including the practice of pharmaceutical care) and United States demographics will have on the need for pharmacy practitioners.

First, the PUA assumes that all dispensing functions are removed from registered pharmacists' control. These functions will likely fall to dispensing technology and pharmacy technicians. Pharmacists perform only cognitive functions, such as drug utilization review and pharmaceutical care activities. The model assumes that all physical distribution and dispensing of prescription drugs would be accomplished through the use of logistics personnel and technology.

Second, the PUA assumes that, of the approximately 300 million persons currently residing in the United States, approximately 10 percent have at least one drug-related problem (DRP) in any given year. For argument's sake, we make the assumption that only these individuals are in need of pharmaceutical care once in a year. Thus, approximately 30 million individuals would need the attention of a pharmaceutical care practitioner yearly. Also, we assume that one practitioner can see ten patients daily, and that each practitioner works a standard five-day workweek for fifty weeks each year. Each pharmacist can thus see 2,500 patients yearly. Combining these figures suggests that 12,000 pharmaceutical care practitioners would be sufficient to meet future needs.

If one were to use another set of assumptions, a different result would be found. For example, let us assume that every resident of the United States requires at least one pharmaceutical care visit yearly. This is reasonable, given that nearly everyone uses at least some kind of prescription or over-the-counter (OTC) product (especially if we include vitamins and herbals). Now, approximately 300 million individuals would need the attention of a pharmaceutical care practitioner yearly. Using the same logic described above, the need for pharmacists would increase tenfold to 120,000 full-time practitioners to provide these services.

The most important variable in this model is the number of patients seen and no longer the number of prescriptions dispensed, as outlined later in the "dispense first" model. This model also suggests that pharmacy practice would be linked with all of a patient's drug-related needs (prescription, OTC, herbals, vitamins, and other therapies that might emerge). Helping patients manage therapy *in a way consistent with the patient's needs and wants* would emerge as the dominant mission of pharmacy. In this model, pharmacists might not focus as much on being "responsible for all of a patient's drug-related needs" but rather be responsible *to* the patient to meet needs as defined by the patient (www.concordance.org).[72]

"Virtual Visits" Model

The Institute of Medicine (IOM) recently issued a report, called "Crossing the Quality Chasm," that calls for a redesign of the health care system. The IOM report cites many areas where the present "system" is deficient. Four different levels were identified that frame what changes need to occur, starting with the experience of patients and communities, the microsystems of care, health care organizations, and the health care environment.[73] If this system redesign were to occur, where would pharmacy fit? What would happen to pharmacy? How could pharmacy support a redesign that focuses on and supports the experience of patients? How does the pharmaceutical care model support this change?

This discussion will focus on pharmacy as a microsystem of care that supports the experience of patients. Pharmacy exists in a microsystem of care as defined by a small team of people that has a local information center (computer record systems), a client (patient) population, and a defined set of work processes.[74] Donald Berwick proposed ten rules to frame how microsystems can be effectively enhanced.[75] The rules contrast the present system with how a new system would be designed. Applying these rules to pharmacy should position the profession to be integrated in a new design.

Basis of Care

Current system: Care is based primarily on visits.

New system: Care is based on continuous healing relationships. The pharmaceutical care model requires that pharmacists establish therapeutic relationships with the patients. These relationships serve as pharmacy's foundation. Pharmaceutical care promotes the patients' participation in the therapeutic process.[76] Pharmaceutical care is not just delivered when a patient is in the pharmacy, it is delivered over the phone, Internet, or whatever the prevailing communication method is. Pharmacists are proactive in assuring that health-promotion activities (immunization, smoking cessation) occur. Patients can access their whole interdisciplinary health care team through "virtual visits."

Customized Care

Current system: Professional autonomy drives variability.

New system: Care is customized according to patients' needs and values. To deliver care that is customized requires that pharmacists establish the therapeutic relationship and they understand patient needs. Pharmacists need to actively provide care that enhances the health of patients, such as managing risks of taking medicines through preventing, identifying, and resolving drug-related problems.[77]

Control of Care

Current system: Professionals control care.

New System: The patient is the source of control. Pharmaceutical care should be available twenty-four hours a day, seven days a week. This availability would not necessarily be dependent on the physical setting of a pharmacy. Technologies, including the Internet and telepharmacy, would be used to ensure that pharmacists are available when and where the patients need their services. A system in which "virtual visits" are reimbursed would emerge.

Information Control

Current system: Information is a record.

New system: Knowledge is shared freely. Patients would have direct access to their pharmacy records if necessary through a direct link to pharmacy computer systems. In conjunction with other care providers, pharmacists would provide electronic care plans that include diagnostic, pharmaceutical care, and health-promotion activities directly to patients. Policy and technology related to assuring patient privacy would be important, debatable issues under the new system.

Decision Making

Current system: Decision making is based on training and experience.

New system: Decision making is based on evidence. Pharmacists can no longer be passive in meeting their continuing education requirements and will have to increase the number of hours required to keep current. Pharmacists would provide consistent care across the profession without substantial variability.

Safety

Current system: "Do no harm" is an individual responsibility.

New system: Safety is a system property. Pharmacists would be required to report error rates in filling, adverse reactions to medications, and drug interactions resulting in adverse events. Pharmacy will have to develop new systems that facilitate quality improvement, to minimize errors that are created and identify errors created by prescribers and payers.

Secrecy

Current system: Secrecy is necessary.

New system: Transparency is necessary. The electronic pharmacy record would be developed so it would not matter what pharmacy, grocery, or health-foods store a prescription, OTC, or herbal product was purchased. The information would be available to patients, pharmacists, pharmacies, and prescribers. Again, policy and technology related to assuring patient privacy would be important, debatable issues under the new system.

Needs

Current system: The system reacts to needs.

New system: Needs are anticipated. A system would be developed that identified and alerted the patient about overuse and underuse of medications. Pharmacists would contact a patient to determine if newly prescribed medications were safe, effective, and convenient. The pharmacist would have a system that would anticipate patient needs.

Cost Factors

Current system: Cost reduction is sought.

New system: Waste is continually decreased. Waste in terms of patient time, worker productivity, product effectiveness, and rework related to drug-related misadventuring, morbidity, and mortality would be focus points.[78]

Cooperation

Current system: Preference is given to professional roles over the system.

New system: Cooperation among clinicians is a priority. A new standard of intra- and interprofessional collegiality among physicians, nurses, pharmacists, and other health care providers will be expected. Education, licensure, and practice environments would be affected under this new system.

To meet the challenges of the "quality chasm" report will require a complete retooling of how pharmacy is viewed and practiced.[79] Berwick points out that the health care organizations and health care environment will not likely encourage this extent of change.[80] However, pharmacy would need to be at the table when discussions occur about how the health care system will change or be left out again.

"Dispense First" Model

As one thinks toward the future one is encouraged to think "outside the box." For pharmacy that exercise, although intriguing, is fraught with problems. The reality is that today and in the near future (next ten to fifteen years) the pharmacist will continue to be a central figure in the medication-distribution process. The numbers of prescriptions written and filled are projected to continue to grow at an exponential rate.[81] That growth, along with the growth of pharmacy outlets and decentralization of regulatory authority, dictate that pharmacists will continue to play a prominent role in product distribution.

The marketplace reality is that the prescription customer wants quick, efficient service. Convenience has been identified as the essential patronage motive of the prescription customer for over thirty years and will continue to be into the future.[82,83] Commercial enterprises incapable of meeting their patrons' expectations will simply not survive. There has been, and continues to be, the expectation that pharmacy should move toward a patron-centered or pharmaceutical care type of practice, yet there is no evidence that the public wants that level of care from a pharmacist.[84] On the other hand, there is ample evidence that patrons expect the right drug and right dose with little wait. First things first—we must ensure a safe and efficient drug distribution system.

The most immediate need is to focus on the technical requirements of the distribution process and consider how the introduction of automation technology can improve efficiency. For the medication distribution systems to meet the future demand a variety of "helper" functionaries must be in place. These "helper" functionaries may include individuals (i.e., pharmacy technicians) and/or logic-driven automated dispensing systems. It can be expected that these "helper" systems will be highly reliable and replace a substantial portion of the current activities of pharmacists.

The reliance on pharmacy technicians in these systems brings into question the training process, which in today's environment is often on-the-job-training. Clearly, standards for training and expectations of persons functioning in these roles must be developed and put into place. The establishment of training standards and outcome expectations will help ensure competence, yet not dictate the mode or source of delivery. Community/technical schools or corporate pharmacy operations may deliver technician-training programs.

The education system for pharmacists must be considered as well. Colleges of pharmacy must focus a substantial portion of education toward the management of people and technology. Consideration should be given to the development of a limited-practice degree in pharmacy. The program would be a four-year BS degree in pharmacy with a balance of pharmaceutical sciences, patient communication/counseling content, and management sciences—including personnel, technical, and financial. Graduates of these programs would be granted a limited-practice license, with their scope of practice limited to the distributive arena.

For some, these ideas may appear heretical. Why has education moved toward a doctoral program? Are graduates of these programs overeducated and not needed in the system? In many cases, doctoral graduates are overeducated for the distributive function. As the number of distributive positions grows, pharmacy graduates educated for a patient care role increasingly fill them. In the long term, this will lead to apathy and job dissatisfaction. At the same time, the health care system needs the patient-focused/clinical expertise the doctoral degree provides. Population-based pharmacy care, which is delivered or supported by managed care systems and other large systems (hospitals, clinic systems, long-term care, etc.), requires the expertise of doctoral-trained pharmacists. Pharmaceutical care services provided to individuals is needed today and the need will grow; again, this level of care does require pharmacists with advanced training. The health care system does need the advanced training of doctoral pharmacists, but not all pharmacists require this level of education. In population-based systems, a few highly educated pharmacists affect many lives through rational product selection and provider education. At the individual patient level, care can be provided to those who need or want that level of care without being physically present in a local community-based pharmacy. As outlined earlier in the "patient as unit of analysis" model, perhaps only tens of thousands of doctoral-trained pharmacists would be needed for such functions. The bulk of pharmacists and other helper functionaries (hundreds of thousands needed) would need training in pharmaceutical distribution systems and not patient care. The "dispense first" model might arguably be the dominant pharmacy practice model for the next ten to fifteen years.

"Cream Will Rise to the Top" Model

The primary argument for this model of practice suggests that colleges of pharmacy across the United States should produce pharmacy graduates at a rate greater than the marketplace demand. In doing this, the "cream will rise to the top" through competition for the best pharmacist jobs. Today's demand for pharmacists has outpaced the supply. Education mandates have resulted in pharmacy graduates with skills and employment opportunities as never before. At no other time in history have a greater proportion of pharmacists entered nontraditional roles.

In 2002, approximately 10 percent of licensed pharmacists worked in settings outside of dispensing, compounding, distributive, consulting, and practice/care arenas. Pharmacy benefit companies, health maintenance organizations, investment companies, and biomedical research and development ventures are only a few of the types of entities clamoring to hire our pharmacists. The proportion of pharmacists who work in nondispensing functions is expected to grow.[85]

The American population is aging at an alarming rate. The resultant challenges to health care providers are obvious. Older individuals often have multiple chronic disorders that are managed with medications. Prescriptions for these medications have increased at an exponential rate while the supply of pharmacists has maintained a linear growth. Although alternative methods of medication distribution are evolving, these novel methods of providing medications are inadequate to meet the demand. State statutes and governing board of pharmacy rules also have hampered the use of support personnel.

Short supply and increased demand for pharmacists have driven marketplace value of pharmacists to skyrocket. Between 1997 and 2001, the average salary of a Minnesota pharmacist rose 47 percent. Higher salaries and better benefit packages in urban areas place small rural pharmacies at a disadvantage. A number of characteristics within the marketplace, types of pharmacists being supplied by schools of pharmacy, changes in the demographics of America, and the resultant short supply of pharmacists combine to severely alter/affect pharmacy in rural areas. At the same time, large chain retail pharmacies are continuing to open new stores. As an example, during 2002 Walgreens opened a new pharmacy at a rate of one every seventeen hours. Rural independent pharmacists are having difficulty attracting employees or buyers of their establishments and are closing their doors. At one point, Minnesota pharmacy data showed that 330 (95 percent) of 347 openings for pharmacists in Minnesota were in rural areas. In Minnesota, rural areas account for only one-third of the total population.

If colleges of pharmacy were to produce pharmacists at a rate greater than demand, the trickle-down effect would occur. Salaries would decline and the small rural pharmacy owner would be better prepared to compete with pharmacies in larger urban areas. Pharmacists would be more likely to find a type of employment that better matched their skill level. Pharmacists in an excess-supply marketplace that are unable to meet a particular skill level will be required to seek a more appropriate employment-skill match. Those unable to maintain their skills would be forced from employment. Survival of the fittest forces would likely result in a stronger profession. Continued restriction of the number of graduates from colleges of pharmacy would only foster mediocrity. Future models of pharmacy practice could let the marketplace determine who should remain licensed. Competition for pharmacist jobs that would result from the oversupply of pharmacists would help define pharmacy practice based on the value that pharmacists provide in a competitive marketplace.

More than One Model Might Dominate the Profession

To determine which model might dominate, we suggest that it will be useful to watch trends in three areas (3 Ts): technicians, technology, and transitions in practice.[86] An example of what is currently being proposed about technicians and technology is a white paper published in 2003 and endorsed by twelve organizations in pharmacy.[87] According to the white paper,

> When pharmacists limit their direct involvement in the technical aspects of dispensing, delegate this responsibility to pharmacy technicians working under their supervision, and increase the use of automated dispensing technology, they can fully concentrate on the services for which they are uniquely educated and trained.[88]

Pedersen, Schneider, and Scheckelhoff also focused on technicians and technology as areas for improvement in hospital settings.[89] They suggested

> increased reliance on technicians and technology to optimize the use of scarce and expensive pharmacist time. Specific technologies that are underutilized included pharmacy-linked point-of-care dispensing cabinets, computer-generated MARs (medication administration records), and bar-code-based bedside drug administration documentation systems.

Regarding transitions in pharmacy practice, the Holland-Nimmo Practice Change Model can be an analytical tool and a framework for action. Their model consists of three basic components: (1) practice environment, (2) learning resources, and (3) motivational strategies.[90] Holland and Nimmo argued that no single component or combination of any two components is sufficient to bring about a decision to change practice and make it happen. All three elements must be functioning at the same time, like the rings in a three-ring circus. To maximize the potential for individual pharmacists to change their practice, three things are needed: (1) creation of an environment conducive to the new form of practice, (2) identification of learning resources and skills to be acquired, and (3) motivation of individual practitioners to change.

We would argue that technicians, technology, and transitions in practice are areas that might provide hints about which models are likely to dominate the profession in the future and provide some indication about when a tipping point might be reached for new ideas. However, present terminology and definitions will be outdated and irrelevant in the future. New, unforeseen terms and definitions will emerge over time. Just as the terms *computer punch card, microfiche, carbon paper, dot-matrix printer, slide projector,* and *floppy disk* came and went, technology and terms we use today in pharmacy will come and go. New vocabularies and new paradigms will be needed as the future of pharmacy unfolds.

Another difficulty in looking to the future is that we will not experience just one tipping point and reach a new steady state of practice. New ideas and constant change await us. Anticipating tipping points and new models of practice can provide competitive advantages for only short periods of time until the next idea is adopted.

Historian Greg Higby described transitions in pharmacy practice over the past fifty years as "count and pour" practice, the clinical pharmacy era, and pharmaceutical care.[91] We suggest that, in the near future (next ten to fifteen years), the pharmacy profession will consist of mixed models and one or more models might dominate in the short term. During such a period of mixed models and transition, it will be important to understand and monitor the rate of adoption and rate of discontinuance of various models.

SUMMARY

We have proposed a monitoring approach that uses diffusion of innovations theory and the tipping point principle as we look to the future of pharmacy. This approach lends itself to not only monitoring what might occur in the future but also considers the *rate of adoption* for new innovations. We believe that rate of adoption (including the rate of discontinuance) is an important study domain. It is often important to identify the tipping point at which a new innovation is adopted (or discontinued) at a comparatively quick rate so that the timing of corresponding actions can be made in the health care system. Once a tipping point is reached, a great deal production capacity is required. Just anticipating these tipping points in pharmacy practice would help make strategic planning decisions about pharmacy infrastructure, technology, workforce, education, and policy more accurate, certain, and adaptable.

Resources are scarce, so an understanding of the most appropriate timing of making changes in pharmacy practice can lead to the cost-effective use of limited resources for improving patient care. Also, by continually monitoring aspects of the diffusion of innovations in pharmacy and health care, we contend that better decisions can be made as we look to, shape, and experience pharmacy's future.

NOTES

1. Doucette, W.R., Schommer, J.C., and Wiederholt, J.B. The political economy of pharmaceutical marketing channels: A conceptual framework. *Clinical Therapeutics* 1993; 15(4): 739-751.

2. Higby, G.J. From compounding to caring: An abridged history of American pharmacy. In C.H. Knowlton and R.P. Penna (Eds.), *Pharmaceutical care* (New York: Chapman & Hall, 1996), pp. 18-45.

3. Ibid.

4. Elliott, E.C. *The general report of the pharmaceutical survey: 1946-1949* (Washington, DC: American Pharmaceutical Association, 1950).

5. Brodie, D.C. and Benson, R.A. The evolution of the clinical pharmacy concept. *Drug Intelligence and Clinical Pharmacy* 1976; 10: 507.

6. *Pharmacy manpower project* (Ann Arbor, MI: Vector Research, 1993).

7. Higby, G. History of pharmacy from compounding to caring. In Knowlton, C. and Penna, R. (Eds.) *Pharmaceutical care* (Chapter 2) (New York: Van Nostrand Reinhold, 1995).

8. Buerki, R.A. *The challenge of ethics in pharmacy practice* (Madison, WI: American Institute of the History of Pharmacy, 1985, p. 47).

9. Higby, History of pharmacy from compounding to caring.

10. Hepler, C.D. and Strand, L.M. Opportunities and responsibilities in pharmaceutical care. *American Journal of Hospital Pharmacy* 1990; 47: 533-549, p. 533.

11. Manasse, H.R. Medication use in an imperfect world: Drug misadventuring as an issue of public policy, Part 1. *American Journal of Hospital Pharmacy* 1989; 46: 929-944.

12. Manasse, H.R. Medication use in an imperfect world: Drug misadventuring as an issue of public policy, Part 2. *American Journal of Hospital Pharmacy* 1989; 46: 1141-1152.

13. Hepler and Strand, Opportunities and responsibilities in pharmaceutical care.

14. Schommer, J.C. The roles of pharmacists, patients, and contextual cues in pharmacist-patient communication. Unpublished doctoral dissertation, University of Wisconsin–Madison, 1992.

15. National Council on Patient Information and Education. October is "Talk About Prescriptions" month. *Talk About Prescriptions Month Newsletter* 1991; October 1: insert.

16. National Council on Patient Information and Education. Smart medicines need smart patients. *Talk About Prescriptions Month Newsletter* 1990; October 1: 1.

17. Perrin, F.V. Improving communication with your patients. *Drug Topics* 1988; 132(9): 48, 50, 52, 54, 56.

18. Ibid.

19. American Pharmaceutical Association. When adults take medicine: Improper use a national health problem. *Pharmacy Update* 1990; October 1: 5-6.

20. Johnson, J.A. and Bootman, L. Drug-related morbidity and mortality: A cost-of-illness model. *Archives of Internal Medicine* 1995; 155: 1949-1956.

21. Ernst, F.R. and Grizzle, A.J. Drug-related morbidity and mortality: Updating the cost-of-illness model. *Journal of the American Pharmaceutical Association* 2001; 41(2): 192-199.

22. Hepler and Strand, Opportunities and responsibilities in pharmaceutical care.

23. Cipolle, R.J., Strand, L.M., and Morley, P.C. *Pharmaceutical care practice* (New York: McGraw-Hill, 1998), pp. 341-342.

24. Hepler and Strand, Opportunities and responsibilities in pharmaceutical care.

25. Brushwood, D.B. The pharmacist's duty to warn: Toward a knowledge-based model of professional responsibility. *Drake Law Review* 1991; 40: 1-60.

26. Kessler, D.A. Communicating with patients about their medications. *New England Journal of Medicine* 1991; 325: 1650-1652.

27. Schommer, The roles of pharmacists, patients, and contextual cues.

28. Hatoum, H.T., Catizone, C., Hutchinson, R.A., and Prohit, A. An eleven-year review of the pharmacy literature: Documentation of the value and acceptance of clinical pharmacy. *Drug Intelligence and Clinical Pharmacy* 1986; 20: 33-48.

29. Lipton, H.L., Burns, P.J., Soumerai, S.B., and Chrischilles, E.A. Pharmacists as agents of change for rational drug therapy. *International Journal of Technology Assessment in Health Care* 1995; 11: 485-508.

30. Holland, R.W. and Nimmo, C.M. Transitions in pharmacy practice, part 1: Beyond pharmaceutical care. *American Journal of Health-System Pharmacy* 1999; 56: 1758-1764.

31. Nimmo, C.M. and Holland, R.W. Transitions in pharmacy practice, part 2: Who does what and why. *American Journal of Health-System Pharmacy* 1999; 56: 1981-1987.

32. Holland, R.W. and Nimmo, C.M. Transitions in pharmacy practice, part 3: Effecting change—The three ring circus. *American Journal of Health-System Pharmacy* 1999; 56: 2235-2241.

33. Nimmo, C.M. and Holland, R.W. Transitions in pharmacy practice, part 4: Can a leopard change its spots? *American Journal of Health-System Pharmacy* 1999; 56: 2458-2462.

34. Nimmo, C.M. and Holland, R.W. Transitions in pharmacy practice, part 5: Walking the tightrope of change. *American Journal of Health-System Pharmacy* 2000; 57: 64-72.

35. Cipolle, Strand, and Morley, *Pharmaceutical care practice*.

36. Holland and Nimmo, Transitions in pharmacy practice, part 1; Nimmo and Holland, Transitions in pharmacy practice, part 2; Holland and Nimmo, Transitions in pharmacy practice, part 3; Nimmo and Holland, Transitions in pharmacy practice, part 4; Nimmo and Holland, Transitions in pharmacy practice, part 5.

37. *A profile of older Americans, 2001* (Washington, DC: Administration on Aging, 2001).

38. Adamcik, B.A. The consumers of health care. In J.E. Fincham and A.I. Wertheimer (Eds.), *Pharmacy and the U.S. health care system* (Binghamton, NY: The Haworth Press, 1997), pp. 337-394.

39. Cooksey, J.A., Knapp, K.K., Walton, S.M., and Cultice, J.M. Challenges to the pharmacist profession from escalating pharmaceutical demand. *Health Affairs* 2002; 21(5): 182-188.

40. *The pharmacist workforce: A study of the supply and demand for pharmacists* (Washington, DC: Health Resources Services Administration, 1999).

41. Cooksey et al., Challenges to the pharmacist profession.

42. Fleming, H. No rest for the weary. *Drug Topics* 2000; 143(12): 50-52, 55-56.

43. Kreling, D.H., Mott, D.A., and Wiederholt, J.B. 1999 salary survey. *Journal of the Pharmacy Society of Wisconsin* 2000; January/February: 17-23.

44. Pedersen, C.A. 1999 compensation and labor survey for Ohio pharmacists. *Ohio Pharmacist* 1999; 48(12): 12-17.

45. Pedersen, C.A. and Amick, S.D. 1999 labor market assessment and practice activities for Ohio pharmacists. *Ohio Pharmacist* 2000; 49(1): 12-18.

46. Schommer, J.C., Worley, M.M., Hadsall, R.S., et al. 1999 Minnesota pharmacist compensation and salary survey, part 1: Pharmacists' hourly wages and benefits. *Minnesota Pharmacist* 1999; 53(6): 13-15, 24, 26-28.

47. Schommer, J.C., Worley, M.M., Hadsall, R.S., et al. 1999 Minnesota pharmacist compensation and salary survey, part 2: Pharmacists' work activities. *Minnesota Pharmacist* 2000; 54(2): 17-20, 27-29.

48. Schommer, J.C. and Pedersen, C.A. Pharmacists' work activities in two Midwestern states. *Journal of the American Pharmaceutical Association* 2001; 41(5): 760-762.

49. Sorofman, B.A., Doucette, W.R., Kittisopee, T., et al. 1999 Iowa pharmacist compensation report. *The Journal of the Iowa Pharmacy Association* 2000; 65(1): 30-32.

50. Schommer, J.C., Pedersen, C.A., Doucette, W.R., et al. Community pharmacists' work activities in the United States during 2000. *Journal of the American Pharmaceutical Association* 2002; 42(3): 399-406.

51. Ibid.

52. Schommer and Pedersen, Pharmacists' work activities in two Midwestern states.

53. Ryan, B. and Gross, N. The diffusion of hybrid seed corn in two Iowa communities, *Rural Sociology* 1943; 8: 15-24.

54. Gladwell, M. *The tipping point: How little things can make a big difference* (New York: Little, Brown and Company, 2002).

55. Rogers, E.M. *Diffusion of innovations* (Fourth edition) (New York: The Free Press, 1995).

56. Shetty, S. and Brooks, J. Influence of physician mix and supply on the diffusion of atypical antipsychotic agents. Paper presented at Midwest Pharmacy Administration Conference, July 26, 2002, Ann Arbor, Michigan.

57. Ibid.

58. Gladwell, *The tipping point;* Rogers, *Diffusion of innovations.*

59. Shetty and Brooks, Influence of physician mix and supply.

60. Rogers, *Diffusion of innovations.*

61. Ibid.

62. Ibid.

63. Blumenthal, D. Doctors in a wired world: Can professionalism survive connectivity? *The Milbank Quarterly* 2002; 80(3): 525-546.

64. Ibid.

65. Gladwell, *The tipping point.*

66. Ibid.

67. Ibid.

68. Ibid.

69. Ibid.

70. Ibid.

71. Rogers, *Diffusion of innovations.*

72. Cipolle, Strand, and Morley, *Pharmaceutical care practice.*

73. Committee on Quality of Health Care in America, Institute of Medicine. *Crossing the quality chasm: A new health system for the 21st century* (Washington, DC: National Academies Press, 2001).

74. Berwick, D.M. A user manual for the IOM's quality chasm report. *Health Affairs* 2002; 21(3): 80-85.

75. Ibid.

76. Cipolle, Strand, and Morley, *Pharmaceutical care practice*.

77. Ibid.

78. Manasse, Medication use in an imperfect world, part 1 and part 2; Johnson and Bootman, Drug-related morbidity and mortality; Ernst and Grizzle, Drug-related morbidity and mortality.

79. Committee on Quality of Health Care in America, Institute of Medicine. *Crossing the quality chasm.*

80. Berwick, A user manual.

81. Kreling, D.H., Mott, D.A., Wiederholt, J.B., et al. *Prescription drug trends: A chartbook update* (Menlo Park, CA; Kaiser Family Foundation, 2001).

82. Gagnon, J.P. Factors affecting pharmacy patronage motives: A literature review. *Journal of the American Pharmaceutical Association* 1977; NS17: 556-559, 566.

83. Stergachis, A., Maine, L.L., and Brown, L. The 2001 national pharmacy consumer survey. *Journal of the American Pharmaceutical Association* 2002; 42: 568-576.

84. Schommer, J.C., Pedersen, C.A., Castellanos, W.J., and Gordon, J.A. Pharmacists' and patients' views about the pharmacist's role in health care. Paper presented at the First Annual Deep Portage Conference, February 26, 2002, Hackensack, MN.

85. Knapp, D.A. *Professionally determined need for pharmacy services in 2020.* 2002. Available online at <http://www.aacp.org>.

86. Ibid.

87. Rouse, M.J. White paper on pharmacy technicians 2002: Needed changes can no longer wait. *American Journal of Health-System Pharmacy* 2003; 60(1): 37-51.

88. Ibid.

89. Pedersen, C.A., Schneider, P.J., and Scheckelhoff, D.J. ASHP national survey of pharmacy practice in hospital settings: Dispensing and administration—2002. *American Journal of Health-System Pharmacy* 2003; 60(1): 52-68.

90. Holland and Nimmo, Transitions in pharmacy practice, part 1; Nimmo and Holland, Transitions in pharmacy practice, part 2; Holland and Nimmo, Transitions in pharmacy practice, part 3; Nimmo and Holland, Transitions in pharmacy practice, part 4; Nimmo and Holland, Transitions in pharmacy practice, part 5.

91. Higby, From compounding to caring.

Index

Page numbers followed by the letter "f" indicate figures and those followed by the letter "t" indicate tables.

445

Home health care, 215-216
Hospice care, 216-217
Hospital Statistics, 173
Hospitals
  accreditation, 173, 186-187
  adverse drug events, 406
  AHA. *See* American Hospital
    Association
  *American Journal of Hospital
    Pharmacy,* 99
  American Society of Hospital
    Pharmacists, 97, 120
  basic, 25
  biotechnology impact on costs,
    382-383
  Centers for Medicare & Medicaid
    Services, 173, 184
  challenges, 187-188
  classifications, 173-174
  community, 174, 181t, 183
  competition, 37
  costs, 7
  employed and insured people, 9
  for-profit corporations, 173
  future, 187-188
  government, 181t, 182-183
  history, 7, 169-171
  insurance payments, 36-38
  not-for-profit corporations, 173
  organizational structure, 174-176,
    175f
  osteopathic, 173
  ownership, 180-184
  pharmacy services, 105, 176, 178,
    178f
  regulations, 184, 185f, 186
  requirements if not certified,
    188-189
  rural, 183
  scope, 171-173, 172t
  services, 176, 177f
  staffed beds, 170t
  staffing, 178-180
  types, 173-174
HRSA. *See* Health Resources and
    Services Administration
Human cloning, 150, 387-388
Human Genome Project, 359, 364
Humoral medicine, 283-284
Hurd, Richard S., 357

Hybridoma cells, 365
Hypercompliance, 301f

Idler, E.L., 281
IHS (Indian Health Service), 13
Illich, Ivan, 304
Illness behavior, 276, 278-280, 278f,
    279f
Immunizations. *See* Vaccinations
Immunomodulatory cytokines, 367-369
Immunopharmacology, 102
IMR (infant mortality rate), 4
In vitro fertilization (IVF), 386
Incentives for prescriptions, 161
Income and drug-use compliance, 309
Income as ability to pay, 34
Incongruity, 258
Indemnity plans, 26, 27, 47
Independent licensed practitioners, 179
Independent pharmacy
  decreased ownerships, 87-88
  employee shortage, 437
  practice setting, 105
Independent practice association (IPA),
    48
Indian and Middle Eastern health care,
    285
Indian Health Service (IHS), 13
Individual consumer behavior model,
    269-274, 270f
Infant mortality rate (IMR), 4
Infectious disease
  antibiotics, 7
  tuberculosis, 5, 310
Information and Analysis study, 84
Information control, 433
Information gathering, 269, 271
Ingredient costs, 40, 51-52
In-house pharmacy, 50
Initial compliance, 301f
Injectable drug delivery, 375
Innovation, diffusion, 423-427, 424f,
    430
Institute of Medicine (IOM)
  "Crossing the Quality Chasm"
    report, 431
  drug regimen review, 208
  To Err Is Human, 406
Institutional accreditation, 65

National Association of Boards of
    Pharmacy *(continued)*
National Institute for Standards in
    Pharmacist Credentialing,
    138, 140
Pharmacy Manpower Information
    Project, 82-83
Verified Internet Pharmacy Practice
    Sites (VIPPS) Program, 246
National Association of Chain Drug
    Stores (NACDS)
background, 124-125
demand for pharmacists and, 90
drug distribution, 243
National Institute for Standards in
    Pharmacist Credentialing,
    138, 140
National Association of Mail Service
    Pharmacies (NAMSP), 125
National Association of Retail
    Druggists (NARD), 97, 119
National Center for Health Statistics
    (NCHS), 74
National Commission for Health
    Certifying Agencies, 67-68
National Committee on Quality
    Assurance (NCQA), 186
National Community Pharmacists
    Association (NCPA)
background, 119
curriculum, 97
demand for pharmacists, 90
National Institute for Standards in
    Pharmacist Credentialing,
    138, 140
National Council for Prescription Drug
    Programs (NCPDP), 50
National Health Services Corps
    Programs, 17
National Infant Immunization Week,
    144
National Institute for Health Care
    Management Research and
    Educational Foundation, 199
National Institute for Standards in
    Pharmacist Credentialing
    (NISPC), 138, 140
National Institutes of Health (NIH),
    107, 385
National Nursing Home Survey, 203

National Pharmaceutical Association
    (NPhA), 120-121
National Pharmaceutical Council
    (NPC), 125
National Pharmacists Workforce
    Survey, 74
National practitioner organizations
ACCP. *See* American College of
    Clinical Pharmacy
AMCP. *See* Academy of Managed
    Care Pharmacy
American Association of
    Pharmaceutical Scientists
    (AAPS), 121-122
American College of Apothecaries
    (ACA), 119-120
APhA. *See* American Pharmacists
    Association
ASCP. *See* American Society of
    Consultant Pharmacists
ASHP. *See* American Society of
    Health-System Pharmacists
National Community Pharmacists
    Association (NCPA), 90, 97,
    119
National Pharmaceutical
    Association (NPhA), 120-121
National Quality Forum, 406
National trade organizations
Consumer Healthcare Products
    Association (CHPA), 123
Generic Pharmaceutical
    Association, 124, 380
Healthcare Distribution
    Management Association
    (HDMA), 124, 239
NACDS. *See* National Association
    of Chain Drug Stores
National Pharmaceutical Council
    (NPC), 125
Pharmaceutical Care Management
    Association (PCMA),
    125-126
PhRMA. *See* Pharmaceutical
    Research and Manufacturers
    of America
National Wholesale Druggists'
    Association, 124
Nationalized health care program, 17